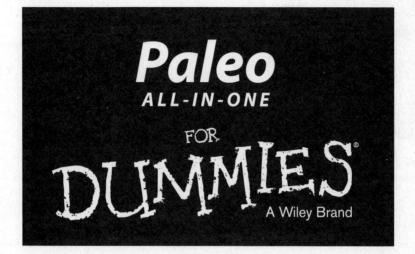

Paleo
ALL-IN-ONE

FOR
DUMMIES

A Wiley Brand

by Patrick Flynn, Adriana Harlan, Melissa Joulwan, and Dr. Kellyann Petrucci

Regina Public Library
BOOK SALE ITEM
Non-Returnable Item

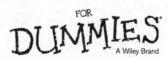

FOR
DUMMIES
A Wiley Brand

Paleo All-In-One For Dummies®

Published by
John Wiley & Sons, Inc.
111 River Street
Hoboken, NJ
07030-5774

www.wiley.com

Copyright © 2015 by John Wiley & Sons, Inc., Hoboken, New Jersey

Media and software compilation copyright © 2015 by John Wiley & Sons, Inc. All rights reserved.

Published simultaneously in Canada

No part of this publication may be reproduced, stored in a retrieval system or transmitted in any form or by any means, electronic, mechanical, photocopying, recording, scanning or otherwise, except as permitted under Sections 107 or 108 of the 1976 United States Copyright Act, without the prior written permission of the Publisher. Requests to the Publisher for permission should be addressed to the Permissions Department, John Wiley & Sons, Inc., 111 River Street, Hoboken, NJ 07030, (201) 748-6011, fax (201) 748-6008, or online at http://www.wiley.com/go/permissions.

Trademarks: Wiley, For Dummies, the Dummies Man logo, Dummies.com, Making Everything Easier, and related trade dress are trademarks or registered trademarks of John Wiley & Sons, Inc., and may not be used without written permission. All other trademarks are the property of their respective owners. John Wiley & Sons, Inc., is not associated with any product or vendor mentioned in this book.

LIMIT OF LIABILITY/DISCLAIMER OF WARRANTY: WHILE THE PUBLISHER AND AUTHOR HAVE USED THEIR BEST EFFORTS IN PREPARING THIS BOOK, THEY MAKE NO REPRESENTATIONS OR WARRANTIES WITH RESPECT TO THE ACCURACY OR COMPLETENESS OF THE CONTENTS OF THIS BOOK AND SPECIFICALLY DISCLAIM ANY IMPLIED WARRANTIES OF MERCHANTABILITY OR FITNESS FOR A PARTICULAR PURPOSE. NO WARRANTY MAY BE CREATED OR EXTENDED BY SALES REPRESENTATIVES OR WRITTEN SALES MATERIALS. THE ADVICE AND STRATEGIES CONTAINED HEREIN MAY NOT BE SUITABLE FOR YOUR SITUATION. YOU SHOULD CONSULT WITH A PROFESSIONAL WHERE APPROPRIATE. NEITHER THE PUBLISHER NOR THE AUTHOR SHALL BE LIABLE FOR DAMAGES ARISING HEREFROM. SOME OF THE EXERCISES AND DIETARY SUGGESTIONS CONTAINED IN THIS WORK MAY NOT BE APPROPRIATE FOR ALL INDIVIDUALS, AND READERS SHOULD CONSULT WITH A PHYSICIAN BEFORE COMMENCING ANY EXERCISE OR DIETARY PROGRAM.

For general information on our other products and services, please contact our Customer Care Department within the U.S. at 877-762-2974, outside the U.S. at 317-572-3993, or fax 317-572-4002. For technical support, please visit www.wiley.com/techsupport.

Wiley publishes in a variety of print and electronic formats and by print-on-demand. Some material included with standard print versions of this book may not be included in e-books or in print-on-demand. If this book refers to media such as a CD or DVD that is not included in the version you purchased, you may download this material at http://booksupport.wiley.com. For more information about Wiley products, visit www.wiley.com.

Library of Congress Control Number: 2014951013

ISBN: 978-1-119-02277-0 (pbk); ISBN 978-1-119-02278-9 (ebk); ISBN 978-1-119-02279-4 (ebk)

Manufactured in the United States of America

10 9 8 7 6 5 4 3 2 1

Contents at a Glance

Introduction 1

Book I: Getting Started with Paleo 5

Chapter 1: Grasping the What and Why of Paleo 7
Chapter 2: Modern Foods and Your Inner Cave Man 33
Chapter 3: Preparing and Using Your Cave Kitchen 63
Chapter 4: Using Paleo Concepts in Your Fitness Routine.................89
Chapter 5: Making Paleo Practical in a Modern World 113

Book II: Recipes for Every Occasion and Meal............ 137

Chapter 1: Crafting Paleo Breakfasts...139
Chapter 2: Packing Nutrition into Soups and Salads........................157
Chapter 3: The Meat (and More) of the Matter: Paleo Main Dishes.......189
Chapter 4: Paleo Life in the Slow (Cooker) Lane 209
Chapter 5: Vegetable Dishes That Satisfy.....................................227
Chapter 6: Paleo for Kids: Recipes Your Littles Will Love...............245

Book III: Paleo Extras: Snacks, Sauces,
Spice Mixes, and Sweets...................................... 257

Chapter 1: Snacks That Fuel Your Body, Sugar Crash Not Included.......259
Chapter 2: Spicing Up Paleo Cooking with Sauces, Dressings, and Salsas...........275
Chapter 3: Mixing Rubs and Paleo Seasonings 295
Chapter 4: Satisfying Your Sweet Tooth 307

Book IV: Primal Power Moves for a Healthier Body..... 335

Chapter 1: Hinging and Squatting Your Butt and Legs to Primal Perfection 337
Chapter 2: Pushes and Pulls for a Strong, Solid Torso 363
Chapter 3: Carrying Heavy Things and Ab Exercises That Don't Suck....387
Chapter 4: Primal Power Moves for Explosive Athleticism..................411
Chapter 5: Beyond Strength Training and Cardio to Metabolic Conditioning.......425
Chapter 6: Programs for Getting Started — and for Pushing Forward 447

Appendix.. 481

Index 485

Recipes at a Glance

Breakfast Dishes

Almond Banana Pancakes 150
Anytime Waffles 152
Breakfast Sausage Scramble 143
Eggs in Spicy Tomato Sauce 145
Frozen Blueberry Breakfast Bars 154
Grilled Eggs with Homemade Chorizo 146
Huevos Rancheros 142
Lime-Blueberry Poppy Seed Coffee Cake 153
Machacado and Eggs 148
Mini Cinnamon Pancakes 149
Morning Honey Muffins 151
Pizza Frittata 141
Thai Rolled Omelet 144

Soups and Stews

Bacon Butternut Squash Soup 169
Beef Bone Broth 211
Cheater Pork Stew 217
Chicken Fennel Soup 168
Coconut Curry Chowder 164
Curried Cream of Broccoli Soup 167
Deep Healing Chicken Broth 161
Hearty Chili 174
Immune-Building Vegetable Broth 162
Provençal Veggie Soup 170
Roasted Red Pepper and Sweet Potato Soup 225
Teriyaki-Turkey Meatball Soup 172
Thai Butternut Squash Soup 173
Tomato Fennel Soup 171
Turkey Spinach Soup 166
Watermelon Soup 175

Salads

Avocado and Egg Salad 177
Chinese Chicken Salad 186

♻ Chopped Salad with Tahini Dressing.. 184

♻ Classic Cole Slaw.. 188

Curried Chicken Salad... 179

Kale with a Kick Salad 176

Mango and Fennel Chicken Salad 180

Simple Crab Salad 181

♻ Turkish Chopped Salad 182

♻ Tuscan Spinach Salad 178

♻ Vietnamese Cucumber Salad 185

Waldorf Tuna Salad 183

Main Dishes

Chicken Cacciatora... 213

Chicken Fingers.. 193

Citrus Carnitas 197

Club Sandwich Salad 195

Coconut Shrimp with Sweet and Spicy Sauce 203

Creamy Baked Scallops... 204

Creamy Red Shrimp and Tomato Curry.. 224

Easy Chicken Curry with Cabbage.. 223

Grilled Buffalo Shrimp 202

Kalua Shredded Pork 216

Leafy Tacos... 192

♻ Lunchbox Stuffed Peppers 250

Macadamia Nut Crusted Mahi-Mahi 206

Mango Coconut Chipotle Chicken 214

Meatloaf 220

Olive-Oil Braised Albacore 207

Orange Shrimp and Beef with Broccoli... 194

Pineapple and Mango Sweet Heat Chicken Wings... 219

Pineapple Pork Ribs 218

Roasted Oysters... 205

Salmon a L'Afrique du Nord 208

Sausage-Stuffed Peppers 221

Slow Cooker BBQ Pulled Pork 215

Slow Cooker Moroccan Apricot Chicken 222

Slow Cooker Pork and Sauerkraut 212

Slow-Roasted Rack of Lamb.. 200

Spicy Stuffed Eggplant 201
Tandoori Chicken Thighs 199
Thai Green Curry Chicken 198
Winter Squash and Sausage Hash 196

Vegetables and Side Dishes

☼ Brussels Sprouts with Cranberries and Almonds 241
☼ Cauliflower Rice 234
☼ Cocoa Cauliflower 235
☼ Creamy Kale 230
☼ Creamy Spiced Broccoli 238
☼ Italian Broccoli 239
☼ Kimchi 242
☼ Lemon Cucumber Noodles with Cumin 244
☼ Mashed Cauliflower 233
Parsnip Hash Browns 251
Sautéed Kale with Bacon and Mushrooms 252
☼ Sautéed Kohlrabi 240
☼ Sesame Kale 229
☼ Spaghetti Squash Fritters 232
☼ Spiced Sweet Potato Fries 247
☼ Sweet Potato Shoestring Fries 231
☼ Vegetable Latkes 243
☼ Zucchini Pasta with Fire-Roasted Tomato Sauce 236

Sauces, Dressings, and Salsas

☼ Basil and Walnut Pesto 292
☼ Cashew Butter Satay Sauce 278
☼ Cilantro Vinaigrette 286
☼ Classic Stir-Fry Sauce 281
☼ Cooked Olive Oil Mayo 288
☼ Cucumber Avocado Salsa 293
☼ Ghee 277
☼ Mark's Daily Apple Ketchup 289
☼ Moroccan Dipping Sauce 279
☼ Olive Oil Mayo 287
☼ Orange Coconut Marinade 291
☼ Paleo Ranch Dressing 284

⟳ Smooth and Creamy Avocado Dressing 283
⟳ Sri Lankan Curry Sauce 280
⟳ Sweet and Spicy Vinaigrette 285
⟳ Tangy BBQ Sauce 290
⟳ Tangy Carrot and Ginger Salad Dressing 282

Sweets and Desserts

⟳ Almond Cookies with Cinnamon Glaze 310
⟳ Avocado Chocolate Bread 328
⟳ Banana Cacao Muffins 322
⟳ Berries and Whipped Coconut Cream 332
⟳ Blueberry Espresso Brownies 326
Chocolate Bacon Brownie Muffins 323
⟳ Chocolate Chip Cookie Dough Granola Bars 314
⟳ Chocolate Ice Cream 330
⟳ Chocolate-Strawberry Crumble Bars 316
⟳ Chocolate Zucchini Bread 327
⟳ Cinnamon Chocolate Chip Muffins with Honey Frosting 320
⟳ Classic Apple Crisp 315
⟳ Coco-Mango Ice Cream 331
⟳ Coconut Chocolate Chip Cookies 313
⟳ Cranberry Ginger Cookies 309
⟳ Fudge Bombs 272
⟳ Lemon Brownies with Coconut Lemon Glaze 324
Maple Bacon Ice Cream 329
⟳ OMG Chocolate Chip Cookies 312
⟳ Pumpkin Cranberry Scones 317
⟳ Pumpkin Pie Muffins 318
⟳ Pumpkin Poppers 319
⟳ Raspberry Cheesecake Bites 254
⟳ Raspberry Peppermint Sorbet 253
⟳ Star Fruit Magic Wands 256
⟳ Tropical Mango Parfait 269

Snacks

⟳ Avocado Cups 268
Barbecue-Flavored Kale Chips 248
⟳ Cocoa-Cinnamon Coconut Chips 273

♻ Crispy Kale Chips...261
♻ Fried Sage Leaves...265
♻ Ginger-Fried Pears..271
♻ Grilled Spiced Peaches..270
Meatball Poppers..266
♻ Nutty Fruit Stackers..274
♻ Roasted Rosemary Almonds..262
♻ Seaweed with a Kick..267
♻ Southwest Deviled Eggs...263
♻ Sweet Potato Chips...264

Spices

♻ Dukkah..301
♻ Everything Seafood Seasoning..299
♻ Flame Out Blend...304
♻ Garam Masala..302
♻ Gremolata..305
♻ Grilling Spice Rub..297
♻ Italian Seasoning..300
♻ Morning Spice...303
♻ Succulent Steak Seasoning...298

Table of Contents

Introduction *1*

   About This Book 1
   Foolish Assumptions 2
   Icons Used in This Book 3
   Beyond the Book 4
   Where to Go from Here 4

Book 1: Getting Started with Paleo *5*

Chapter 1: Grasping the What and Why of Paleo 7

   It's a Lifestyle, Not a Diet 8
      Enjoying foods that make up the Paleo diet 9
      Taking a cue from our ancestors 10
      Living the way we were designed 10
   Glimpsing the Science Behind the Lifestyle 11
   Curing Modern Ailments with Prehistoric Practices 13
      Losing weight on the Paleo diet 14
      Clearing up gut and skin issues 15
      Getting a good night's sleep 16
      Stabilizing blood sugar 16
      Reducing chronic inflammation 17
   Stealing Moves from Cave Men: The Paleo Fitness Difference 18
      Three principles of Paleo fitness 19
      Keeping it simple: The secret to a good fitness program 19
   Undergoing the Paleo Transformation 20
      Identifying why Paleo works better than other approaches 20
      Switching on your healthy genes with Paleo 20
   Creating a Paleo Lifestyle 21
      Shifting your belief system 22
      Summing up the lifestyle with a few basic guidelines 22
      Minimizing the effects of stress with a Paleo diet 26
   Practicing Paleo Fitness: Movement by Design 28
      Making exercise a requirement, not an option 29
      Keeping your modern-day body strong and lean 30
      Doing what you love 31
      Improving your framework 31

Chapter 2: Modern Foods and Your Inner Cave Man 33

   Getting Familiar with the "Yes" and "No" Foods of the Paleo Diet 34
      100% Paleo-approved: Checking out the Paleo "yes" list 34
      Paleo no-nos: Watching out for foods on the "no" list 38

The Truth about Common Foods 42
    Slaying the sugar demon.. 43
    Making the case for high-quality fats 43
    Fitting fruit into the Paleo plan 44
    Realizing that eggs are A-OK (and cholesterol isn't so bad).......... 45
    Making happy hour truly happy 45
Figuring Out How Much You Can (and Should) Eat 47
    Understanding why a calorie isn't just a calorie 47
    Trying the eat-until-satisfied approach.................................... 48
    Measuring your food at a glance... 49
Supercharging Your Body with the Power of Paleo Foods 50
    Getting the nourishment you need.. 50
    Creating healthy cells.. 51
    Balancing your pH 52
    Identifying food allergies and sensitivities 52
Capturing Your Personal Before and After Makeover 53
Building the Foundation for Success: The 30-Day Reset 54
    Developing a habit with 30 days 55
    Renewing your system 55
    Mastering the plan... 56
    Understanding your body's transformation............................. 58
    Battling the sugar demon.. 58
    The rules for your first 30 days 60
    Dear Diary: Guidelines for 30 days of journaling 61

Chapter 3: Preparing and Using Your Cave Kitchen **63**
Rethinking What You Know about Nutrition 64
    The flawed USDA Food Guide Pyramid 64
    The Paleo pyramid... 66
The Paleo Big Three: Animal Proteins, Natural Fats,
    Complex Carbohydrates 69
    Paleo proteins and why animals matter 70
    Friendly fats and why they're essential 72
    Complex carbs and why they're king.. 74
Getting Rid of the Foods that Don't Fit 75
    Cleansing the pantry 75
    Clearing out the refrigerator and freezer................................. 77
Refilling Your Kitchen with Paleo Foods 78
    Picking Paleo-smart protein 78
    Grabbing Paleo-smart produce 79
    Spicing things up.. 80
    Allowing Paleo-smart fats 81
    Packing a Paleo-smart pantry... 82
    Sipping Paleo-smart drinks... 83

Cooking Smart to Retain Flavor and Nutrition.............................84
    Paleo-smart cooking methods....................................84
    Keeping healthy fats healthy: Smoke points 86

Chapter 4: Using Paleo Concepts in Your Fitness Routine.........89
Cultivating Strength 90
    Knowing what strength really is 90
    Getting stronger to fix just about everything...............90
    Developing strength as a skill 92
    Realizing there's more to fitness than strength............93
Moving Every Day..93
Breathing the Way You Were Meant To 94
Knowing What Compels You...96
    Identifying your primal motivators 96
    Setting goals that stick....................................97
Training the Primal Patterns Primarily...........................98
    Pushing..98
    Pulling..99
    Hinging 99
    Squatting...100
    Carrying..101
    Walking and sprinting 102
Keeping Your Conditioning Inefficient...........................103
    Conditioning for strength or fat loss.....................103
    Comparing efficiency and effectiveness 104
Doing the Least You Have to Do..................................105
The Big Seven: Tracking Your Progress with Health Markers.......106
    Body composition..106
    Strength..107
    Blood pressure..108
    Blood sugar markers 108
    C-reactive protein 109
    Cholesterol and triglycerides.............................110
    pH (acid-base balance) 112

Chapter 5: Making Paleo Practical in a Modern World..........113
Dealing with Potential Pitfalls.................................113
    Clearing diet-related hurdles.............................114
    Accelerating through common roadblocks to living Paleo....115
    Incorporating Paleo into vegetarian and vegan lifestyles .118
Dining Out and Traveling..119
    Choosing the right restaurant.............................120
    Making informed choices...................................120
    Managing the restaurant menu 121
    Planning for Paleo on the road............................121

Enjoying Special Occasions..124
    Planning ahead for social events 124
    Eating Paleo during celebrations and holidays 125
    Indulging with pleasure...128
Transitioning the Family...129
    Teaching kids the "why" behind the "what" 129
    Providing tasty, nutritious treats...130
    Managing mealtimes...132

Book II: Recipes for Every Occasion and Meal 137

Chapter 1: Crafting Paleo Breakfasts 139
Expanding Your Breakfast Options 139
Enjoying Paleo-Friendly, Grain-Free Goodies......................................140

Chapter 2: Packing Nutrition into Soups and Salads 157
Making Your Own Savory Soups, and Buying Wisely
    When You Can't...158
Seizing the Versatility of the Salad 160

Chapter 3: The Meat (and More) of the Matter: Paleo Main Dishes. 189
Building Paleo Meals from Top-Quality Meats.....................................189
Buying Fresh Fish for Fab Dishes 191

Chapter 4: Paleo Life in the Slow (Cooker) Lane 209
Getting the Scoop on Slow Cooking 209

Chapter 5: Vegetable Dishes That Satisfy .227
Evolving Past Starches: Paleo-Friendly Hot Side Dishes 228

Chapter 6: Paleo for Kids: Recipes Your Littles Will Love 245
Packing Kid-Friendly Paleo Lunches...245

Book III: Paleo Extras: Snacks, Sauces, Spice Mixes, and Sweets 257

Chapter 1: Snacks That Fuel Your Body, Sugar Crash Not Included. 259
Making Sure Your Snacks Are Healthy..259

**Chapter 2: Spicing Up Paleo Cooking with Sauces,
Dressings, and Salsas**. 275
  Making Your Own Dressings and Condiments 275
  Adding Flavor with Sugar-Free Spice Blends 276

Chapter 3: Mixing Rubs and Paleo Seasonings 295
  Tapping the Healing Power of Spices. 295

Chapter 4: Satisfying Your Sweet Tooth 307
  Spotting Sugar in Its Sneakiest Forms. 308

Book IV: Primal Power Moves for a Healthier Body *335*

**Chapter 1: Hinging and Squatting Your Butt and Legs
to Primal Perfection** 337
  The Lowdown on Hinges 337
    Using your hips in the hinge. 338
    Counting the benefits of a strong hinge. 339
  Beginner Hinging Exercises. 339
    The dead lift. 339
    The single-leg dead lift 341
  Intermediate Hinging Exercises 343
    The swing. 343
    The one-arm swing 345
  Advanced Hinging Exercises 346
    The clean. 347
    The snatch 349
  The Lowdown on Squats 350
    Getting to the truth about squatting 351
    Exploring the benefits of a deep squat. 351
  Beginner Squatting Exercises. 352
    The goblet squat 352
    The bodyweight squat. 354
    The goblet lunge 355
  Intermediate Squatting Exercises. 356
    The racked squat 356
    The racked lunge 358
  Advanced Squatting Exercises. 359
    The front squat. 359
    The pistol squat 360

Chapter 2: Pushes and Pulls for a Strong, Solid Torso **363**

All about the Primal Pushes..363
    Reaping the benefits of the big pushes...364
    Practicing strength...364
Beginner Pushes..365
    The push-up..365
    The military press..367
Intermediate Pushes...368
    The one-arm push-up...368
    The bench press..369
    The dip...372
Advanced Pushes...373
    The one-arm one-leg push-up..373
    The handstand push-up..373
All about the Primal Pulls...375
    Balancing out with pulls..376
    Recognizing the many benefits of pulling.....................................376
Beginner Pulls..377
    The bodyweight row...377
    The chin-up...378
Intermediate Pulls...379
    The one-arm row...380
    The pull-up..381
Advanced Pulls...382
    The L-sit pull-up/chin-up...382
    The muscle-up...383
    The one-arm chin-up..385

**Chapter 3: Carrying Heavy Things and Ab Exercises
That Don't Suck.** **387**

Mastering the Art of the Loaded Carry..388
    Focusing on an everyday activity...388
    Carrying heavy things for strength and fitness.............................388
Beginner Carries..389
    The farmer's carry...389
    The waiter's carry..391
Intermediate Carries...392
    The racked carry..392
    The two-arm waiter's carry...393
Advanced Carries: The Bottoms-Up Carry...394
Getting the Abs of Your Dreams...396
Beginner Ab Exercises...397
    The four-point plank..397
    The V-up...397
    The windmill...399

Intermediate Ab Exercises..400
The hanging knee raise 401
The two-point plank..402
Advanced Ab Exercises 403
The hanging leg raise 403
The windshield wiper..405
An All-Around Paleo Exercise: The Turkish Get-Up 406

Chapter 4: Primal Power Moves for Explosive Athleticism........411
Understanding Primal Power 412
Your need for speed 412
The benefits of power training...412
Beginner Power Moves 413
The push press...413
The broad jump..415
Intermediate Power Moves 416
The jerk...417
The box jump 418
Advanced Power Moves 420
The double jerk 420
The double snatch 422

**Chapter 5: Beyond Strength Training and
Cardio to Metabolic Conditioning...........................425**
Introducing Primal Strength Training...426
Defining strength training...426
Acknowledging the benefits of lifting heavy things......................427
Determining how heavy is heavy enough 428
Gaining Strength Without Gaining Weight.....................................429
Tensing (and relaxing) muscles to develop strength....................429
Combining heavy weight and low reps 430
Deciding on your training frequency...430
Working the best strength-building exercises 431
Moving Past Chronic Cardio Syndrome...432
Facing the little-known drawbacks of excessive cardio................433
Doing what you love..433
Getting more out of your cardio with fasting................................434
Developing the Recipe for a Good Exercise Program...........................435
Simple...435
Sensible...436
Reasonable..436
Introducing Metabolic Conditioning...437
Discovering the benefits of metabolic conditioning 438
Switching on your fat-burning furnace..439
Getting results in just 15 minutes 439

Turbocharging Fat Loss with Complexes 440
    Starting with basic bodyweight complexes 441
    Taking it up a notch with kettlebell complexes 443

**Chapter 6: Programs for Getting Started —
and for Pushing Forward 451**
    Beginning at the Beginning: The 21-Day Primal Quick Start 448
    Gearing Up for the 21-Day Program 448
        Start with a warm-up 449
        Get ready for some repetition 454
        Be prepared to lift heavy 454
        Expect to improve your conditioning 455
    Your 21-Day Primal Quick Start 455
    From Average to Elite: The 90-Day Primal Body Transformation 459
    Building a Balanced 90-Day Program 460
        Strength-training exercises 461
        Metabolic conditioning 464
        Your daily warm-up 464
        Your weekly schedule 465
    Your 90-Day Primal Body Transformation 465

Appendix *481*

Index *485*

Introduction

A ny Paleo aficionado will agree that your Paleo journey starts with food. Discovering the "yes" and "no" Paleo foods, converting your kitchen into a primal one, and creating your own Paleo meals can help you lose weight, boost immunity, fight aging, heal conditions, and perform better.

But living Paleo isn't a "diet" in the traditional sense but a way of thinking about health and fitness — one that's based on eating and moving like your ancestors did. This means loading up on some foods and avoiding others. It also means heavy lifting, sprinting, and other movements that the conveniences of modern day have made largely irrelevant.

Whenever someone comes along with a "new and exciting" exercise program, it's generally all wrong. When it comes to fitness, a new way of doing something is rarely a better way of doing something. It's almost invariably the exchange of one nuisance for another. The same is true of what you eat. This book shows you what you need to live a lifestyle that supports your health with all the information, tips, and recipes you need to feel alive, vibrant, and nourished the Paleo way.

About This Book

Adopting the Paleo lifestyle may seem overwhelming at first, so *Paleo All-in-One For Dummies* is organized in a way that makes the benefits of eating and exercising Paleo easy to understand. Use this book as both a reference and a cookbook; if you need to check on whether a food is a Paleo yes or no, you can find that information easily. If you're creating a menu for a dinner party and want to go all Paleo, you can pick your recipes and get to work. If Paleo is new to you, you can start with the foundational information and get to know Paleo superfoods, how Paleo eating can improve how you feel, and how you can get started with a cleansing 30-Day Reset. You can find out exactly what it means to work out Paleo, the benefits you reap from doing so, and all the exercises you need to build a solid workout program. (For good measure, you also get 90 days' worth of workouts to follow.)

Cooking is a big part of the Paleo equation. The recipes in this book will keep you well fed from breakfast through dinner, with healthy snacks in between. Here are some specific recipe-related conventions that apply throughout the book:

- ✔ Temperatures are given in degrees Fahrenheit.
- ✔ All eggs are large unless noted otherwise.
- ✔ All water is filtered so all the toxic elements are removed.
- ✔ All bacon is free of nitrates, casein, gluten, and antibiotics.
- ✔ All pepper is freshly ground black pepper unless otherwise noted.
- ✔ All butter is grass-fed and organic. (If you can't find grass-fed butter, though, you can substitute conventional organic butter.) You may also replace any butter with *ghee* (clarified butter).
- ✔ All salt is unprocessed. Good sources for unprocessed salt include Selina Naturally brand Celtic sea salt (www.celticseasalt.com) and Real Salt brand sea salt (http://realsalt.com).

At the end of many recipes, you'll see a note indicating that the recipe has been vetted by the team at Whole9 (http://whole9life.com) and is considered acceptable for a cleansing 30-day Paleo launch, which in this book is called the 30-Day Reset Paleo cleanse. These recipes don't include any added sugars (real or artificial), grains, legumes, or dairy. They replace butter with clarified butter (ghee). If a recipe includes a processed food (such as chicken broth, bacon, or tomato paste), you should choose brands that don't contain off-limits ingredients such as sugar, soy, additives, or preservatives.

So that this book is as practical as possible (because that's what it's really about, right?), it includes web addresses for sources of products and other information. Some web addresses may break across two lines of text. If you're reading this book in print and want to visit one of these web pages, simply key in the address exactly as it's noted in the text, pretending as though the line break doesn't exist. If you're reading this text as an e-book, you've got it easy — just click the web address to be taken directly to the web page.

Foolish Assumptions

As we wrote this book, we made the following assumptions about you:

- ✔ You want to change your diet, lose weight, improve your fitness, or manage some type of medical condition and have heard about the Paleo diet.
- ✔ You want to stop eating processed and unhealthy foods to feel younger, healthier, happier, and more vibrant.

✔ You're open to the idea of making lifestyle changes — avoiding certain foods, making sleep a priority, reducing stress — to enhance your quality of life.

✔ You want to encourage yourself to continue the Paleo lifestyle by finding great-tasting recipes that are easy to make.

✔ You're adopting a level of commitment to Paleo that has you craving an all-around useful guidebook that has everything you could possibly need to jump back into your kitchen — and into your life.

✔ You want to be healthier, leaner, stronger, or more productive. Or perhaps you want to be all of these things.

✔ You've tried exercise programs in the past and haven't been satisfied with the results or have been frustrated with the process.

✔ You have control over your food choices and those of your family, and you want to help your loved ones enjoy a healthy Paleo lifestyle, too.

Note: We recommend that you get your doctor's approval before beginning any exercise program, whether you're a novice or a veteran to fitness.

Icons Used in This Book

To make this book easier to navigate, the following icons help you find key information about the Paleo lifestyle and Paleo cooking.

 This icon indicates practical information that can help you in your quest for improving health and fitness, adopting a Paleo diet, or making one of the recipes.

 When you see this icon, you know that the information that follows is important enough to read twice!

 This icon highlights information that may be detrimental to your success or physical well-being if you ignore it.

 This icon gives you a heads-up that what you're reading is more in-depth or technical than what you need to get a basic grasp on the main topic at hand.

Beyond the Book

In addition to all the material, resources, and recipes you can find in the book you're reading right now, this product also comes with some access-anywhere goodies on the web. Check out the eCheat Sheet at www.dummies.com/cheatsheet/paleoaio for details on Paleo superfoods, ideas for getting your kids to eat their Paleo veggies, and advice for eating Paleo while you're traveling.

You can also go online to see the proper method for performing many of the Paleo exercises included in Book IV. The videos linked to at www.dummies.com/extras/paleoaio show you how to position and move your body correctly, thereby reducing the chance of injury from using the incorrect form. At www.dummies.com/extras/paleoaio, you can also read about supplements that may be beneficial to your health and protein-filled foods that are suitable for packing in your kid's lunchbox.

Where to Go from Here

This book is organized so you can read it in the way that makes the most sense to you; feel free to jump around to the information that's most relevant to you right now. You can use the table of contents to find the broad categories of subjects or use the index to look up specific information.

Do you want to know more about the Paleo superfoods so you can get started on the Paleo path? Start with Chapter 2 of Book I. Feeling hungry and want to get started on the recipes? Feel free to jump right into the recipes in Books II and III. Can't wait to get an exercise high? Book IV has the exercises that will get you there.

And if you're not sure where to begin, read Book I. It gives you the basic information you need to understand why and how eating and living Paleo can help you improve your health and quality of life.

Book I
Getting Started with Paleo

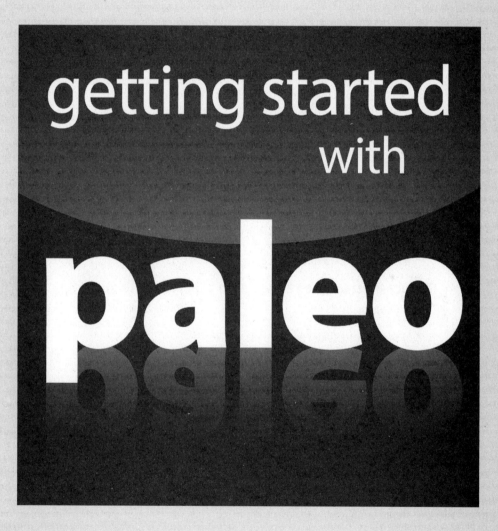

Visit www.dummies.com for free access to great Dummies content online.

Contents at a Glance

Chapter 1: Grasping the What and Why of Paleo 7

It's a Lifestyle, Not a Diet..8
Glimpsing the Science Behind the Lifestyle..11
Curing Modern Ailments with Prehistoric Practices...............................13
Stealing Moves from Cave Men: The Paleo Fitness Difference 18
Undergoing the Paleo Transformation..20
Creating a Paleo Lifestyle...21
Practicing Paleo Fitness: Movement by Design......................................28

Chapter 2: Modern Foods and Your Inner Cave Man 33

Getting Familiar with the "Yes" and "No" Foods of the Paleo Diet..........34
The Truth about Common Foods 42
Figuring Out How Much You Can (and Should) Eat................................47
Supercharging Your Body with the Power of Paleo Foods 50
Capturing Your Personal Before and After Makeover 53
Building the Foundation for Success: The 30-Day Reset........................54

Chapter 3: Preparing and Using Your Cave Kitchen 63

Rethinking What You Know about Nutrition...64
The Paleo Big Three: Animal Proteins, Natural Fats, Complex Carbohydrates 69
Getting Rid of the Foods that Don't Fit..75
Refilling Your Kitchen with Paleo Foods...78
Cooking Smart to Retain Flavor and Nutrition..84

Chapter 4: Using Paleo Concepts in Your Fitness Routine 89

Cultivating Strength..90
Moving Every Day...93
Breathing the Way You Were Meant To...94
Knowing What Compels You..96
Training the Primal Patterns Primarily 98
Keeping Your Conditioning Inefficient..103
Doing the Least You Have to Do...105
The Big Seven: Tracking Your Progress with Health Markers 106

Chapter 5: Making Paleo Practical in a Modern World 113

Dealing with Potential Pitfalls..113
Dining Out and Traveling 119
Enjoying Special Occasions..124
Transitioning the Family...129

Chapter 1

Grasping the What and Why of Paleo

In This Chapter

▶ Explaining the foundations of the Paleo diet and why it works

▶ Digging into the scientific foundation of the lifestyle

▶ Looking and feeling better by following the Paleo lifestyle

▶ Bringing the exercise component into your Paleo program

▶ Finding out about the Paleo transformation

▶ Being sensible about moving your body

*P*aleo is the answer. If you've suffered with weight problems or health issues, you're in for a treat. Every aspect of your health improves when you incorporate Paleo principles into your life. Your body starts to transform right before your eyes, and suddenly, your outlook is optimistic.

Your eyes brighten, your skin takes on a completely different sheen, and your wrinkles start to fade. You begin to shed body fat as you watch your stomach get flatter and flatter. Your muscle tone improves, your hair gets silky, your teeth seem stronger. Your mood elevates, and you begin to notice that you feel happier. Your body begins to calm, releasing anxiety and tension. You start to forget what it feels like to have aches and pains, and your entire body seems to lose the bloated feeling it's been carrying around for far too long. You begin to be more than just *present* in life; you begin to start really *living* life. For some, it's the first time in a very long time.

You'd be hard-pressed to find a more excited group of people than those who have transformed their lives to living Paleo. What you find in the pages of this book is an easy-to-follow nutritional blueprint and fitness program that actually exists and works — and when you adopt this plan, everything gets easier.

In this chapter, you discover some foundational Paleo principles, including the answers to questions about how the Paleo diet came to be, the foods that make up the Paleo diet, the science behind Paleo success, and how living Paleo will soon have you looking and feeling better than ever.

Living Paleo takes you from a place of hopelessness to hope. So what are you waiting for? Dig in!

It's a Lifestyle, Not a Diet

Living Paleo takes the mystery out of eating. It's simplicity at its finest, which is one of the reasons eating Paleo foods works well for so many. When you eat simply (but deliciously), you get results.

Many eating plans, programs, and products give you lots of rules and may even require special foods, which makes understanding these plans and staying committed to them even harder. The biggest missing element in other plans is the core ingredient for long-term success — *health*. Most programs don't move you toward health either biologically or behaviorally. If your cells aren't getting healthier and your behavior is expected to change in strict ways only for the short term, the entire purpose is lost. You don't discover how to eat and live for the *rest of your life*.

Paleo is different; Paleo is based on simple, easy-to-understand nutritional principles. Eating Paleo takes away all the confusion and is natural to implement. It's something you can stick with for a long time.

Paleo is the abbreviation for *Paleolithic*. The Paleo diet refers to foods consumed during the Paleolithic era, the time from about 2.5 million years ago up to 10,000 BC.

A lot of people start the Paleo diet to get a killer body. And living Paleo is a great way to move toward your ideal body, but what most people experience is even more powerful. Living Paleo literally changes their lives for the better. If you've had aches and pains, fatigue, skin issues, menstrual problems, chronic inflammation, digestive complaints, weight gain, depression, fertility problems, autoimmune struggles, diabetes, or cardiovascular disease, you're going to love living Paleo.

The hormone-modulating, anti-inflammatory, nutrient-dense properties of the Paleo lifestyle help regulate all the systems and functions of the body. Your body resets at a higher functioning level, so you'll not only look better eating Paleo, but you'll also feel better. Living Paleo supports the healing and prevention of many chronic diseases. And thanks to the nutrition-packed foods of the Paleo diet, you start sporting a much stronger cellular system, and with that comes healing and transformation.

Enjoying foods that make up the Paleo diet

When you think Paleo foods, think grassroots — simple, back-to-nature foods filled with nutrients that bring you back to life. Paleo foods are what you are *designed* to eat. They're the foods that your body digests and absorbs efficiently. Paleo foods have the most positive impact on all the structures and functions of your body.

The foundational Paleo foods include lean meats, seafood, vegetables, fruits, nuts, seeds, and naturally occurring healthy fats — those that have always been found in animals and plants. Our hunter-gatherer ancestors survived on these foods. In the Paleolithic era, no one planted crops, and no factories churned out industrialized foods. Our ancestors didn't have access to grains, sugars, starches, legumes, dairy, processed foods, or oils — and autopsies show that they were better for it. They may not have had the convenience of a one-minute meal, but our ancestors had far higher levels of health and didn't suffer from the modern-day diseases we do today.

Changes in everyday foods and in food processing have fundamentally altered modern diets. Paleo foods differ nutritionally in several ways, such as their ability to do the following:

- ✔ Balance blood sugar and keep your overall sugar load down
- ✔ Create a favorable fatty-acid balance (omega-6 to omega-3 balance)
- ✔ Balance macronutrients (proteins, fats, and carbohydrates)
- ✔ Provide adequate amounts of trace nutrients (minerals)
- ✔ Promote and maintain acid-base balance (how acid and alkaline your blood is)
- ✔ Add robust amounts of fiber to your daily plate (for intestinal health)

The fact that modern-day foods aren't working is rather obvious. People are sicker and fatter than ever and are more confused about what to eat and how to live than in any other time in history. But living Paleo cuts through the confusion and clarifies what foods move you toward health.

When you begin eating Paleo, your body sheds unhealthy cells. You peel away layers of fat; you become leaner, stronger, and healthier.

Taking a cue from our ancestors

Our bodies haven't changed much since before agricultural society. Our body's needs now are similar to what they were during Paleolithic times, before the dawn of agriculture.

Humans have been shaped and molded over a hundred thousand generations. What our bodies were designed to eat then, they are designed to eat now. In other words, our genes are still stuck in the hunter-gatherer's time, even though we're living in the modern world. Our genes simply haven't caught up to the modern-day divergence.

About 10,000 years ago, the birth of *agriculture* changed the way people lived. Hunter-gatherers became attracted to a new way of life based on a routine and settled existence that centered around agriculture and the breeding of animals.

The tidal wave of change happened again a few hundred years ago with the *Industrial Revolution*. The impact that this technological progress has had on human biology is huge. Some of these advancements have provided safety and convenience. But some of these man-made environmental changes have caused a pandemic of human suffering and diseases that were unknown to our ancestors.

Autopsies show that the hunter-gatherers were some of the healthiest people to walk the earth. Using their lifestyle as our template, we can strike a balance between modern-day living and our grassroots beginning.

Living the way we were designed

If you've tried other eating plans and haven't been successful long term or if you've been trying to get well and are making little headway, you're probably carrying the wrong road map. Here's why: The missing link is probably that you're not eating the foods that you're *designed* to eat or living the lifestyle you're designed to live.

Our genes have changed very little since Paleolithic times. In fact, according to medical anthropologist S. Boyd Eaton, MD, 99.99 percent of our genes were formed before the development of agriculture. This is big. That means that our hunter-gatherer ancestors programmed our genes. How they ate is our nutritional blueprint, how they moved is the blueprint for our physiology, and how they lived is the blueprint for the lifestyle we should strive to lead.

You don't need to live life as a science experiment, trying to reenact everything our ancestors did or see the world through Paleo goggles. You just need to understand how your genes were programmed and try to model that as closely as you can. When you model the Paleo lifestyle, your struggles will be greatly reduced.

As humans, our bodies are the result of an optimal design that has been shaped and molded by nature. To look and feel your absolute best, you have to do what it's designed to do. *Paleo All-in-One For Dummies* is your reference guide to show you how to live according to your nature.

Living Paleo is about getting you healthy. When your cells are healthy, everything falls into place. You feel better, look better, and lose weight. What makes Paleo different from everything else is that the nutrient-dense foods are just one piece of the puzzle. The way you live *outside* of the kitchen has as much to do with how you look and feel as the foods you eat.

Traditional diets provide food rules, and that's where they end. You follow the rules, hope to get results, and hope that the results stick. This pattern is often the recipe for disappointment and frustration because eventually the rules stop and your life takes over. You haven't made lifestyle changes that support lasting results.

Paleo considers why you eat, when you eat, how you eat, and other factors in your life that influence how you feel, such as amount and quality of sleep, stress levels, sunlight, movement, supplementation, and your thoughts. It's a lifelong change that's fairly simple to make and has lasting, positive consequences, unlike a diet that's meant as a short-term solution to lose a few pounds, which ultimately leads to frustration and hopelessness.

In the end, your habits and patterns are responsible for how you look and feel. Living Paleo gives you the lifestyle patterns and strategies that go well beyond a flash-in-the-pan diet. You figure out how to make the lifestyle changes that have lasting, positive effects.

Genetically, you can live for 120 years. The key is creating healthy lifestyle patterns so your body expresses health and vitality and doesn't express disease or obesity. That's what living Paleo is all about.

Glimpsing the Science Behind the Lifestyle

Yes, the excitement and results of living Paleo are awesome. But knowing that some of the most respected leaders in the field, as well as some of the most brilliant researchers, have found evidence for why Paleo foods and Paleo living work well is a great reassurance.

Here are some facts from leading Paleolithic researchers S. Boyd Eaton, MD, and M. Konner, PhD, cited in the *New England Journal of Medicine* ("Paleolithic nutrition: a consideration of its nature and current implications." 1985: N. Eng. J. Med. 321, 283–289):

- "The human genetic constitution has changed relatively little in the past 40,000 years."

- "The development of agriculture 10,000 years ago has had a minimal influence on our genes."

- "The Industrial Revolution, agribusiness, and modern food-processing techniques have occurred too recently to have any evolutionary effect at all."

- "Physicians and nutritionists are increasingly convinced that the dietary habits adopted by Western society over the past 100 years make an important etiologic contribution to coronary heart disease, hypertension, diabetes, and some types of cancer."

- "These conditions have emerged as dominant health problems only in the past century and are virtually unknown among the few surviving hunter-gatherer populations whose way of life and eating habits most closely resemble pre-agricultural human beings."

Here's some compelling research from Dr. Loren Cordain (*The Paleo Diet* [Wiley]), professor in the Health and Exercise Science Department at Colorado State University and one of the top global researchers in the area of evolutionary medicine:

- "DNA evidence shows genetically humans have hardly changed at all (to be specific, the human genome has changed less than 0.02% in 40,000 years)."

- "Nature determined what our bodies needed thousands of years before civilization developed, before people started farming and raising livestock."

- "In other words, built into our genes is a blueprint for optimal nutrition — a plan that spells out the foods that make us healthy, lean, and fit." (The *blueprint* is Paleo foods.)

Finally, Rainer J Klement and Ulrike Kämmerer discuss the striking benefits and prevention of cancer with a Paleo diet in *Nutrition & Metabolism* ("Is there a role for carbohydrate restriction in the treatment and prevention of cancer." October 2011. 8[75]):

✔ "Cancer is *very* rare among uncivilized hunter-gatherer societies."

✔ "The switch from the 'cave man's diet' consisting of fat, meat, occasionally roots, berries, and other sources of carbohydrates to a nutrition dominated by easily digested carbohydrates derived mainly from grains as a staple food, would have occurred too recently to induce major adoptions in our gene encoding and metabolic pathways." (In other words, our bodies don't have the genetic wiring for adapting to grains.)

✔ "[In a cave man–like diet,] carbohydrate restriction is not only limited to avoiding sugar and other high glucose foods, but also to a reduced intake of grains. Grains can induce inflammation in susceptible individuals due to their content of omega-6 fatty acids, lectins, and gluten."

✔ "Paleolithic-type diets, that by definition exclude grain products, have been shown to improve glycemic control and cardiovascular risk factors more effectively than typically recommended low-fat diets rich in whole grains. These diets are not necessarily low carbohydrate diets, but focus on replacing high glycemic index modern foods with fruits and vegetables, in this way reducing the total glycemic [sugar] load. *This brings us back to our initial perception of cancer as a disease of civilization that has been rare among hunter-gatherer societies until they adopted our Western lifestyle.*"

Many anthropologists and health care providers recognize that the hunter-gatherers represent a *reference standard* for modern-day nutrition and a model way of eating to get well and stay well. When you see the results *and* the research, you begin to understand why.

Curing Modern Ailments with Prehistoric Practices

Modern-day ailments have become pandemic. Everyone knows someone who's wrestling with diabetes, cancer, or an autoimmune disease. To be in one's 60s and not be on medication is remarkable. Even worse, the diagnosis of chronic childhood diseases has almost quadrupled over the past four decades.

Think about it. With all the modern drugs and all the surgeries, we're not getting any better. You can't possibly look at the data on our supposed health care model and think that what we're doing is working. In fact, in a two-part series published in the *Annals of Internal Medicine,* Dr. Elliot Fisher, professor of medicine at Dartmouth University, came to the following conclusion: "Our study suggests that perhaps one-third of medical spending is now devoted to services that don't appear to improve health or quality of care — and may makes things worse."

What that means is staggering. Here's some perspective: We're spending annually about $1.4 trillion a year on health care that's proven to be ineffective! So that's $4 billion per day down the drain! Then there's the issue of not only having ineffective treatments but also having adverse effects from the treatments. Either way you look at it, *it's not the answer.*

So the question becomes, what *is* the answer? How do we get well and stay well? We need to understand how we got into this mess in the first place. We're not sick because of bad genes or rotten luck. Most of our modern-day ailments were born out of *bad choices.* If we want to get well and stay well and avoid the circus of reactive health care, we have to get in the right paradigm and learn to make *smart choices* and *prevent* disease before it starts.

Putting real food first, like eating Paleo foods that you're designed to eat, is one of the smartest things you'll ever do to get well and stay well. The following sections explore other benefits of living Paleo.

Losing weight on the Paleo diet

If your goal is to lose weight, you've come to the right place. When you eat a well-planned Paleo diet (this doesn't include copious amounts of Paleo cookies, bars, muffins, and so on), your body naturally loses body fat until you've reached your ideal weight. When you get healthy, everything in your body recalibrates, including your weight. What's so great about eating Paleo is that you lose stored fat because you're actually using that stored fat for energy. Your body transforms in a way it may never have before, and you begin to look — and feel — lean and toned.

Here are some of the reasons you lose weight by eating Paleo:

- ✔ You're eating foods with a high-nutrient density without all the garbage calories.
- ✔ You lose the *bloat* (dump excess water retention).
- ✔ You reduce food sensitivities by healing your gut.
- ✔ You eat foods that help you maintain a healthy blood sugar.
- ✔ You eat foods that regulate your hormones along with the signals associated with hormones.
- ✔ You burn stored fat, thanks to the proteins and fat in the food you eat.
- ✔ You feel more satiated because of the healthy fats you're eating.

✔ You eat nutrient-dense foods, creating healthy cells, and weight loss is a natural byproduct.

✔ You have more energy eating Paleo, so you tend to move more and have more efficient workouts.

✔ You use stored fat for energy instead of sugary carbohydrates, which is a more efficient fat-burning pathway.

✔ You eat foods with a high fiber content, which encourages weight loss.

Living Paleo is about getting you to optimal health and keeping you there. The weight loss is a wonderful bonus!

Clearing up gut and skin issues

Eating Paleo is like an internal spring cleaning. You feel healthy from the inside out. All the grains, sugars, starches, legumes, and poorly prepared, refined, processed, and denatured foods have created havoc in your intestines. Over time, this means inflammation and *leaky gut*.

Your intestinal walls are lined with these armed guards (immune cells). As long as these cells and good bacteria are there lying over your intestines, you're good to go. Nothing can get in or out. Your body is in a health lockdown. When your gut becomes damaged or perforated by the inflammation caused by the foods you eat or the medications you take, it becomes leaky and porous. The structures of the intestines become damaged, and your armed guards are killed in action. You can't absorb nutrients the same way. Undigested food and bacteria flow into your body where they don't belong and aren't recognized. When undigested food and bacteria flow into your bloodstream, your body screams, "Attack!" like it would with any foreign invader. Your body literally attacks itself instead of protecting itself, as it's designed to do, and you get autoimmune problems, chronic disease, unexplained fatigue, intestinal distress, and hypersensitivities. Not a whole lotta fun.

Interestingly enough, a damaged gut causes skin problems as well. A direct link exists between intestinal health and the health of your skin. If you have acne, rashes, eczema, psoriasis, or poor skin tone, a leaky gut may be the culprit. If you want beautiful skin, it's an inside job, and it starts with putting real food first.

The upside here is a leaky gut isn't hard to fix. It's completely reversible, and when eating Paleo foods, you're well on your way!

Getting a good night's sleep

One of the most motivating factors to give Paleo a spin is the improvement to your sleep cycle. After you're adjusted to Paleo and hit your Paleo stride, you'll find your sleep is deeper and more restful.

Here are some of the reasons you sleep like a baby when you start living Paleo:

- ✔ You're getting foods loaded with minerals, which are grounding and calming to your body.
- ✔ When your blood sugars are more balanced, like they are with Paleo foods, you don't get that blood sugar dip in the middle of the night, causing your body to release hormones to restore blood sugar, which disturbs sleep.
- ✔ A lot of Paleo foods contain B vitamins, which are great for calming nerves and balancing the nervous system for restful sleep.
- ✔ Some Paleo foods, like eggs, turkey, nuts, fish, and some fruits, contain an essential amino acid called *tryptophan,* which helps promote sleep.
- ✔ When eating Paleo, your body naturally regulates hormones and signals associated with hormones that, in turn, help you sleep better.
- ✔ When you create healthy cells like you do when eating Paleo, all the systems and functions in your body run smoother, including sleep cycles.
- ✔ You have more energy eating Paleo, so you run your battery down naturally with activity, rather than with sugary foods and carbohydrate crashes, leading to more restful sleep.

If you have sleep issues, let Paleo be your all-natural sleep aid. It works — with no nasty side effects!

Stabilizing blood sugar

What may be most astonishing about eating Paleo is its powerful ability to manage blood sugar, which is one of the most compelling and worthwhile reasons to make the switch. Managing blood sugar is essential for disease control, energy level, and how youthful you look and feel.

People with diabetes or pre-diabetes or those who feel a little out of kilter with their blood sugar benefit tremendously when eating Paleo. By eating mainly non-starchy vegetables and moderate amounts of fruit with minimal

TIP

starchy foods, you can dramatically lower blood sugar load. Lean proteins and healthy fats round out the Paleo diet to further control blood sugar.

High blood sugars are a thing of the past when eating Paleo. Work with a health care provider who knows you and your situation and prepare to be amazed!

Reducing chronic inflammation

When you think inflammation, you probably think "ouch!" because the inflammation you've probably heard about or experienced firsthand is the kind of inflammation that makes you feel all-over aches, pains, swelling, fatigue, or just plain discomfort.

One kind of inflammation is actually a good thing; it's called *acute inflammation,* or short-term inflammation. This inflammation is a natural part of your body's healing process and one of the "trump cards" your body hands out to give you a healing push. When you get an illness, like the flu, or physical trauma, like a shoulder injury, your body goes into action immediately by calling on your immune system for healing. The inflammation that ensues is there to protect the damage already done and make sure it doesn't get any worse.

So how does this good thing (your healing push) get out of hand and cause you trouble? If your intestines have those pesky little perforations called leaky gut (see the earlier section "Clearing up gut and skin issues"), foods are going to squeak through the holes to the other side of your intestinal wall into your bloodstream where they don't belong and aren't recognized. When your body goes into overdrive to fight off these foreign invaders, you have chronic inflammation.

Whatever overloads your immune system can cause this overreaction and inflammation. Here are some of the immune system stressors:

- Unhealthy foods (packaged, processed, refined, or foods denatured in any way)
- Foods containing gluten
- Toxic overload (everything from environmental toxins to toxic cleaning products)
- Excessive stress
- Overload of medications (especially NSAIDs) or antibiotics
- Sleep deprivation
- Too much exercise training

You can see from this list that many of these immune stressors are lifestyle choices, including the foods you eat. When you eat Paleo foods, you make a huge difference in *controlling* and *preventing* the long-term inflammation that can lead to a lot of misery.

Here are some of the conditions that are caused by chronic inflammation:

- Arthritis
- Asthma and allergies
- Autoimmune diseases, like celiac disease
- Cardiovascular disease
- Diabetes
- Intestinal inflammatory disease, like Crohn's disease
- Thyroid dysfunction

Eating Paleo does an outstanding job at keeping your immune system strong and inflammation at bay.

Stealing Moves from Cave Men: The Paleo Fitness Difference

The cave man was perhaps a perfect role model for health and exercise because he didn't try to improve something that was virtually faultless. He followed his genetic programming: He moved how he was meant to move and ate how he was meant to eat. He was fit and healthy.

In the domain of exercise today, fads come (and just as often go) like pimples on a teenybopper. Most of these crazes are, at best, useless, but quite a few have even grown to be dangerous.

Most popular fitness programs make people move but fail to first show them how to do so. Many make the conventional assumption that people just know how to move, or that they know how to move well. However, for most, quality movement is like writing cursive — an elegant skill that gets sloppy without practice.

Three principles of Paleo fitness

Not all movement is good for you, and more exercise isn't necessarily better. The principles of Paleo fitness give you basic directives for making the most of your fitness routine:

✔ The first principle of Paleo fitness states that the most basic and appropriate function of exercise should be to condition for something other than exercise. Whether that something is a sport is of small significance. Exercise should be a means to health. Exercise should promote health and vitality — and never, under any circumstance, should it ever detract from that.

✔ The second principle of Paleo fitness states that exercise is best served in small to moderate doses, which is to say just enough to get the job done and not a smidgeon more. But again, conventional practices overlook this detail, made clear by the number of people who spend hours every day trudging on treadmills and spinning on bicycles. Practices that create a chronic state of stress on the body are ill suited for sustainable bodily profits, not to mention wholly ineffective for long-term weight loss.

✔ The third principle of Paleo fitness states that exercise should promote beautiful movement and stimulate a positive hormonal response. Just as trudging on the treadmill is equal to committing biomechanical treason, so is crushing yourself day in and day out by lifting weights.

With Paleo fitness, you marry beautiful movement with beautiful food, which results in a strong, beautiful body.

Keeping it simple: The secret to a good fitness program

Any exercise (and nutrition) program will improve in direct proportion to the number of things that you can keep out of it that don't need to be there. In other words, the secret to a good exercise program is to strip it down to the fewest possible parts — the fundamentals — and leave it at that. Paleo fitness is all about simplicity.

The fundamentals of Paleo are simple and proven effective. All you have to do is follow a simple diet of meats, eggs, fish, veggies, nuts, seeds, and *some* fruit. Then move often and move beautifully, lift heavy every couple of days, and occasionally run for your life (just not on a treadmill).

The secret is to practice strength selectively. About 20 tried-and-true exercises — which probably amounts to less than 5 percent of all the exercises out there — are guaranteed to get you 95 percent of all the results you could ever want.

Undergoing the Paleo Transformation

You live longer, stronger, and more healthfully when you start eating and living Paleo because you move toward health. When you're truly healthy, your immune system is solid, protective, and strong. Your body works for you, not against you, and transformation happens.

People usually start Paleo to lose weight. Then layers and layers begin to peel back. Their waists get smaller, their skin and eyes glisten, and their hair may get shinier. They notice conditions healing, and before long, they get the most amazing part of the transformation — a mental, spiritual kind of change. They start thinking more clearly and enjoying a more positive outlook. Paleo reboots the body by flooding it with vitamins and minerals. This healing is possible for anyone who decides to commit to living Paleo!

Identifying why Paleo works better than other approaches

Paleo is more effective than other approaches because it centers on the food that works best with your body. Most important, Paleo foods have one purpose, which is what truly defines Paleo: to nourish the body and get you healthy.

That's right, the objective behind eating Paleo is to get you healthy. Period. Everything else that comes along the way just follows the natural progression. It's against natural law not to lose weight, boost immunity, fight aging, heal conditions, and perform better when you're healthy.

Switching on your healthy genes with Paleo

You're in the driver's seat of your health. Your lifestyle choices and the environment in which you choose to live have the biggest impact on the quality of your life. This science is called *epigenetics*. If you feel as though your genes are the reason you can't lose weight or get well, no matter how much Paleo food you eat, you can erase all that thinking. Epigenetics is proof that how we look and feel is the result of our choices. Think of epigenetics as your ambassador of health. Epigenetics sends messages to your genome (genes) telling it to flick on the switch of health — or not — depending on your lifestyle choices.

If you're living Paleo, your body will flip the switch to health, and your genes will express this choice. You'll be healthy, lean, strong, and energetic. If you aren't making healthy choices, your genes will express sickness, fatigue, or obesity.

A Paleo diet and lifestyle create the raw material your genes need to flip the switch to health. You find that you look and feel your best — naturally.

Creating a Paleo Lifestyle

Eating Paleo foods is exciting. It's a simple approach to eating that has gained so much traction in mainstream media because of its landmark success in helping people lose weight and get healthy. But that's just the beginning of the story.

Paleo is a lifestyle, not a flash-in-the-pan, red-carpet diet with the entire focus on getting the weight off. That's the magic of Paleo: It does get the weight off, but it does so by creating healthier cells. When you create healthier cells, you naturally lose weight, boost your immunity, heal your body, and fight aging. You literally get healthier from the inside out when you live a Paleo lifestyle. It's against natural law not to.

Putting real food first is the foundation. However, Paleo considers all influences on your body, even those that happen outside the kitchen. Your relationship with food and how your food makes you feel, how much you eat, your movement, your exposure to sunlight, supplementation, your stress levels, and your thoughts all matter. Each of these variables creates the building blocks for the positive, long-lasting effects of living Paleo.

Ultimately, your habits and patterns are the defining factor of your success in losing weight, healing your body, boosting your immunity, and aging gracefully. The following sections give you the lifestyle strategies that have positive, lasting effects, allowing you to live your life by the optimal design shaped and molded by nature.

Shifting your belief system

Wrapping your head around Paleo living means changing your belief system, or *paradigm*. You may be used to some of the following beliefs about eating, which Paleo debunks:

- Cow's milk is the best way to get your calcium.
- Beans offer the benefits of superimmunity and fiber.
- Grains and whole grains are an essential part of a healthy diet.
- Soy is a superfood.
- A slab of meat and a baked potato make up the perfect meal.
- If you want to balance your blood sugar, grab a cheese stick.
- Fruit is healthy, so eat as much as you want.
- Red meat is really bad for you and will make your heart explode.
- Fat is evil.
- You should eat eggs in strict moderation because they raise your cholesterol.
- Vegetarian-based diets are the healthiest.

These statements may have been a big part of your life, so the Paleo principles may take you by surprise. Until, of course, you see the cold hard truth: the undisputable results.

Will you make the paradigm changes necessary to live your healthiest life? Some people may need to make only small changes, but others may need to make bigger changes. Shifting your belief system requires a conscious choice to embrace health. Your choices — not bad genes or bad luck — determine your health.

Adjusting your belief system so you constantly work toward choosing health may be one of the best gifts you can give yourself. When your body gets the raw material it requires to function at its best, the magic starts to happen.

Summing up the lifestyle with a few basic guidelines

Your habits create your destiny, and that plays out profoundly in your physiology. Like it or not, the human body is designed to live a certain way, and the more we stray from nature's blueprint, the more we suffer.

The environment you choose to live in and stay in determines whether you create a healthy body or an unhealthy body, so choose an environment that lets your body function the way it was designed. The following sections point out a few major guidelines for creating a Paleo-conducive environment (don't worry; none of them involves moving to a cave).

Sticking to the 80-percent rule

To get long-lasting results, you can benefit from spending at least 30 days eating a strict Paleo diet (see Book I, Chapter 2). After that, the 80-percent rule keeps you in check both physically and healthwise. The *80-percent rule* means that if you adhere to Paleo principles at least 80 percent of the time, you'll experience the benefits of Paleo. If you eat poorly, you'll feel bad. What you eat is like the foundation of a house, and you must build a healthy framework to build a solid house. That said, you do have a little life leeway; you can adjust the rule to fit your personal needs.

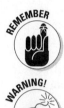

This 80-percent rule assumes that you're not trying to heal yourself of an illness or lose considerable weight. If you are, you may need to be 90 percent compliant or more for a while.

The 80-percent rule isn't a license to fill 20 percent of your diet with crummy processed foods or go to town on cookies, pancakes, bread, or muffins — even if they're Paleo! Sugar is still sugar, and too much of it is going to send you right back to needing a 30-day Paleo cleanse.

Some people choose to eat Paleo 90 or even 100 percent of the time, which is very powerful. Others feel that eating Paleo even 80 percent of the time causes constant cravings. It really comes down to food choices and what works best for you in your life.

Getting more — and better — sleep

Quality sleep is essential for losing weight and being healthy. One of the most priceless factors when eating and living a healthy lifestyle is improvement to your sleep cycle. After your body adjusts to eating cleaner, more nutrient-dense foods, you find your sleep is deeper and more restful.

Maybe you have trouble falling asleep, or you wake in the middle of the night, unable to drift back to sleep. No matter what the scenario, eating Paleo foods can completely change the quality and duration of your sleep. You find good reasons for this benefit in the earlier section "Getting a good night's sleep."

Becoming more social

No matter where you fall on the social spectrum, one thing is for certain: Your body is healthiest when you take some time out to be a part of a community or socialize. Humans aren't designed to be alone for an extended period. Your social blueprint is wired to spend time around others, enjoying yourself.

Although some time alone is definitely beneficial, be sure to actively include social time as another path to wellness. Joining a community or group of people with like-minded interests can really make a difference in your life.

You may be thinking, "But I'm busy enough already!" Just remember that you're better at everything else you do when you satisfy your soul's innate desire for connection!

Spending time outdoors

One of the most important shifts in your health is to spend time outdoors so you get sunshine. When sunlight hits the skin, a process begins that leads to the creation and activation of vitamin D.

To make radical changes in your future health, be clear about this point: Sunlight is a nutrient. When your body creates vitamin D, your body fights colds and the flu better as well as osteoporosis, cancer, heart disease, depression, and a host of other conditions. When you're outdoors getting sun and vitamin D, your body also produces more of the feel-good hormone serotonin, which helps you relax.

Regular sun exposure is grossly understated as a vitally important barrier to disease. You may worry about sun-related skin damage and skin cancers, but intermittent sun exposure actually increases your odds because you have a greater chance of burning, and burning is what causes your risk factors to go up. Regular exposure to the sun protects against skin cancers.

How much exposure you need to get your dose of vitamin D depends on how dark your skin is and environmental factors such as how close you live to the equator or what time of day you're in the sun. The average person usually needs about 20 minutes daily of sunshine at peak times. The darker your skin, the more exposure you need.

Start practicing the *slow immersion* process without sunscreen so you can benefit from vitamin D. When you get frequent short periods of exposure, you build a protective layer. Build up your tolerance on a regular basis gradually and early in the spring to prep your skin for the stronger summer sun. Try to get sun earlier in the morning when you have less chance of burning and overheating.

Reprogramming your mind-set

How you think is really what defines you. Understanding your mind-set is essential if you want to embrace wellness.

Major influences in your life — whether they were your parents, teachers, preachers, or whoever — programmed your current belief systems, which in turn create your reality. In fact, most of your programming (your unconscious thought) is wired in your brain by the time you're 18. Here's where it gets really interesting: Your unconscious mind is responsible for about 95 percent of your thoughts during the course of a day. Therefore, the programming you received as a youngster is still guiding you through life today.

You may not have had any say in how you were programmed when you were younger, but you do now! You can reprogram your thoughts to be healthier and more positive. Having positive thoughts is an essential piece of living healthfully and aging well.

 One the best ways to reprogram your mind is by using positive *affirmations* (statements of conviction) and journaling. You have to override all the negative affirmations that you replay in your mind by repeating your positive affirmations over and over. You begin to become aware that you really do create your reality. Start by journaling your affirmations in a notebook and saying them out loud in the morning (before your mind has time to fight back). Use the present tense as if your affirmations were already happening, such as "I *am* lean, strong, and healthy, and every day I'm creating what I want." Say them with intention and with complete clarity — don't rush through them. Write and say your affirmations over and over until your physiology believes you. Soon your affirmations will become part of you!

Taking a technology timeout

Computers, smartphones, and other handheld devices are super convenient, but shutting down once in a while is important — your cells benefit from the break. Here's why: Electricity goes hand in hand with electromagnetic fields (EMFs). When something is plugged in but not used, it generates electrical fields, or low frequency electromagnetic waves. The EMFs create an invisible pollution called *electrosmog*.

Technology has gained a lot of traction over the last 50 years, spawning a multitude of new inventions that all require electricity. Everywhere you go, you find electrical poles, wires, substations, transformers, and the hidden wires in the walls of every building. All this electricity creates a dangerous electrical environment and places new stresses on your cells, similar to the ones produced by heavy metals or toxic chemicals.

You can't live in a bubble, but you can take some steps to reduce your exposure:

- ✔ **Remove yourself from the source as much as possible.** Make sure you aren't sleeping near a lot of wiring or electronic devices.

- ✔ **Eat foods that naturally shield your body.** Protect yourself against cellular damage by eating Paleo foods such as grass-fed beef, blueberries, asparagus, cinnamon, artichokes, garlic, olive oil, wild salmon, sea vegetables (nori), and walnuts. These choices are all superfoods for your cells.

- ✔ **Schedule a shutdown day.** Take one day per week and completely remove yourself from all electronics. Completely unplug.

Minimizing the effects of stress with a Paleo diet

What many people don't know is that stress not only makes you sick but also makes you fat. Society tends to equate weight problems with gorging on food, but the roots often go much deeper than that. Some people eat because they're hungry for something more in their life — like balance. Being under stress causes them to crave unhealthy foods without even realizing it.

When you find food clarity and begin to dig into some of the recipes in Books II and III, your body starts normalizing. You create nutrient sufficiency and begin to regulate your hormones. You begin to gain the energy and the strength to deal with your stressors and create a better life.

Examining your body under stress

Almost everything you do rises and falls on how much stress that activity places on your body. Some stress is short term and can be positive (called *eustress*) if it gives you that short burst of adrenaline to move you closer to your purpose. For example, the stress of meeting deadlines to finish a book and share our nutritional message creates excitement and catalyzes us to move forward.

Your body isn't designed for constant, ongoing stress. Your stress hormones are in place to deal with short-term stress (such as being chased by a tiger). Long-term stress is adverse to your physiology and dangerous to your health. Balance really is the key.

Your body changes under constant stress. Stress makes you heavy, makes your hair thin, ages your skin, and deteriorates all the structures and functions of your body. No wonder stress is a major contributor to illness, disease, and an unhappy life. Countless diseases (such as heart disease, high blood pressure, and irritable bowel syndrome) stem from your body having to deal with chronic stress.

Understanding how stress affects food choices

Here's information that can change your life: Sugar and fat are the main ingredients of stress hormones, so when you're under stress, you crave more sugar and fat than you do under normal conditions. That's why many people start stress eating; they're trying to find a slower pace. In that way, *stress eating* is really a form of self-medication.

You're actually hard-wired to eat sugar and fat. Ideally, however, you'd follow your nutritional blueprint and get your fat and sugar from wild game, nuts, fruits, and vegetables like your ancestors did, not from all the refined sugary carbohydrates around today.

Ever notice when you crave sugar and fat the most? Dollars to donuts, it's when you're stressed. That's because of *serotonin* (or, rather, a lack of it). This hormone is a stress buffer; when your body is in balance, serotonin is released and offsets the activity in your body that leads to anxiety and depression. If you're constantly under stress, though, your body can't keep up with demand.

That's when you start feeling a mess. You eventually have increased stress hormones (such as *cortisol*) and decreased serotonin — a terrible combination. You become anxious, irritable, tired, and unhappy. You get changes in your appetite for — you guessed it — sugar and fat. It ends up being a vicious cycle that leads to even more stress.

Eating Paleo is a great way to step off the roller coaster. The fats that are part of the Paleo diet are all healthy fats, and the lower-sugar nature of the diet is really helpful in breaking negative eating patterns. For more tips on easing stress, check out the following section.

Finding stress solutions

When you bring your stress level down, you quell your cravings for sugar and fat. The answer to reducing stress is to have balance between work/stress and play/relaxation. So often, the people seeking weight-loss management are heavy because their lives have gotten out of balance. They have too much stress and not enough tools to relax their bodies and bring them back to an even keel.

Living Paleo is about your choices. Ask yourself these questions before you make any decision: "Is this decision going to add a lot of stress in my life? Is it going to simplify my life or bring complexity to it?" Stress follows complexity. Learning to say "no" is one of the best stress-management tools you can develop!

Here are some suggested techniques to help you decompress. Make one of these options, or another healthy stress-management technique you enjoy, part of your lifestyle:

- **Chiropractic:** Analyzes the body for nerve interference that occurs as a result of life's stresses. Many people feel immediately calmer after treatment. The later section "Improving your framework" has more info on incorporating chiropractic care into your life.

- **Massage:** Decreases the stress hormone cortisol and the hormones that can cause aggressive behavior.

- **Yoga and meditation:** Provide mental calmness, improved breathing, increased energy, and immunity.

- **Energy work:** Taps into that force within your body that gives you deep healing and strength. Chinese medicine, acupuncture, Qi Gong, Reiki, and Emotional Freedom Techniques (EFT) are just some of the techniques that center their healing on your body's life force (also called *prana, chi,* or *Qi*).

- **Exercise:** Boosts metabolism and changes the way your body responds to stress. Exercise is one of the most powerful things you can do to reverse stress, depression, anxiety, cravings, or negative eating patterns. But be careful — too much exercise is a stressor also.

Probably the best way to find a practitioner or a technique that may be right for you is to ask a holistic practitioner (holistic MD, naturopath, or chiropractor) who knows your history for her recommendations. These folks are often well connected to other practitioners in natural health and can recommend techniques and individual practitioners that suit your needs. If you don't know any such practitioners, ask around; people love to share this kind of information. You can also find a Paleo practitioner at http://paleophysiciansnetwork.com/doctors.

Practicing Paleo Fitness: Movement by Design

If you could take a miracle pill every day that would decrease your incidence for almost every disease, help you look better, moderate your cravings, and allow far less stress on your body, would you take it? Well, you already have this miracle pill; it's called exercise!

Movement is a big part of living Paleo because it keeps your body healthy and makes all the structures and functions in your body work better. One of the best ways to stimulate your brain and hormones to produce pleasure is through exercise, so movement is great for elevating your mood as well. The following sections give you an overview of exercise's role in a Paleo lifestyle.

Making exercise a requirement, not an option

Exercise offers too many benefits for Paleo practitioners to ignore it. Your cells require exercise in order to be healthy; if you're deficient in anything that's required for healthy cell function, your overall health eventually suffers.

Here's the good news: Just as a deficiency in exercise can make you sick and obese, the reverse can work as well. You can use exercise to create healthy cells and robust health and even use it in place of some medications to heal your body and help fight aging.

Here are some of the medications that regular exercise may help you avoid:

- **Cold and flu meds:** The average adult has two or three colds or flu viruses each year. But if you're active, studies suggest that you'll have fewer colds than those who aren't.

- **Cholesterol meds:** Being active boosts your good cholesterol and reduces unhealthy triglycerides, keeping a clear pathway for blood to flow naturally and preventing conditions like diabetes, stroke, and heart disease.

- **Antidepressants:** If you work out three times per week hard enough to sweat, the activity can reduce depression just as well as an antidepressant can. The connections made between nerve cells while exercising behave as a natural antidepressant.

- **Respiratory/asthma meds:** When you exercise, your breathing becomes deeper, allowing more oxygen and nutrients to become more readily available.

- **Digestive aids:** Exercise stimulates your digestive juices, which creates movement through your bowels and helps prevent constipation.

- **Alzheimer's meds:** The *Archives of Neurology* published a report indicating that a daily walk or run may lower the risk of Alzheimer's disease or tame its impact.

- **Sedatives:** During exercise, your body releases chemicals called *endorphins*. These chemicals act as a sedative and create feelings of happiness and joy. Endorphins also decrease the perception of pain.

Keeping your modern-day body strong and lean

Existing in a world that you weren't designed for is certainly a challenge. Lifestyle patterns have moved away from what the human species requires to genetically express health and toward what causes it to express illness (sitting too much, sleeping too little, eating processed foods — the list goes on). How do you exist in this world and come out on the other end healthy, strong, and vibrant?

That's where living Paleo comes in. Your hunter-gatherer ancestors lived healthier lives. Regardless of what they died from, they were free from chronic illness and were healthy, fit, and full of vitality. They didn't have the maladies of modern civilization, such as heart attacks, strokes, diabetes, hypertension, and obesity. They were lean and strong.

The good news is you can mimic some of the lifestyle patterns of your ancestors and change the way you move by incorporating exercise into your everyday life.

Paleolithic peoples moved constantly and worked hard. Being physical was the center of their existence. If they wanted to eat, they had to work for it. If they wanted shelter, they had to work for it. They needed remarkable amounts of energy to provide their own clothing and even to prepare for bedtime. They were active and kept a vigorous pace.

That's where a big part of today's problems come in. With all the modern-day conveniences and affluence, people have gotten fat and lazy. In the Western world, people don't need to work for survival. Life in the wild may seem dangerous and unpredictable, but a modern-day sedentary life has just as many risks and uncertainties.

If you incorporate natural, functional movements like walking, crawling, sprinting, twisting, climbing, pushing, pulling, squatting, lifting, and throwing into your exercise routine, you train your body to use all of your muscles. This training helps you perform everything better (which is why these actions are often called *functional* movements). Whether you're chasing after kids or working as a professional athlete, a doctor, or an office worker, everything you do improves. Understanding natural movements is an important step in transforming your body into a lean, strong, modern-day physique.

High-intensity workouts that are shorter and faster get you strong and fit more quickly. This strategy allows your body to release growth hormone, which keeps you young. Your body puts on muscle, burns fat, and becomes metabolically conditioned. In fact, doing short bursts of exercise followed by rest is far better at getting you fit than all that long, stretched-out exercise that takes forever. That's good news — the exercise you need takes less time to be more effective! Short bursts of exercise not only give you fast results but also are way more practical for your busy life! Always think intensity, not time, when it comes to exercise.

Consider adding some high-intensity, natural movement into your routine two to three times per week, and watch your body transform into a leaner, stronger, younger, and healthier one!

Doing what you love

You need movement every day. About one hour should do it. That sounds like a lot, but remember, everything counts. Walking to your car, chasing after your kids, walking through the grocery store — it all matters.

Making time for about 20 minutes of high-intensity training two to three times per week is important for putting on muscle — which is one of the healthiest, most youth-promoting things you can do. The rest of the time, find movement you enjoy so you keep on keeping on! If you like to do yoga, hit the mat. If you like to hike, go for a hike. The idea is to keep moving so you get an hour a day.

Make sure you exercise at a slower pace at least one day a week so you give your body the downtime it needs. Just because you move at a slower pace doesn't mean it's not effective. This slower movement helps with daily stress, weight maintenance, blood sugar control, muscle tone, joint health, improved fat metabolism, a stronger immune system, and increased energy. As long as you're doing your high-intensity training and eating Paleo foods, you still benefit from slower movements.

Improving your framework

If you like to run, jump, push, pull, or lift anything, take care of your spine. It has one of the most important jobs of all the structures in your body: to protect your spinal column and allow you to bear weight. Your spine truly is the framework of your body; without it, you'd be like a jellyfish.

Hands down, the most effective way to care for your spine is chiropractic care combined with exercise and spinal stretching. This combination is extraordinary for getting results. Many high-performers and high-profile people use chiropractic care as part of their best practices.

Add chiropractic care and spinal stretching to your exercise routine for better posture and a healthier spine. You'll even notice improvements in your stress levels and immune system.

Chapter 2

Modern Foods and Your Inner Cave Man

In This Chapter

▶ Understanding what you can and can't eat on the Paleo diet

▶ Uncovering surprising truths about common foods

▶ Knowing when to put down your fork (or lettuce wrap)

▶ Forming healthy Paleo habits with the 30-Day Reset

You're about to realize that the Paleo diet — with the throwback name and cave-man roots — is far more natural, easy to follow, and delicious than you may at first imagine. Paleo eating is all about enjoying natural foods. So forget about feeling like you're on a diet or focusing on giving up favorite foods, because when you make the transition to the Paleo diet, something kind of magical happens.

This chapter is devoted to helping you clear the clutter and confusion about how and what to eat on the Paleo plan. You figure out which foods are Paleo approved and which ones need to be banished from your kitchen — but in exchange for the ones taken away, you get the green light on some surprisingly healthful foods that you can include in your everyday diet. In this chapter, you also discover how to build your perfect Paleo plate and see how Paleo-approved foods can make you more energetic, help you think more clearly, and make you feel better than ever. You also get the encouragement you need to start fresh with the 30-Day Reset, which takes your body on an admittedly challenging journey from sluggish and carb fueled to efficient.

Getting Familiar with the "Yes" and "No" Foods of the Paleo Diet

Eating Paleo is a lifestyle approach to nutrition, not a short-term diet. Although eating Paleo will help you lose weight and will increase your muscle mass, both of which lead to a leaner physique, the Paleo "diet" is about even more than that. Before you can enjoy all the benefits of the Paleo diet, though, you have to understand a few Paleo food rules.

The "yes" and "no" lists for Paleo eating include foods that help you with two major accomplishments: reducing inflammation inside your body and slaying the sugar demon that can trick you into making poor food choices, which can make you overweight and undernourished as well as leave you tired, cranky, and craving more sugar.

Book I, Chapter 3, shows you all the nutritional aspects of Paleo-approved foods. In the following sections, you find out about the foods that will make up the majority of your meals (and those you should leave out) so you can immediately see that eating Paleo isn't about deprivation or denial; Paleo eating is really about feeding your body and mind with real, whole foods that supply essential building blocks, energy, vitamins, and minerals.

100% Paleo-approved: Checking out the Paleo "yes" list

The Paleo "yes" list is made up of nutrient-dense foods — proteins, vegetables, fruits, and fats — that any human, at any time in human history, would recognize as food. With these four basic food types outlined in the following sections, you can power your body with all the healthy fats, vitamins, and minerals it needs to be lean, strong, and healthy. To kick these Paleo foods up a notch, the section includes some staples and pantry items that make preparing Paleo foods easy, fun, versatile, and absolutely delicious. It also clues you in on some Paleo-approved drinks that will keep you healthy and keep the sugar demon away.

Powerful Paleo proteins

The Paleo diet focuses on animal proteins from high-quality sources. Surely, you'll find a lot of your favorites on this list:

- Beef
- Bison
- Chicken
- Duck
- Eggs
- Elk
- Fish
- Goat
- Lamb
- Nitrite- and gluten-free deli meats
- Nitrite- and gluten-free sausages
- Organ meats
- Pork
- Pheasant
- Quail
- Shellfish
- Turkey
- Veal
- Venison
- Wild boar

Nutrient-rich vegetables

A rainbow of vegetables makes your plate look appetizing and packs a major nutritional punch. Eat at least two servings of the following vegetables at every meal, and enjoy as much variety as possible:

- Acorn squash
- Artichoke
- Arugula
- Asparagus
- Beets
- Bell peppers
- Bok choy
- Broccoli
- Broccoli rabe
- Brussels sprouts
- Butternut squash
- Cabbage
- Carrots
- Cauliflower
- Celery
- Celery root
- Chile peppers
- Cucumber
- Eggplant
- Endive
- Escarole
- Garlic
- Green beans
- Greens (beet, collard, mustard, and turnip)
- Jalapeños

- ✔ Jicama
- ✔ Kale
- ✔ Kohlrabi
- ✔ Leeks
- ✔ Lettuce (all types)
- ✔ Mushrooms
- ✔ Nori (seaweed)
- ✔ Okra
- ✔ Onion
- ✔ Parsnip
- ✔ Plantain
- ✔ Pumpkin
- ✔ Radish
- ✔ Rutabega
- ✔ Shallots
- ✔ Snow peas
- ✔ Spaghetti squash

- ✔ Spinach
- ✔ Sprouts
- ✔ Sugar snap peas
- ✔ Summer squash (zucchini, yellow summer squash, crookneck, marrows, straightneck, scallop, and cocozelles)
- ✔ Sweet potatoes/yams
- ✔ Swiss chard
- ✔ Tomatoes
- ✔ Tomatillos
- ✔ Turnips
- ✔ Watercress
- ✔ Winter squash (butternut and acorn)
- ✔ Yucca
- ✔ Zucchini

Some Paleo-approved vegetables are *nightshade* foods, and these may cause discomfort if you have joint pain, autoimmune conditions, multiple sclerosis, fibromyalgia, or chronic fatigue syndrome. They include bell peppers (green, orange, red, and yellow), chile peppers, jalepeños, eggplant, and tomatoes.

Satisfyingly sweet fruits

Fruit delivers its nutrition with a side serving of sweetness, so vegetables should always be the first produce priority — but one or two servings of fruit per day are satisfying and nutritious; choose any from the following list. As your body becomes balanced and your internal environment becomes cleaner and stronger, you may be able to add more fruit, but at the beginning of your transition to Paleo, sticking to one or two servings is your best strategy.

Limit your consumption of dried fruit; it's easy to overeat, and it lacks the nutrition of fresh fruits while concentrating the sugars. You also have to be aware of the sulfites in some dried fruits, which are toxic. Always opt for no-sugar-added and sulfite-free dried fruit when you indulge, or choose to skip it altogether. Also be cautious of fruit juices and blending fruit into smoothies and sauces because they provide all the sugar of the fruit without the fiber and satiety of eating whole fruits.

- ✔ Apple
- ✔ Apricot
- ✔ Banana
- ✔ Blackberries
- ✔ Blueberries
- ✔ Cantaloupe
- ✔ Cherries
- ✔ Clementine
- ✔ Cranberries, fresh
- ✔ Date, fresh
- ✔ Fig, fresh
- ✔ Grapefruit
- ✔ Grapes
- ✔ Guava
- ✔ Honeydew melon
- ✔ Kiwi
- ✔ Kumquat
- ✔ Lemon

- ✔ Lime
- ✔ Lychee
- ✔ Mandarin orange
- ✔ Mango
- ✔ Nectarine
- ✔ Orange
- ✔ Papaya
- ✔ Peach
- ✔ Pear
- ✔ Pineapple
- ✔ Plum
- ✔ Pomegranate
- ✔ Raspberries
- ✔ Rhubarb
- ✔ Strawberries
- ✔ Tangerine
- ✔ Ugli fruit
- ✔ Watermelon

Enjoy all fruit, but keep in mind that your healthiest options for everyday fruits are ones low in fructose, so choose berries and cherries most often. Dates in particular are very high in sugar.

Tasty essential fats

Fats ensure that you feel satisfied after a meal, and they are vital to the function of your body and brain — plus they taste really, really good. So go ahead and eat some of the following healthy fats with every meal to ensure proper absorption of nutrients and to please your taste buds.

- ✔ Avocado
- ✔ Clarified butter (organic, grass-fed only)
- ✔ Coconut (butter, fresh, flakes, oil, and milk)
- ✔ Nuts and nut butters (almonds, Brazil nuts, cashews, chestnuts, hazelnuts, macadamia nuts, pecans, pistachios, and walnuts)
- ✔ Olives and olive oil
- ✔ Seeds (pumpkin, sesame, sunflower, and pine nuts)

Pantry powerhouses for extra flavor

Herbs and spices add zing to your meals and can take you on a world tour of cuisines. All herbs and spices are Paleo approved; just be sure to check labels for problematic ingredients — you want *pure* spices and extracts with no added sugars, wheat, gluten, or chemicals.

Here are more Paleo-approved flavorings to keep in your pantry:

- ✔ Almond meal
- ✔ Broth and stock (beef, chicken, seafood, and vegetable)
- ✔ Canned tomatoes and tomato paste
- ✔ Coconut aminos (replacement for soy sauce)
- ✔ Coconut flour
- ✔ Curry paste

Paleo-approved liquids for hydration

Wouldn't you prefer to eat your calories in delicious food rather than mindlessly drink them in a sugary beverage? Drinks like sodas, sports drinks, and fruit juices are basically liquid carbohydrates in a bottle. You can unknowingly take in 20 teaspoons of sugar and 300 calories without even thinking about it! And packaged drinks almost always include artificial sweeteners and chemical additives that do you no favors.

Here's the "yes" list of Paleo-approved drinks:

- ✔ Water (preferably filtered)
- ✔ Black coffee
- ✔ Tea (black, herbal, green, and white — check labels for added sugars)

Paleo no-nos: Watching out for foods on the "no" list

Now that you've had a look at the lengthy list of foods you *can* enjoy, it's time to swallow the potentially bad news of the "no" list. You may find some of your favorites on this list, but in Book I, Chapter 3, you discover why these foods are harmful to your health and well-being.

The foods on the "no" list can wreak havoc on your health and sabotage your weight-loss goals. They create hormonal imbalances, trigger inflammation, and make you age more quickly.

Say good-bye to grains and gluten

Grains contain toxic *antinutrients* — substances that prevent your body from absorbing the nutrients it needs and that create autoimmune and digestive irritation — and inflammatory proteins like gluten. They damage your gut lining and cause irritation throughout the body. Many of these grains also cause the body to release insulin, which triggers fat storage. Grains are not only nutritionally unnecessary but can be downright harmful. For many people, they're also problematic for their high carbohydrate content, but even fans of healthier starches generally recommend eating starchy tubers like sweet potatoes rather than grains.

In a paper published in *The American Journal of Clinical Nutrition* in 2005, Dr. Loren Cordain examined 13 nutrients most lacking in the diet. He then ranked seven food groups — whole grains, milk, fruits, vegetables, seafood, lean meats, and nuts/seeds — for each of these 13 vitamins and minerals in 100-calorie samples. He ranked the food 7 to 1, where 7 was the most nutrient-dense and 1 was the lowest. He summed up all the ranked scores to determine the most nutrient-dense foods.

Fresh vegetables were a clear winner, followed by seafood, lean meats, and fruits. Whole grains and milk came in last. Therefore, whenever you choose grains rather than these other foods, your vitamin and mineral content is actually lowered. (For more research, check out Dr. Cordain's website at www.thepaleodiet.com.)

Clearly, our diets don't need grains to be healthy or to provide us with the nutrients we need. Better, more efficient ways exist. So all grains — and the baked goods, flours, and pastas made from them — are at the top of the "no" list.

- ✔ Amaranth
- ✔ Barley
- ✔ Buckwheat
- ✔ Bulgur
- ✔ Corn
- ✔ Millet
- ✔ Oats

- ✔ Quinoa
- ✔ Rice
- ✔ Rye
- ✔ Sorghum
- ✔ Spelt
- ✔ Teff
- ✔ Wheat

Pitch the processed foods

Foods that come in brightly colored boxes or crinkly, vacuum-sealed bags are generally not Paleo approved. Candy, baked goods, junk food, and prepackaged meals are usually loaded with chemicals, additives, sugar, and other ingredients you'll find on the Paleo "no" list. Eating Paleo means eating real, natural food, so foods produced in a lab or factory are out.

Let go of the legumes

Although beans have a reputation for being healthful, they contain many of the same antinutrients that grains do. Even with pre-soaking, sprouting, or fermenting, beans are a high-carbohydrate food that triggers insulin release and are difficult for your body to digest. Keep away from the following legumes:

- ✔ Black beans
- ✔ Broad beans
- ✔ Garbanzo beans (chickpeas)
- ✔ Lentils
- ✔ Lima beans
- ✔ Mung beans
- ✔ Navy beans

- ✔ Peanuts and peanut butter
- ✔ Peas
- ✔ Pinto beans
- ✔ Soybeans, including tofu, tempeh, natto, soy sauce, miso, edamame, and soy milk
- ✔ White beans

Snow peas, sugar snap peas, and green beans are the exception to the no-beans rule because those vegetables are green and are more pod than pea or bean.

Ditch the dairy

Humans are the only species that drink the milk of another animal and the only species that continues to drink milk past the weaning period. Cow's milk is designed to help calves grow quickly so they can sprint away from predators, not for humans to consume throughout their lives. In addition, processed cow's milk contains growth hormones, bacteria, and antibiotics and also produces a strong insulin response. The following dairy products are on the Paleo "no" list:

- ✔ Cheese
- ✔ Cream
- ✔ Half-and-half
- ✔ Ice cream

- ✔ Milk
- ✔ Sour cream
- ✔ Yogurt

One exception to the no-dairy rule is clarified butter from a cow that's organically and grass-fed. This type of butter is an excellent source of healthy fat.

Wipe out white potatoes

White potatoes are like the useless, black sheep of the vegetable family, and they deserve a shady reputation. Because of their high sugar and starch content, they produce a big insulin response, and they also contain antinutrients that can cause intestinal distress.

Be extra careful not to eat potatoes that appear to be turning green because it's an indication of an increased level of *solanine* and *chaconine.* These substances occur in nature to ward off insects, disease, and predators by making the food bitter, which also makes them toxic to you. So if your potatoes taste bitter or are starting to turn green, definitely take them off the menu!

Say "no" to added sugar

Eliminating all sugar from your diet is impossible. After all, the carbohydrates in healthy vegetables and fruits are, essentially, sugar. For optimal health and weight loss, you need to eliminate *added* sugars from your diet, including sugar in all its (deliciously sweet) forms and artificial sweeteners, such as the following:

- Agave
- All other packaged, boxed, or packets of artificial sugars
- Aspartame (NutraSweet or Equal)
- Brown sugar
- Coconut sugar
- Corn syrup
- Dextrose
- High-fructose corn syrup
- Honey
- Maltodextrin
- Maple syrup
- Molasses
- Raw sugar
- Rice syrup
- Sucralose (Splenda)
- Sugar cane
- Stevia
- White sugar

Sugar is sugar is sugar, but after your 30-Day Reset, you can enjoy organic, raw honey from time to time. All types of sugar, including high-quality honey, produce an insulin response in your body. But once in a while, a little raw honey can be a sweet treat as part of a healthy Paleo diet.

Ignore the industrial and seed oils

These oils are often billed as "healthy," but they're not naturally occurring fats, so they require significant processing to become edible. They're prone to turning rancid and creating free radicals in your body, making them very inflammatory.

- Canola oil
- Corn oil
- Cottonseed oil
- Margarine
- Palm kernel oil
- Partially hydrogenated oil
- Peanut oil
- Safflower oil
- Soybean oil
- Sunflower oil
- Trans fats
- Vegetable oil
- Vegetable shortening

Avoid (most) alcoholic beverages

Common sense tells you that drinking alcohol, particularly spirits or beer that contain gluten, isn't going to make you healthier. So generally speaking, alcohol is on the "no" list.

But don't despair. An occasional glass of wine may be a good thing. Find out more in the section "Making happy hour truly happy," later in this chapter.

The Truth about Common Foods

Some favorite foods are the source of confusion, especially on morning TV shows and magazine covers. Is it sugar or fat that's making us fat and unhealthy? Do eggs dangerously raise our cholesterol? Wait, doesn't saturated fat cause heart disease? Is alcohol a bad idea, or should I drink a glass of red wine every day?

The following sections tackle these issues one by one to show you that sugar and its associated insulin cycles are the demons of the food world and how the right fats can actually make you leaner and healthier. In fact, eggs are an excellent source of protein, and you can eat them to your heart's (and health's) content. And, yes, an occasional glass of wine can be part of a Paleo lifestyle.

Slaying the sugar demon

Thanks to processed foods and soft drinks, sugar consumption has reached dangerous proportions. If you're like a typical American, you consume about 165 pounds of sugar every year. Two decades ago, the average American ate just 26 pounds of sugar per person per year. All that sugar has led to an epidemic of lifestyle ailments, including diabetes, cancers, obesity, and heart disease.

But don't think your lack of willpower is solely to blame. Sugar's behavior in the body is insidious and makes resisting the temptation of a sweet treat very difficult. Eating sugar releases insulin in the bloodstream to reduce your level of blood sugar. This increase in insulin can make your blood sugar drop too low, so your brain triggers your body to eat more sugar. The diabolical being who rules this cycle is known as the *sugar demon* (and, yes, he really does exist!).

If you've been trapped in the sugar cycle, you know it can be pretty unpleasant. Physical hunger and mental temptation gnaw at you, compelling you to make poor food choices, which lead to more unhealthy food choices. You feel edgy and cranky before eating, energized for a short time while eating, then sluggish and sleepy after a meal.

The Paleo diet helps you break this cycle to vanquish the sugar demon. To be your leanest, healthiest self, you must break out of the sugar cycle. The most successful way to do that is by eating Paleo-approved foods that stabilize your insulin, reduce inflammation, and increase your food satisfaction.

Making the case for high-quality fats

Fat doesn't make you fat. Go ahead and chew on that for a few minutes.

The media has told you for decades that the key to a leaner body is a low-fat diet and that saturated fats are the cause of heart disease. Both of those assertions are wrong.

Fat, including saturated fat, is essential to your health and, as it turns out, to building a lean, strong body. To access the fat stored in your body for energy, you need to consume fat in your meals so your body can then burn stored fat for energy.

Dietary fat is also crucial in helping your body absorb fat-soluble vitamins, such as vitamins A, D, E, and K. And let's be honest about taste: A little bit of fat makes food more palatable, so you feel more satisfied after eating. A diet that's too low in fat can lead to food cravings that compel you to overeat or make poor food choices.

Additionally, when your body doesn't regularly receive high-quality fat in meals, it can retaliate with dry skin, hair loss, bruising, intolerance to cold, and, in extreme cases, loss of menstruation.

Don't take that wrong: You don't get a free pass to dive face first into a bowl of butter. Instead, it means you can free yourself from a fear of fat. Choose high-quality fats from the "yes" list (see the earlier section, "100% Paleo-approved: Checking out the Paleo 'yes' list") in appropriate quantities to make your meals taste great while doing good things for your body. (Later in this chapter, you find out how much fat is the right amount for you.)

Fitting fruit into the Paleo plan

Fruit provides beneficial plant compounds, fiber, and antioxidant power; however, you must eat fruit in moderation. Fruits contain fructose, which is just another form of sugar, so consuming too much fruit can cause weight gain and may cause blood sugar swings.

When you're just beginning to fight the sugar demon and starting to live Paleo, remember to not let your fruit take over your plate. Reach for vegetables more often than fruits, and keep your fruit intake to about one or two servings per day.

All fruits aren't equal on the health scale. Some have a higher sugar content than others. The more sugar present, the higher the insulin release, and the more insulin that's released, the more fat that will be stored.

Here are a few things to keep in mind about fruit:

- Melons and tropical fruits, like bananas, mango, and pineapple, include higher amounts of natural sugar.
- Fruits that are darker in color — blueberries, raspberries, strawberries, blackberries, and cranberries — have higher amounts of antioxidants and less sugar.
- Eating fruit that's in season is your best bet for nutrition and an appropriate amount of sugar.

Realizing that eggs are A-OK (and cholesterol isn't so bad)

Eggs are just about the perfect food. They're filled with vitamins and minerals, including choline and biotin. *Biotin* helps your body turn the foods you eat into energy, and *choline* helps move cholesterol through your bloodstream. They're both an excellent source of fatty acids and sulfur-containing proteins, which make the walls around your cells healthy.

Many people have eliminated eggs from their shopping list because of worries about high cholesterol and heart disease; the egg yolk, in particular, has been demonized for the natural cholesterol it contains. But the yolk is the prize of the egg. It's loaded with healthy omega-3 fatty acids and nutrients.

The cholesterol fuss is based on the assumption that if you eat cholesterol, you raise your blood levels of cholesterol. But that's simply not true. In fact, egg yolks contain the B vitamin choline, which is a concentrated source of *lecithin* (a natural fat transporter), and naturally keeps cholesterol from entering the bloodstream.

Cholesterol isn't all bad. Your body needs cholesterol to make bile, which breaks down fats. And your brain cells need cholesterol to deliver your body's messages where they need to go.

Almost everyone produces less cholesterol in their bodies when they consume more in food; studies show that dietary cholesterol doesn't have much of an effect on blood cholesterol. When you don't get cholesterol from the food you eat, your liver makes it for you. Moreover, cholesterol isn't a good indicator of heart disease. Dietary cholesterol has very little impact on blood cholesterol.

Making happy hour truly happy

There's an appropriate time to enjoy a moderate amount of alcohol to unwind or to celebrate. Aside from the positive aspects of socializing, some types of alcohol are associated with a lower risk of cardiovascular disease, and they may also reduce the risk of infection with the bacteria that causes ulcers.

Here are a few key factors to help you decide whether you should pop a cork:

- ✔ Alcohol is a toxin to the liver.
- ✔ Alcohol is a drug, which means it's addictive.
- ✔ If losing weight is your goal, remember that your liver can't help you burn fat if it's busy detoxifying alcohol.

Before you pour yourself a glass of something intoxicating, consider your goals and your overall eating habits, and then make smart choices about which type of alcohol you drink.

Steer clear of grain-based drinks that can also include gluten, such as the following:

✔ Beer

✔ Bourbon

✔ Gin (some brands are processed with grain-based alcohol)

✔ Grain-based vodka

✔ Whiskey

To celebrate on special occasions, feel free to choose one of these:

✔ Potato vodka

✔ Red wine

✔ Rum

✔ Sparkling wine

✔ Tequila

✔ White wine

To manage your body's insulin response to the sugars found in alcohol, mix spirits, like tequila or vodka, with soda water, ice, and a squeeze of lemon or lime juice. Avoid fruit juices that are liquid sugar, and avoid tonic water, which is also high in sugar.

When uncorking wine, choose the driest (least sweet) wines possible. The driest reds include Pinot Noir, Cabernet Sauvignon, and Merlot; the driest whites are Sauvignon Blanc and Albarino.

Our hunter-gatherer ancestors occasionally let their hair down when they consumed alcohol while eating fermented grapes. But they didn't sit around the fire doing shots. You can't maintain a high level of health if you drink alcohol frequently or in large quantities. The pleasant buzz that alcohol provides also places stress on your liver, creates a strong insulin response, and dehydrates your cells. Enjoy cocktails in moderation.

During your 30-Day Reset, abstain from alcohol completely. Doing so ensures that you break free of the sugar demon and can make clear-headed food choices. (For more on the first 30 days of living Paleo and the 30-Day Reset, see the section "Building the Foundation for Success: The 30-Day Paleo Reset" later in this chapter.)

Figuring Out How Much You Can (and Should) Eat

Knowing how much to eat is essential to your success in your dietary goals. If you don't eat enough food, your body may lack the nutrition it needs. You can start breaking down muscle or slow your metabolism. But if you eat more than you need, you can gain weight or feel fatigued — and that leads to frustration.

Living Paleo makes it easier than ever to assess how much you need to eat, and when you eat foods from the Paleo "yes" list (see the earlier section "100% Paleo-approved: Checking out the Paleo 'yes' list"), feeling satisfied while giving your body everything it needs to thrive is easy. Your weight will normalize, and you'll feel more vibrant and energetic than ever before. After you develop the ability to know how much food your body needs, which the following sections help you figure out, many of your struggles will be behind you.

Understanding why a calorie isn't just a calorie

Conventional thinking abides by the theory that people become overweight because they habitually eat more calories than they can burn. Under this theory, those extra calories lead to an individual becoming overweight and, eventually, obese. It's a simple equation of calories in, calories out. The amount of calories you eat *does* matter, but there's much more to it than that. Here are two key points you must understand:

- ✔ **All calories aren't created equally.** The most fattening foods in the grocery store aren't the ones that are highest in calories. The most fattening foods you can eat are the foods that wreak havoc on your blood sugar and insulin levels: poor-quality carbohydrates.

- ✔ **The amount of total calories you consume is less important than the quality of the calories you eat.** When you eat concentrated sources of carbohydrates that cause a strong insulin response, you gain weight.

Some examples of carbohydrates that trigger this unfavorable insulin response include grains, dairy, fruit juices, soda, alcohol, sugar, potatoes, and corn — these are all found on the "no" list (see the earlier section "Paleo no-nos: Watching out for foods on the 'no' list").

When you eat carbohydrates from the "yes" list (see the section "100% Paleo-approved: Checking out the Paleo 'yes' list," earlier in this chapter), you regulate your insulin and store less fat. Paleo-approved carbohydrates, like leafy greens and other vegetables, are bound up by fiber, so they elicit a low insulin response and your blood sugar remains low.

Even though a calorie isn't just a calorie, it's still important to eat just the right amount. Luckily, you come equipped with a natural means to figure out how much you need to eat on any given day — and living Paleo will help you tap into that innate calorie meter so you feel satisfied and energetic.

Trying the eat-until-satisfied approach

It seems simple enough: Eat until you're satisfied.

Eating until you're satisfied, however, doesn't mean eating until you're full. If you're a numbers person, *satisfied* is about 70 percent of full — and that means you're not hungry, but you're not stuffed. You feel at ease and satiated, but not stuffed.

It may take some time to get accustomed to this feeling, but after you internalize this concept, knowing when to stop eating gets easier. You can figure out how to really listen to your body's signals, and this awareness leads to eating that feels natural and instinctive.

But for you to receive your body's messages, it needs to send you the right signals. To produce the hormones that are in charge of sending messages to your brain, you have two jobs: (1) You have to get enough sleep, and (2) you have to eat enough food. Lack of sleep leads to a spike in appetite, thus, stimulating the hormone ghrelin and declining the hormone lectin, which tells you when you're full. You also have to make sure you're eating enough food so you're producing enough lectin in the first place!

Your mom's advice was solid: Eat slowly and chew your food. It's not just about good table manners; you need to give your brain time to get the signal from your body that you're full, and that takes about 20 minutes. If you eat too fast, you'll miss the signal. But with smaller bites and leisurely meals that include fiber- and nutrient-dense foods, you'll feel fuller faster. And that's good for your waistline and your health.

Measuring your food at a glance

Portion distortion is common. Most people never realize how much they're eating in a day. Until you get in the swing of things, make sure you pay attention to the portion sizes of what you're eating. After the first 30 days, understanding correct portions becomes second nature, and you automatically know how much should be on your plate. The goal here is to reset your visual imaging.

The amount of food you choose to eat every day is determined by three variables:

✔ Your hunger level

✔ Your energy level

✔ Your exercise/activity level

To build each meal, you need to take those three variables into account and fill your plate with an appropriate portion size of Paleo foods.

With the following at-a-glance guidelines, you can stay on track, whether you're eating in a restaurant, traveling for work or pleasure, or dining with friends — no embarrassing or annoying tools involved. You'll develop a useful lifetime skill that will help you quickly eyeball how much food to grab.

✔ **Protein:** A serving of meat, fish, or poultry should be about the size and thickness of your palm. (That's about 3 to 4 ounces for women, 5 to 6 ounces for men.) Each meal should include a serving of protein.

✔ A serving of eggs is as many as you can easily hold in your hand. (That's about two or three for women, three or four for men.) For egg whites, double the amount of whole eggs.

✔ **Vegetables:** A serving of vegetables should be at least the size of a softball. You can't eat too many vegetables, so fill your plate with at least two or three softballs' worth.

✔ **Fruit:** A serving of fruit is half an individual piece (for example, half an apple, half an orange) or a tennis ball–size serving of berries, grapes, or tropical fruits. (That's about half a cup.)

Eat no more than two servings of fruit per day, and break them up across meals and snacks to distribute your sugar intake. Eating multiple servings in one sitting will release more insulin than if they're broken up throughout the day.

- ✔ **Fat:** A serving of liquid fat should be about the size of a super ball, or typical bouncy ball. (That's about 1 tablespoon.) Each meal should include one to two servings of fat.

  A serving of nuts, seeds, coconut flakes, and olives is about one closed handful. A serving of avocado is one-quarter to one-half of the avocado, depending on its size. A serving of coconut milk is one-third of the can.

Supercharging Your Body with the Power of Paleo Foods

When living Paleo, it feels as if someone plugged you back into your energy source! All of a sudden, the magic starts to happen. You feel thinner, your skin looks better, and your eyes glisten. Hormonally, things start to "shift." You sleep better, PMS disappears, acne goes away, wrinkles fade, and you actually feel like exercising. You feel like playing with your kids; you feel like cooking that meal for your family. Your life goes from a bunch of "I have to" to a bunch of "I want to!"

There are reasons for this change. Your body begins to come alive, often flooded with nutrition for the first time in years. You're also eating energy-producing foods. Many people have had such a nutritionally devoid diet for so long that they don't even remember what it's like to feel consistently good for long stretches of time! They haven't had food that's alive, so their body perks up in every way when it starts to get what it needs.

Other reasons Paleo works for so many is because people know they're eating in a way that their body is designed, but they're also getting healthier by being more alkaline, releasing toxins, and eating notoriously low-allergen foods. The following sections show you the power of Paleo.

Getting the nourishment you need

Paleo foods create *nutritional sufficiency* — the point when your body is balanced with all its vitamins, minerals, and essential fats. Many people live in the state of *deficiency,* not getting the nourishment they need, because they aren't getting their macronutrients in the right quantity or the right quality.

The hunter-gatherers' nutrition came from macronutrients but in different quantities and a much higher quality than today's typical consumption. Their foods came from wild game, fish, vegetables, fruits, and nuts. Here's the breakdown of our ancestors' macronutrients:

- ✔ Protein: 20 to 35 percent
- ✔ Carbohydrates: 25 to 40 percent
- ✔ Fat: 30 to 45 percent

Modern diet, on the other hand, consists of marbled grain-fed conventional meats, grains, sugar and artificial sweeteners, and rancid fats:

- ✔ Protein: 15 to 20 percent
- ✔ Carbohydrates: 45 to 55 percent
- ✔ Fat: 35 to 40 percent

Creating healthy cells

Nutrition is addressed mainly from a biological perspective. Your body is viewed as structural with biochemical and bio-available nutrients. These vitamins and other nutrients are essential to your health and well-being.

But food also has an electrical component, based on its mineral composition. Your food basically has a life force from this electrical component. Cellular metabolism is dependent on biochemical reactions, but it also depends on the capacitance (the ability to store a charge) of the body.

Everything in life has a vibration or frequency attached to it. Seemingly solid objects are molecules, atoms, and particles floating, vibrating, and rotating. Our world is definitely vibrational, so our food has different energies, or charges, attached to it, just like any object.

When your food is healthy, vibrant, and alive (like healthy meats, vegetables, fruits, and healthy fats), it holds a better charge. When your food is processed, overcooked, microwaved, or depleted of nutrients, the charge is weak.

Eating Paleo naturally encourages healthier nutrition from both a biochemical and a molecular standpoint. Health comes down to the cells, and your living Paleo plan will create healthy cells. Incorporating fresh raw vegetables that are filled with energy and life into your daily diet can increase cellular health.

Balancing your pH

One of the most challenging health issues people have today is that they don't have a pH that's conducive to health. Your pH is the acid-base balance of your body — literally, how acidic or alkaline you are. It's as important as your body temperature. Just as your body works to keep a tight control on temperature, it does the same in regard to pH.

Unfortunately, most people are on the acidic side of the pendulum, which is a major stressor to the body. Your body will be in a constant fight to stay healthy and regulate your level by taking minerals, like calcium and magnesium, from your bones and dumping them into your bloodstream.

How do you get acidic? Dietary choices, such as processed foods, dairy, grains, and sugary drinks, cause acidity in your body. You may be on the acidic side if you have any of the following symptoms:

- ✔ Aches and pains
- ✔ Arthritis
- ✔ Fatigue
- ✔ Headaches
- ✔ Inflammation

- ✔ Low immunity
- ✔ Muscle cramps
- ✔ PMS
- ✔ Skin disorders

If you want to test your pH, you can find test strips at any pharmacy. These strips test your acidity by using a urine or saliva sample. A normal reading is about 7.4. Anything below that, and you start to get into the more acidic range.

Identifying food allergies and sensitivities

How do you know whether you have a food allergy or sensitivity? Right off the bat, be aware that a difference exists between a full-blown food allergy and a food sensitivity. If you have a true food allergy, even a tiny bit of the offending food can cause a quick, severe reaction, called *anaphylaxis*. Some of the symptoms are swelling, tingling, breathing problems, and sudden low blood pressure. This is a life-threatening condition for which you should seek medical treatment.

Food sensitivities, on the other hand, come on slowly, and you can eat some of the offending food and be fine. You won't get a sudden severe reaction; however, you do experience discomfort and symptoms over time. When you have food sensitivities, one of the biggest problems is that your body is repeatedly exposed to a food that causes increased stress on the immune system. This constant exposure can trigger autoimmune diseases and, eventually, affect other body organs. This exposure can cause rapid aging and discomfort.

How do you know whether you have food sensitivities? Here are some of the symptoms:

- Acne
- Arthritis
- Attention deficit disorder
- Autoimmune problems
- Bloating
- Depression
- Fatigue
- Food cravings

- Irritable bowel
- Migraines
- Sinus drainage
- Skin disorders
- Skin rashes
- Stomach cramps
- Weight gain

To find out whether you have a food sensitivity, try an elimination/provocation test: Eliminate the suspected foods from your diet for 30 days. If you feel better, you may in fact be sensitive. Slowly (and carefully) add them back in one at a time to see which one may be the culprit. A great time to implement this test is during the 30-Day Reset (see the upcoming section "Building the Foundation for Success: The 30-Day Reset").

Following are the most common food allergens:

- Eggs
- Fish
- Milk
- Peanuts

- Shellfish
- Soy
- Tree nuts
- Wheat

Isn't it great to know that half the list doesn't even include Paleo-approved foods! The reason for that is because living Paleo has very low sensitivity foods, making it a great eating plan for those with a lot of food sensitivities.

Capturing Your Personal Before and After Makeover

One of the most important things you can do for yourself is to capture your brilliance and bravery. A common refrain from people who live a Paleo life-style is "I really wish I had a picture of myself before I started Paleo." You will transform — and you'll want to capture your transformation. Here are a few tools you can use to document your transformation:

- **Photos:** Take a picture of yourself standing against a plain background and wearing something revealing like a bathing suit. If you want the date documented, hold a newspaper or magazine in your hand. Be sure to get photos from all angles. Don't settle for a poor quality photo and just be done with it. Take the time to get some good shots of yourself. You will be so glad you did.

- **Blind measurements:** Another fantastic tool is *blind measurements*. Here's how it works: You take a piece of yarn and wrap it around the body part you want to measure. Cut the yarn when you're done and label the piece of yarn with the date and the body part you measured. In four to six weeks, take that same piece of yarn and measure the same body part to see the difference. Whatever excess yarn you have, cut it off and keep it in a baggie. Keep all these little pieces of yarn as a visual reminder of your success. You end up with something more valuable than just a number. You have these tangible pieces of yarn to remind you of all the inches you ditched!

- **The emperor's new clothes:** Your clothing will start to fit differently as you progress on your living Paleo path. You can find plenty of newfound Paleo people out there shopping for new clothes. It kind of goes with the territory. Relish this moment because, odds are, you won't be digging in those green bags for your old clothes any time soon.

Building the Foundation for Success: The 30-Day Reset

The 30-Day Reset is the foundation of your Paleo program. When you get past these 30 days, everything gets easier. Everything starts to fall into place. The magic starts to happen.

In the following sections, you find out why the reset lasts 30 days (and not 23 or 28, for example). Also, you discover what's happening to your cells during the 30-Day Reset that makes such startling improvements happen for you. You also get a master plan to help you walk through your days with certainty. Half the battle of doing anything new is facing the unexpected. Find out what you can expect during your transformation so you can prepare in the best possible way.

The brain versus the tongue (what you know you should eat versus what you crave) is an interesting battle, but it's easy to decode and deal with when you know that's what's happening. Explore the ins and outs of this battle and what it means for you during these 30 days.

Developing a habit with 30 days

The reason the reset lasts 30 days is because it's a good start to developing a habit. Dropping some of your favorite foods and cutting out packaged, processed foods with sugar isn't an easy battle. In fact, you may want to cry in your ice-cream bowl for a while.

You may not be completely automatic in your responses after 30 days; however, this time frame will go a long way in starting you off in the right direction.

It has most likely taken you a long while to develop your eating habits, and it will take some time before you can erase those old habits and form new ones. Just know that after 30 days, most everyone feels considerably better, and cravings are greatly diminished. The longer you've depended on sugary foods, the more difficult it may be to retrain your taste buds to natural sweetness again.

It also takes about 21 days for your intestinal cells to turn over, which helps you get through this process a little easier as your body renews with good raw material.

Renewing your system

During the 30-Day Reset, you're improving the caliber of your cells. Keep in mind that you're only as healthy as your cells. When you eat foods that are denatured, packaged, and processed, you're poisoning your cells. When people are lean and healthy and have a youthful, vibrant appearance, they have cells that are free of waste.

By eating the cleansing Paleo-approved foods, waste leaves through the following *detox organs:*

- ✔ **Kidney:** Toxins leave through adequate fluid intake.
- ✔ **Liver:** The liver eliminates or neutralizes toxins as they pass.
- ✔ **Lungs:** Toxins leave as you exhale.
- ✔ **Intestines:** Toxins leave through stool elimination.
- ✔ **Skin:** Toxins leave through sweating.

As you eat foods full of nutrition and drink plenty of water, the toxins start to flood out of your body, and nutrients enter. Your cells start to regenerate and exude health.

You can do a few things during this time to move waste along. Here are some suggestions to help rid your body of toxins:

✔ **Get sweaty.** Sweat is a great carrier of waste. Sweating through exercise or sauna is a great way to eliminate toxins. The toxins leave through your kidneys, so be sure to drink extra fluids while you sweat.

✔ **Jump.** Mini trampolines called *rebounders* squeeze waste matters from cells as you bounce lightly. Rebounding is one of the healthiest exercises you can do for your cells and for elimination of toxins.

✔ **Brush.** Dry brushing cleanses your skin, which is important because your skin is your largest organ and an eliminator of toxins. Through dry brushing, waste is lifted, which allows your body to take in more oxygen through the skin. It also stimulates the lymphatic system, which is your body's drainage system, so you have clear pathways to eliminate effectively. Brush your legs and arms first then your upper torso in circular strokes. Dry brush before exercise or showering for best results. Be sure to purchase a natural bristle brush, which you can find in most stores for about $8 to $10.

✔ **Eat.** Add some raw vegetables to your plate daily. This is a great way to move food through your colon and help your intestines in the elimination process.

✔ **Drink.** Plenty of water keeps you hydrated and helps move and flush toxins from your system.

✔ **Breathe.** Yoga breathing is simple but powerful. Because your lungs are eliminative organs as well, when you exhale, you release toxins. Most people usually take shallow breaths, but when you take the time to inhale and exhale deeply, you get more oxygen in and toxins out. Yoga is a fantastic addition to the 30-Day Reset and beyond for detoxification as well as health benefits.

The process of ridding your body of this waste is like magic. When you start giving your cells fewer toxins and begin flooding them with nutrition, you can see and feel the difference in your weight, energy levels, skin, and overall health. Your cravings start to diminish, and your body naturally desires healthier foods as your taste begins to change.

Mastering the plan

Now that you know the *why* behind the 30-Day Reset, you're ready to begin implementation. For the most successful journey possible during your 30 days, here are some guidelines to follow:

1. **Make the decision to move forward with the 30-Day Reset.**

   Grab a calendar and mark off the 30 days. Don't wait too long! Don't give yourself time to back out — just mark it down and get going.

2. **Tell people in your tribe what you're up to.**

   Ask for their support during this time, and explain that you need to put more focus on yourself for the next 30 days. Make sure they know how important this is to you. Another bonus to doing this is that as soon as you tell people, it helps you be more accountable to the plan, which will push you along when you need the strength to keep going.

3. **Start your positive reprograming through affirmations.**

   Remember to try to do these internal self-scripts first thing in the morning and say them loud and clear (refer to Book I, Chapter 1, for more about affirmations). A good plan is to say your affirmations in the morning as soon as your feet hit the floor. Hang them in your bathroom or somewhere you're sure to see them. You may want to try journaling at night. Journal your thoughts in a positive tone as if they're already happening, such as "I am feeling healthier, thinner, and more vibrant than I ever have."

4. **Clear the decks.**

   Go through your kitchen with a trash bag and get rid of foods that aren't part of your 30-day plan. Stock your kitchen with all the wonderful Paleo-approved foods that kick off this chapter.

5. **Get organized.**

   Make sure you have the ingredients and the equipment you need to plan the foods you want. Get as many resources as you can get your hands on to help you prepare meals or give you snack ideas. Try to keep it as simple as possible when you first start. The recipes in this book will give you some great ideas!

In addition to the steps in the master plan, you can do the following things to keep your spirits up and promote a healthy mind and body:

- ✔ **Move every day.** The more you move, the more you'll start feeling the healing effects of your 30-Day Reset. High-intensity exercise, walking, yoga — no matter what you do, it helps toxins leave your body and keep your mind clear. Make sure you adjust your food accordingly.

- ✔ **Set aside 20 minutes for meditation every day.** You have a lot of options to help you meditate, but the important thing is to be still, calm, and quiet for 20 minutes each day. This practice will start to balance and rejuvenate you.

- ✔ **Get a weekly massage and chiropractic adjustment.** This is a great way to start calming your nervous system and to help your body detox. When your nervous system works better, your organs work better; when your organs work better, they detox more readily and effectively.

At the end of your 30 days, celebrate! You just accomplished a major milestone. Give yourself a pat on the back.

Understanding your body's transformation

You may feel pretty lousy during the first few weeks transitioning to Paleo. But with this book, you're equipped with so much knowledge about implementing these first 30 days that you're way ahead of the game.

Some people experience mental fuzziness, fatigue, headaches, moodiness, shakiness, and are just plain out of it. Your body is conquering carbs and detoxing, so it takes a while for your body to adjust. Although your body may be looking better, sometimes it takes a while for the rest of you to catch up. Some call these symptoms "the carb flu," which is the nasty transition that your body goes through when going from a high-carb to a lower-carb diet. Even though living Paleo isn't considered a low-carb diet, it's naturally lower in carbs, so your body is making that transition.

During this transition process, your body needs glucose (sugar) for the brain, muscles, cells, and so on. Until you started living Paleo, glucose was easy to access from all the sugary carbohydrates you may have been eating. Now your body has to create glucose from fats and proteins, which isn't as easily done. It will happen, though, soon enough, and you'll start feeling better and your body will run more efficiently because of it.

Try some extra healthy fats like coconut and lots of water to calm the effects of the carb flu.

Some people feel few symptoms during this transition period; others get a heavy dose. But just remember: It's worth it on the other side, so hang tight!

Battling the sugar demon

When you're going through the first 30 days, you're breaking food habits and cravings. The toughest of these to break is cravings for sugary foods. The sugar demon will constantly tap you on the back, trying to get you to eat your bagel, pasta, or bowl of cereal. This guy will try to justify why it's no big deal to have a bowl of oatmeal or a sandwich.

Your mind will rationalize why you need to stop what you're doing and hit the bagel barn. What your brain thinks it wants isn't always what your body needs, and you need the strength to have a clear understanding of what's happening.

How do you know whether you have a sugar addiction? If eating sugar makes all your symptoms magically go away for a while or if you can't go long without sugary foods, you're probably addicted.

When you have a craving, your body is usually looking for a quick burst of something to make it feel better. Often, that "something" is a brain chemical called *serotonin*. This chemical affects mood, specifically happiness and well-being. The higher the levels, the happier you feel. When serotonin levels drop, your body screams out for a change. It's looking for that feel-good chemical to alter its present brain chemistry. That's one of the reasons so many people are in the vicious cycle of eating sweets and high-carb foods. Often, people self-medicate with sugary carbohydrate foods, looking for something to make them feel good and change their state of mind.

The following factors can lower serotonin levels:

✔ **Stress:** One of the biggest reasons so many people who are stressed out have a weight problem is that they're looking for ways to pull their serotonin back up, and sugary carbohydrates often fill the bill.

✔ **Lack of sunlight:** Sunlight plays a role in the synthesis and regulation of serotonin. If you work in an office or are indoors a lot, the lack of sunlight can cause your serotonin levels to drop.

✔ **Natural aging:** This natural process can drop serotonin.

To really help your cravings on an ongoing basis and to rid yourself of the sugar demon once and for all, you have to be in the practice of maintaining your serotonin levels. Always strive for healthy ways to elevate your serotonin levels. To balance serotonin, do the following:

✔ **Eat Paleo foods.** This is one of the best things you can do for your serotonin levels. The high-fiber fruits and vegetables, Paleo proteins, and non-processed foods are all foods your brain loves. Paleo-approved foods are the perfect intervention for low serotonin levels.

✔ **Exercise.** Exercise is an amazing tool for altering brain chemistry and serotonin levels. For more on incorporating Paleo exercises into your life, see Book IV.

✔ **Think good thoughts.** Try to focus on keeping your thoughts happy and positive. This habit will do your serotonin levels a lot of good! Thinking positively is a very powerful tool for keeping your mood naturally elevated.

The sugar demon is *not* hanging around because you lack willpower or because you're weak. People who manage to be content with wrapping their protein in lettuce instead of bread aren't stronger, nor do they hold some special gift of willpower. Most likely, they've managed to slay their sugar demon. Their body is no longer screaming for sweets, and they truly are content doing without. When you follow the steps we've given you, you'll also be free of this demon and at peace with your lettuce wraps.

After you go through your 30-Day Reset, you'll feel the sugar demon start to distance itself. Before long, you'll be rid of that bugger once and for all! The key is to stay onboard and understand what's happening to your body.

The more knowledge you have through living Paleo, the harder it will be for the sugar demon to talk you into a trip to the bakery.

The rules for your first 30 days

To reap the rewards of living Paleo, you don't need to be perfect. In fact, if you follow the Paleo guidelines 80 to 90 percent of the time, you'll enjoy the majority of the benefits and vastly improve your health. However, during the 30-Day Reset, you need to follow the Paleo guidelines stringently. To put it in plain language: There's no cheating during the 30-Day Reset. To really detox and heal your body, you need to grit your teeth and get through the 30 days with no slip-ups, no compromises, no excuses, and no gray areas. Doing so isn't always easy, but you're tougher than any loaf of bread or bowl of pasta. You can outsmart a doughnut, and you can absolutely triumph over happy hour.

Ready to jump in? Here are the guidelines for your 30-day immersion into living Paleo:

- **Omit the foods on the "no" list.** The purpose of the 30-Day Reset is to remove inflammatory foods from your plate, which means you need to avoid consuming processed foods, all grains, vegetable and seed oils, soy, legumes, added sugars, dairy, and alcohol.

- **Embrace the foods on the "yes" list.** The good news is that you can eat until you're satisfied from these food groups: all animal proteins, vegetables, fruits, and naturally occurring fats.

- **Stay hydrated.** Your body needs water to help you detox, and drinking plenty of water can also help you manage your appetite. Get yourself a BPA-free water bottle and commit to drinking fresh water throughout the day. You'll feel more energetic, your skin will look refreshed, and you'll quickly figure out how to distinguish between thirst and hunger.

- **Get moving!** The 30-Day Reset is an excellent time to add movement to your routine. Even 30 minutes of walking every day can make a remarkable difference in your metabolism, your stress level, and your mood.

- **Practice eyeballing portions.** The 30-Day Reset is a great time to practice your portion skills. It may take a few weeks to understand your body's hunger and satisfaction signals, but as you break the sugar cycle and the toxins leave your body, your hormonal systems begin to function correctly, and eating "right" becomes effortless.

- **Record your "before" you.** The earlier section "Capturing Your Personal Before and After Makeover" explains ways you can document your personal "before," so you can celebrate your Paleo improvements. Try any or all of the recommendations in that section, and then get ready to make note of the changes at the end of the 30 days.

Although you may be tempted to weigh yourself during your 30-Day Reset, resist. Instead, take your measurements or weigh yourself before starting the 30 days, and then forget about *results* and keep your focus on how you *feel* along the way. The 30-Day Reset is a liberating experience that helps you create healthy new habits and may change your relationship with the food you eat. Banish the scale for a month and free yourself to learn and grow.

Dear Diary: Guidelines for 30 days of journaling

Keeping a journal during the 30-Day Reset can be a valuable tool to help you learn from the experience and identify challenges or issues specific to you and your body so you can make corrections. Your journal is all about you, so you can treat it like a diary to capture your entire emotional experience during your 30-Day Reset, or you can view it as more of a scientific document in which you simply record data from your day. Here are some suggestions for the kind of information to include so your review at the end of the 30-Day Reset is helpful and informative.

- **Foods you eat:** Document everything you put into your mouth — especially if you find yourself eating between meals. Doing so helps you identify triggers that may spark your appetite and compel you to eat when you're not hungry. Making note of the quantities you eat, at least in the beginning, can also be helpful. Knowing how much you eat helps you see the connections between your intake and your hunger.

- **Where, when, and how you eat:** Focusing on and savoring your food go a long way toward appetite control and satisfaction. Do you feel differently when you eat standing in front of the fridge or on the run versus when you eat at the dining table? Do you eat more or less when dining with others? That kind of information can help you banish negative old habits and create positive new ones.

- **Cravings:** Especially during the first week or two of the 30-Day Reset, you may experience cravings for specific foods. Your journal can be an effective tool in helping you overcome those cravings. It's essential to your long-term success that you not surrender to the cravings during the 30-Day Reset. Make note of the craving in your journal, and do something to distract yourself from the craving, such as drink a glass of water, go for a walk, or call a friend. If you're truly hungry, a small snack of fat and protein can help curb cravings, particularly if the craving is for sugar.

- **Amount and quality of sleep:** Sleep is vital to your health and can be affected by the foods you eat. Keep track of when you go to sleep, when you wake up, and the overall quality of your sleep. You may find that certain foods or other behaviors influence your sleep patterns.

✔ **Activity:** Tracking your activity — both formal exercise, like a walk or run, a fitness class, strength training, or playing a sport, and casual activity, like gardening or playing with a pet — can provide valuable insight into your energy levels and caloric needs.

✔ **Mood and stress levels:** Food is a powerful mood adjuster, and, especially during the 30-Day Reset, you'll feel the difference when you make the switch from the standard high-carb diet to a Paleo lifestyle. Just make note of when you feel upbeat and energetic or cranky, stressed, or moody. Later, you may be able to draw conclusions from these notes that can help you adjust your eating, exercise, and sleep habits.

✔ **Other goals:** Although you don't want to take on too much at once, the 30-Day Reset can be an excellent time to add in other good habits. Have you always wanted to start a meditation practice? The 30-Day Reset is a fine time to add that into your routine, and you can track your progress in your journal. Other good goals may be watching less TV, drinking a specific number of glasses of water per day, cutting out caffeine, going to bed 30 minutes earlier than usual, and so on. Use the 30 days to dial in your healthiest habits, and use the journal to keep track of your new behaviors and how they make you feel.

Chapter 3

Preparing and Using Your Cave Kitchen

In This Chapter

▶ Taking a new approach to your diet

▶ Understanding proteins, fats, and carbohydrates

▶ Tossing the foods that don't fit

▶ Filling the fridge and pantry with Paleo foods

▶ Looking into Paleo-friendly cooking methods

*P*aleo nutrition is the cornerstone of living Paleo, and it puts real food first. Based on high-quality proteins, fats, and carbohydrates, Paleo nutrition ensures that you'll eat all the nutrients you need, so you build a better you with every bite. By following the Paleo nutrition plan, you create a new relationship with food, and eating nutritiously becomes effortless.

In this chapter, you discover how proteins, fats, and carbs make you healthier, and you see why the Paleo food pyramid makes more sense and feels more natural than any other nutrition "rules" ever have.

Understanding the nutrition side of things doesn't do you a lot of good, though, without solid execution. That means getting your fanny in the kitchen — the most important thing you can do to make living Paleo stick. Cooking Paleo meals probably isn't as hard or as time-consuming as you may think, so don't let this misconception get in the way of your success.

Before you get into the kitchen, though, you have to get your kitchen into Paleo shape. Whether you're an experienced cook or just finding your way around the kitchen, in this chapter you can find advice on how to equip your kitchen with the tools you need and use the best Paleo-friendly cooking methods to keep you and your family well nourished.

Rethinking What You Know about Nutrition

In 1992, the Department of Agriculture created the USDA Food Guide Pyramid. When it came to what to eat and how much, many families, schools, organizations, and nutritionists came to rely on this pyramid as the gold standard. This, unfortunately, was a big mistake. Since adopting the USDA's pyramid, we've become more unhealthy, more overweight, and definitely more confused than ever. In 2010, another attempt was made to get America back on track. The pyramid was retired, and along came the USDA MyPlate — with more confusion and misinformation. However, hope exists. It comes down to eating by design, by making your meals come from food choices that your body understands.

The following sections challenge the USDA's plate and retire it with the pyramid, introducing the most effective eating guide you'll find, the Paleo pyramid. It's decisive, scientifically founded, and super easy to implement! You'll enjoy figuring out why this way of eating is the answer for modern-day cave women and men and how your concerns will be answered once and for all.

The flawed USDA Food Guide Pyramid

The advice about good nutrition can be very confusing. Just browse the magazine covers at the checkout stand to see all the conflict: low-carb, no-carb, low-fat, vegetarian, vegan, no fruit. What's next — no food? No air?

The USDA Food Guide Pyramid can take much of the blame, even though it's been several years since the pyramid was the prevailing guideline for how to eat. Here are some of the biggest problems with the food pyramid:

✔ The base of the food pyramid is cereal, bread, and pasta — and a lot of it, to the tune of 6 to 11 servings per day. These processed carbs are unfavorable sources of energy and, more important, your body does *not* require these foods to operate efficiently. Additionally, antinutrients are found in whole grains, called *phytic acid* and *lectins*.

   • Phytic acid binds to minerals, making them unavailable for you to use. This means that the more whole grains you eat, the less able your body is to take advantage of minerals like calcium, magnesium, and zinc.

- Lectins may cause even more trouble. These tricky guys bind to insulin receptors, which can lead to insulin problems, are linked to inflammatory problems, and damage your gut defenses that line your intestines. When you damage this lining, it allows food particles to enter into the blood system and lymph system, where they don't belong. Digestion becomes compromised along with your immune system — not very appetizing!

The USDA food pyramid identifies whole grains as a good source of fiber. Here's the real skinny: non-starchy veggies and fruits often have more than double the amount of fiber as grains. With the Paleo plan, you have no recommended daily allowance (RDA) for breads, pasta, and cereals. In fact, not only does your body not require these grains, but also your insulin and blood sugar management is better — so you're healthier and happier — without them.

✔ The food pyramid identifies dairy as a key component of good nutrition, but cow's milk is the number-one food allergen for humans. That's because cow's milk isn't intended for human consumption; it's the perfect food for transforming calves into very large cows. Your body just doesn't know what to do with milk — and ailments like digestive disturbance, acne, insulin resistance, and allergic reactions are the result.

Studies show that milk isn't as protective to bone tissue as once thought — and contrary to popular belief, milk does *not* reduce bone fractures! To form and maintain strong bones, your body needs to be in pH balance; the fruits and vegetables in the Paleo diet put it right where it needs to be.

✔ The food pyramid missteps with protein, too. Dried beans and peas can't be eaten interchangeably with animal proteins like meat, poultry, fish, and eggs. Beans and legumes have poor digestibility and don't pack the same complete protein punch as animal sources. In fact, beans and legumes averaged about 20 to 25 percent lower than animal protein ratings in a protein quality index published by the Food and Agriculture Organization/World Health Organization.

Beans and legumes contain about three times less protein than animal sources — and the incomplete proteins found in legumes are difficult for your body to digest.

In 2010, the USDA developed the next generation of food guidelines called MyPlate, shown in Figure 3-1. These guidelines suffer from the same challenges as the food pyramid: Whole grains and dairy are still included requirements for health. The plate approach doesn't solve the old problems. Instead, our actual plates should represent what we've discovered from evolutionary science.

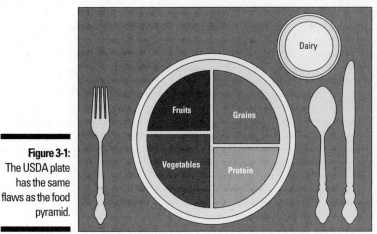

Illustration © U.S. Department of Agriculture

Figure 3-1:
The USDA plate has the same flaws as the food pyramid.

The Paleo pyramid

So the USDA food pyramid had major problems, and the new USDA MyPlate didn't correct those problems. However, the Paleo food pyramid, which you can see in Figure 3-2, is built on simple, real foods that are close to their natural state. When you create meals with the healthy building blocks of the Paleo pyramid, weight loss is effortless, and vibrant good health is a natural side effect.

Here's what good health looks like:

- **The Base:** Meat, fish, fowl, and eggs
- **Level Two:** Low-starch and low-sugar vegetables and fruits
- **Level Three:** Naturally occurring fats and oils
- **The Top:** Paleo-friendly snacks and desserts made with nuts, dried fruit, coconut flour, and nut flours

When you eat the foods that make up the Paleo pyramid, you're free from confusion — and free to eat real food. When you choose Paleo foods, you choose a plan that works with your genetics to bring out the best in everything you do. You'll soon find that the nutrient-rich foods have everything you need to become healthier and stronger and to fight aging.

The next sections go into detail about how following the Paleo pyramid gives you enough fiber, calcium, and all the vitamins and minerals your body needs for its structures and functions to flourish. The nutrients listed in these sections are ones you definitely *won't* be missing when you start living Paleo.

The Paleo Pyramid

The Top
Paleo-friendly snacks and desserts made with nuts, dried fruit, coconut flour, and nut flours

Level Three
Naturally occurring fats and oils — nuts, seeds, coconut oil, macadamia oil, nut butters (like almond butter), grass-fed butter, and ghee

Level Two
Low-starch and low-sugar vegetables and fruits (berries, lemons, and limes)

The Base
Protein: The foundation of the Paleo Pyramid includes meat, fish, fowl, and eggs

© John Wiley & Sons, Inc.

Figure 3-2:
The Paleo pyramid in all its glory.

Yes, you'll get enough fiber

You've probably been hammered with the idea that you need to eat plenty of fiber. And, yes, fiber plays an important role in healthy nutrition. It helps stabilize blood sugar levels while lowering blood cholesterol. Fiber helps you feel more full, so food cravings are reduced, and it helps you build a stronger immune system with fewer hormonal imbalances. It also acts like a scrub brush for your colon to help keep it clean and healthy.

Based on all of that, you may be worried that if you eliminate whole grains from your diet, you'll be short on your fiber requirements. But when you enjoy appropriate quantities of vegetables and fruits, you get all the fiber you need from natural, *digestible* sources.

You may be surprised to realize that the foods you've been taught are high in fiber — whole-grain bread, whole-grain pasta, brown rice — aren't the health foods they've been advertised to be. Your best sources of fiber, in just the right amounts to keep you healthy, are fresh vegetables; fresh fruit; and, in moderation, dried fruit, nuts, and seeds.

Yes, you'll get enough calcium

You probably already know that your body needs calcium to form strong bones and teeth. And like most Americans, you've been taught to believe that drinking milk is essential for getting enough calcium. But dairy can be a major source of inflammation. Instead, get your calcium from high-quality sources like plants, sardines, seafood, and some nuts.

Here are some good options for calcium that are easy for your body to absorb:

✔ **Plant sources:**

- Bok choy and cabbage
- Collard, mustard, and turnip greens
- Green beans
- Kale
- Seaweed, like kelp and dulse
- Spinach
- Watercress

✔ **Seafood sources:**

- Canned mackerel
- Salmon (with bones)
- Sardines (with bones)
- Shrimp

✔ **Fat sources:**

- Nut and seed butters: almond, sesame, sunflower
- Nuts: almonds, cashews, Brazil nuts, chestnuts
- Seeds: sesame, sunflower

✔ **Other sources:**

- Dried dates
- Dried figs
- Olives

If you eat plenty of leafy green vegetables and complement your meals with other calcium-rich choices, you don't need dairy or calcium supplements to meet your calcium requirements.

Yes, you'll get enough vitamins and minerals

Nutrients work synergistically in your body — the vitamins and minerals cooperate to keep you healthy. When you have a vitamin or mineral deficiency, merely supplementing with the one that's falling short won't correct the imbalance.

A healthy diet is the best way to supply your body with the balance of vitamins and minerals it needs. When you eat an abundance of vegetables and fruits, as well as high-quality protein and fat, the nutrients in those foods work together to keep your body functioning well.

No, you don't need whole grains and dairy

Many of us were taught that healthy meals must incorporate some whole grains, legumes, and dairy to be complete and to ensure adequate doses of vitamins and minerals. The truth is that grains and legumes include substances called *antinutrients* that are actually detrimental to your health. In the short-term, they can cause digestive distress and bloating; in the long-term, they can permanently damage your digestive system, which leads to internal inflammation.

And forget what you've heard about milk doing the body good. Once you've been weaned from your mother, you're not designed to consume milk in any of its forms. (Sorry, cheese and yogurt!) Cow's milk is evolved to nourish cows, not humans — and the pasteurization and homogenization processes further obliterate any potentially nutritious components of dairy.

The truth is that grains, dairy, and beans are more damaging than rewarding and don't add value to investments in your nutritional bank.

Real food always equals real nutrition. Your health is determined by your nutrient intake, and the Paleo pyramid supplies all the nutrients you need in delicious, natural packaging.

The Paleo Big Three: Animal Proteins, Natural Fats, Complex Carbohydrates

The nutritional building blocks of proteins, fats, and carbohydrates — the *Paleo Big Three* — are known as *macronutrients*. Understanding them is essential to knowing how the Paleo diet works.

As historical and anthropological records show, in the Paleolithic era (about 2.6 million years ago), hunter-gatherers of the time had many of the attributes that you're probably looking to gain. They were incredibly healthy, lean, fit, and strong. Much of this was undoubtedly attributed to what they ate. So when you eat as they did, you can expect many of the same benefits. To move forward, then, you must look backward to gather wisdom and use it as your own nutritional guideline.

The first step to forming these new nutritional guidelines is to follow the recipe for nutrition that our ancestors took by eating the macronutrients they ate. Evidence suggests that hunter-gatherers ate no dairy, no cereal grains, no refined sugars, and few fatty meats. Instead, they feasted on the Paleo Big Three: wild, lean animals; naturally occurring fats, especially the healthy omega-3 fats found in cold-water fish; and non-starchy, wild fruits and vegetables.

The Paleo Big Three play an essential role in fueling your body:

- ✔ **Protein** builds and repairs you, increasing lean muscle mass and reducing body fat. Adequate protein supports your physique and ensures that your appetite is satisfied.

- ✔ **Fat** is essential and not the enemy. Naturally occurring fats are vital to the health of your cells and, therefore, your entire body. When you enjoy fats from both animal and plant sources, you fight illnesses caused by inflammation and keep your body in balance. Fat also contributes to feelings of fullness so that overeating becomes a thing of the past.

- ✔ Complex **carbohydrates** supply energy. All carbohydrates are eventually turned into a form of sugar called *glucose* — and glucose is what your brain and your cells use for fuel. But just as high-quality gas serves your car's engine better, your body runs best on the carbohydrates found in vegetables and fruits, rather than processed, starchy carbs, like bread, pasta, and sugary treats.

When you're planning your meals, think about the Paleo Big Three and ask yourself, "Will my plate include lean protein, healthy fats, and complex carbs?" Also, think about whether your feast would have been welcome on a hunter-gatherer's table.

Paleo proteins and why animals matter

Humans are omnivores. That means that people have a meat-eating heritage and evolved to subsist on meat and plants. Anthropologists agree that our earliest ancestors were meat eaters, and scientists estimate that our genes are 99.9 percent the same as they were back then. Meat provides us with protein, essential fatty acids, and vitamins — just as it did for our hunter-gatherer ancestors.

Our ancestors ate as much as 3 pounds of protein a day! The meat they ate gave them an abundance of protein, essential fatty acids, and vitamins. It allowed them to build strong muscle and to store the fuel they needed for long walks and short bursts of energy (to, say, outrun a predator or take down dinner).

For modern cave men and women, we recommend that you invest in the highest-quality protein sources you can afford. Here are a few helpful tips:

- ✔ **Happy animals are healthy animals.** And eating healthy animals makes you healthier. As much as possible, choose lean, grass-fed, and free-range meat. You earn bonus points for good health if it's also organic, and it should always be free of antibiotics and other fillers. Beef, buffalo, game, lamb, goat, turkey, chicken, and fish/seafood are all good sources.

- ✔ **Conventional can be okay, too.** If a tight budget means you need to buy store-bought, conventional meat, you can still vastly improve your health. Choose lean cuts and trim visible fat before cooking, and then drain as much of the released fat as you can after cooking.

- ✔ **Go fishing!** Another valuable protein source to pile on your plate is wild-caught, sustainable fish. Your best bets are fattier, cold-water fish like salmon, sardines, mackerel, cod, and herring. Tuna packed in water is also a good choice. Check out the Monterey Bay Aquarium Seafood Watch (www.montereybayaquarium.org/cr/seafoodwatch.aspx) for more recommendations and a helpful mobile app.

- ✔ **Scramble up some eggs.** Eggs are a Paleo protein powerhouse. Rich in many key nutrients, especially fat-soluble vitamins A and D, egg yolk is also loaded with folate — a B vitamin that's super brain food. Look for organic, pastured eggs with omega-3 for the best fatty acid profile. (Eggs are one food where you shouldn't settle for conventional production methods.)

- ✔ **Get wild!** Wild animal meat — venison, rabbit, bear, wild-caught fish, even wild boar — is an excellent choice. It's very lean and full of healthy omega-3 fats. If you're going to splurge a bit on your food bill — or really imitate hunter-gatherers and do the hunting yourself — choosing wild animal meat is a wise way to do it.

 Animal proteins help you reduce excess body fat, build lean muscle, and feed your brain with the nutrients it needs for peak performance. Incorporating adequate animal protein in your Paleo approach will vastly improve your health and well-being.

Friendly fats and why they're essential

If the term *friendly fats* seems like an oxymoron, this section is for you! Your brain may have been hijacked by low-fat, no-fat thinking, but humans are evolved to eat naturally occurring fats (called *fatty acids*) to build their best bodies. In other words, fat is your friend.

Essential fats are those fats that your body can't produce on its own. These fats, important for all systems of the body, must be obtained through the food you eat. Your skin, heart, lungs, nervous system, brain, and all internal organs are improved and maintained by eating fatty acids. Plus, fats make food taste good and help you feel satisfied. What's friendlier than that?

The two essential fats are known as *omega-3* and *omega-6 fatty acids.* You've probably heard about omega-3 in relation to heart health, but these fatty acids are inflammation busters and also aid in other conditions, including diabetes, some cancers, skin disorders, arthritis, cholesterol, and depression.

Getting the right ratio of omega-3 and omega-6 fats

Omega-3 fatty acids are found in animal sources, such as the following:

- ✔ **Cold-water fish** like salmon, sardines, herring, mackerel, and black cod
- ✔ **Wild game** like venison, bear, rabbit, and boar

Omega-6 fatty acids are found in unfavorable sources, such as canola oil, corn oil, and other processed fats known as industrial oils, which are best avoided. But omega-6 fatty acids are also found *naturally* and more health-fully in the following nuts and seeds and the oils extracted from them:

✔ Almonds	✔ Pecans
✔ Brazil nuts	✔ Pistachios
✔ Cashews	✔ Sesame seeds
✔ Hazelnuts	✔ Sunflower seeds
✔ Macadamia nuts	✔ Walnuts

Our number-one pick for nuts is macadamia nuts. With a ratio of 6:3, they're definitely Paleo approved (and delicious).

Wondering what a healthy omega-6 to omega-3 ratio looks like? It's 1:1. Unfortunately, the ratio of omega-6 to omega-3 in the modern diet is between 15:1 and 22:1 — that means that most people are consuming far too much omega-6 fatty acid. About 15 to 20 times too much!

How did this happen? Non-Paleo-friendly fats are used to produce many processed foods found on supermarket shelves, and those types of oils are used almost exclusively in restaurants. Additionally, modern grain-fed meat supply means that the conventionally grown meat is also high in omega-6 fats. The critical balance of omega-6 to omega-3 fatty acids is teetering the wrong way.

Avoiding unhealthy fats

Here are some common fats that aren't Paleo-friendly. These refined oils have very unbalanced fatty acid ratios — corn oil is 57:1! These fats are also sensitive to the damaging effects of heat and are often rancid on the store shelves before you even add them to your grocery cart. Your body isn't adapted to process these oils, and they should be eliminated from your kitchen and your plate.

- Canola oil
- Corn oil
- Cottonseed oil
- Margarine
- Palm kernel oil
- Partially hydrogenated oil

- Peanut oil
- Safflower oil
- Soybean oil
- Sunflower oil
- Trans fats (hydrogenated oils)
- Vegetable shortening

These fats can cause more inflammation in the body. Inflammation causes illness, premature aging, and weight gain. These fats are not naturally occurring, and when you eat fake fat, you get fat, inflamed, and sick.

Eating healthy, natural fats

Here are some smart, healthy choices for friendly fats:

- **Monounsaturated fats:** Monounsaturated fats (MUFA) are liquid at room temperature and solidify when chilled. Good sources include green or black olives, olive oil, macadamia nuts, macadamia oil, avocado, and avocado oil. These fats aren't recommended for cooking because heat can oxidize them, turning them from friend to foe. Use MUFAs on salads, or drizzle them on cooked foods.

- **Saturated fats:** Saturated fats have suffered an unfair reputation as a heart disease villain. The truth is that saturated fats have been an important and beneficial part of the human diet since our cave-man ancestors gnawed on a nice, fatty chop. Saturated fat is solid at room temperature, and our favorite source is coconut. Coconut oil is ideal for cooking because it can withstand higher temperatures. Coconut flakes, coconut milk, and coconut butter are also delicious, healthful options. You should also feel free to indulge in the luscious fat found in organic, grass-fed, pastured meats and poultry, eggs, and wild-caught fish.

✔ **Polyunsaturated fats:** Polyunsaturated fats (PUFA), found primarily in nuts and seeds, are higher in omega-6 fatty acids and should be consumed in moderation. The best choices for PUFAs are almonds and almond butter, Brazil nuts, cashews and cashew butter, pistachios, and pecans.

When you enjoy Paleo-friendly fats, all your body systems function more optimally, and you fight fit, ready to ward off many modern ailments, like cancer, autoimmune diseases, neurological problems, heart disease, obesity, and a host of other issues that deficiency brings. Fake fat makes you fat — natural fats help you thrive.

Complex carbs and why they're king

To understand carbohydrates' role in your body function, you need to know a little about glucose and insulin. Carbs are your body's go-to source for quick energy. Your body transforms all carbohydrates — from whole-grain bread to broccoli florets — into glucose, and your brain and cells use glucose as a primary fuel source. Activities like reading this book, running a mile, or hugging your kids are all made possible by glucose.

Insulin is a hormone that helps your body store fat for later energy use. If you want to control the accumulation and reduction of body fat, you need to control insulin — and to do that, you need to eat the right kinds of carbohydrates. Knowing which carbs to eat is critical because the sources you choose directly dictate your insulin level. When insulin production is under control, weight loss and optimal health are the result.

The best carbohydrate sources are local, organically grown fruits and vegetables. Choose fruits and non-starchy vegetables in all the colors of the rainbow to cover the full spectrum of nutrients. Dark-colored fruits, such as blackberries and blueberries, are packed with antioxidants, and deeply colored veggies, like carrots and kale, are loaded with vitamins and minerals.

Here are some delicious examples of non-starchy vegetables:

✔ Asparagus

✔ Broccoli

✔ Brussels sprouts

✔ Cabbage

✔ Cauliflower

✔ Eggplant

✔ Onions

✔ Peppers

✔ Spaghetti squash

✔ Summer squash

✔ Tomatoes

✔ Vegetable greens: kale, collard greens, Swiss chard, mustard greens, spinach, and so on

✔ Zucchini

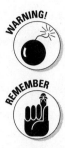

Steer clear of starch- and sugar-laden carbohydrates sources like white potatoes, rice, corn, breads (including whole grain), cereals, pasta, fruit juices, and sodas. These sugars are instantly absorbed and will affect your blood sugar insulin levels in a flash.

The Paleo approach is not a low-carb diet but a healthy-carb plan. When you drop unhealthy refined carbohydrates and replace them with vegetables and fruits, you begin to live the Paleo way.

Getting Rid of the Foods that Don't Fit

Your commitment to living Paleo begins with changing your eating habits, so it's time to create an environment for success: the Paleo kitchen.

People often talk about using a detox to cleanse their bodies so they work more efficiently. Well, think of creating a Paleo-smart kitchen in the same way: You're cleansing your kitchen so it works more efficiently for you and your family. It may be a little uncomfortable at first, but when you're on the other side, you'll have an uncluttered food life and love how you feel.

Look at your calendar and pick a day to give your kitchen a Paleo cleanout. If you wait too long, you'll lose your momentum, so plan time soon. And actually mark it in your calendar because when you schedule something, it becomes real. Otherwise, it's just a thought.

When you first walk in your kitchen to make the Paleo transformation, take a long, hard look. Now visualize your kitchen filled with Paleo-approved foods that provide you and your family with deep nutrition, foods that help you lose weight, boost immunity, and fight aging. Take a moment to experience how that feels in your body. Then put on some music you love and get yourself into a happy state.

Although you may be tempted to keep some foods "just in case" or "for the kids or guests," resist. This book is filled with strategies for success, and keeping non-Paleo foods hanging around while you're trying to make the switch isn't a good strategy.

Cleansing the pantry

Open those pantry doors and just do it! As the late motivational speaker Zig Ziglar said, if you keep doing what you're doing, you'll keep getting what you're getting. Well, you're not going to be getting what you've been getting anymore. If you've been tired, battled certain health conditions, struggled with your weight, or just want to look and feel your best, here's where you start.

Grab a trash bag and a box. The trash bag is obvious; the box is so you can set aside unopened foods to donate to your local food bank or shelter. Some people in your community are striving for calories, and you can help them by sending over a care package of your unopened non-Paleo foods.

Check the labels on your pantry items as you sort them to confirm whether they're keepable, but just a fair warning that you'll have to give most the heave-ho.

Say good-bye to the following:

- Foods with flour, including breads, pasta, crackers, chips, and cookies.

- Breakfast cereals, including granola and oatmeal.

- Foods with grains and whole grains, including wheat, barley, rye, oats, spelt, corn, and quinoa.

- Refined processed fats, such as margarine; vegetable shortening; and canola (rapeseed), soybean, grapeseed, sunflower, safflower, corn, vegetable, and peanut oils.

- Foods with hydrogenated or partially hydrogenated oils, including cookies, snack foods, and buttery spreads such as Earth Balance.

- Foods with artificial sweeteners, specifically Acesulfame K (Sweet One), aspartame (Equal and NutraSweet), saccharin (Sweet'N Low), sucralose (Splenda), stevia, and those containing erythritol (such as Truvia).

- Foods with soy, including soy, teriyaki, and hoisin sauces. Some tuna fish is packed in soy, so check labels.

- Commercial condiments with sugars and artificial ingredients, such as ketchup, BBQ sauce, sweet and sour sauces, and bottled salad dressings and marinades.

- Foods with cornstarch and other food starches.

- All sugars except for raw honey and pure maple syrup, dark chocolate, and cocoa powder.

    Less-processed, natural sweeteners like raw honey and pure maple syrup can stay, but don't eat them during your 30-Day Paleo cleanse (which you find out about in Book I, Chapter 2).

- Packaged processed foods, including microwavable meals or food bars (check all processed foods carefully because most have additives and gluten).

- Sauces, soups, and stews (most have thickened flours).

- Dressings (most are thickened with flour).

✔ Canned foods with sugars and additives, including canned fruits packed in syrup.

✔ Jam and jelly.

✔ Sweetened nut or seed butters.

Clearing out the refrigerator and freezer

Emptying out the refrigerator and freezer can get dicey because you may feel like you're wasting the opened jars and containers. Those bottles of this and that all lined up along your refrigerator door make you inclined to think, "I'll wait to see whether this Paleo thing is really worth its salt." When these doubts strike, remember that you're cleansing your refrigerator. Keeping non-Paleo foods isn't part of the plan.

The following are the items you need to chuck:

✔ Any leftovers that aren't part of your healthy food plan.

✔ Commercial dressings and sauces.

✔ Dairy products, including butter, margarine, milk, cheese, cream, half-and-half, flavored creamers, yogurt, ice cream, and frozen yogurt.

✔ All soy frankenfoods, such as vegetarian burgers, hot dogs, and chicken nuggets. (*Frankenfoods* are processed foods that are made to look like a certain food product but are really made from wheat.) Pitch any tofu as well.

✔ Fruit juices or other sweetened beverages, including soda, sports drinks, or teas.

✔ Lunchmeats, sausage, and bacon that contain gluten, nitrites, soy, or sweeteners.

✔ Commercial condiments or pickled foods with sugars and artificial ingredients.

✔ Frozen waffles, pizza, macaroni, or other frozen meals.

✔ Popsicles and frozen fruit bars with sugar and artificial ingredients.

What's left in your refrigerator should be eggs, unprocessed meats, fresh fruits, vegetables, and condiments that don't contain sugar or other artificial ingredients.

If you decide to have a sweet, you're better off going out and getting a single serving rather than keeping it in your house. That way, after you eat it, you're done, and you're not tempted by it lingering in the kitchen.

Refilling Your Kitchen with Paleo Foods

You decided to take action and committed to a healthy life by clearing out the old and making way for the new. The foods you'll be restocking your kitchen with are full of nutrients and bursting with flavor. They're the foods your body was designed to eat. Enjoy making these foods your base and get excited about your healthy, vibrant future.

Picking Paleo-smart protein

When you read or hear that animal proteins aren't good for you, often the *quality* of that protein is what's in question, not the protein source. Factory-farmed meat is less healthy than meat from animals raised humanely and sustainably. When you can, your best option is always to get meat from organic, pasture-raised, antibiotic-free sources. In fact, if you're going to strain the food budget somewhere, protein is the place. If doing so isn't in the budget right now, though, don't stress. Buying the leanest cuts you can find, removing the skin on poultry and the excess fat on red meat before cooking, and removing and draining excess fat after cooking are great strategies for making conventional meats as healthy as possible.

The difference between grass-fed and pasture-raised really has to do with the animal. *Grass-fed* meat comes from animals that have lived on carefully managed pastures all their lives. When they are indoors during the winter, they are fed hay, but no grain whatsoever. *Pasture-raised* or *pastured* animals are omnivorous animals such as pigs and chickens that cannot exist exclusively on a diet of grass. They are kept on a fresh, clean pasture, and their diet is supplemented with some kind of grain. Bottom line: Beef and lamb are grass-fed; pigs and chickens are pastured.

Follow this advice for purchasing the best Paleo proteins your food budget allows:

- ✔ **Beef:** Grass-fed, organic, antibiotic- and hormone-free beef provides you with the best balance of omega-6 fatty acid to omega-3 fatty acid ratios. In fact, when you buy grass-fed, you can eat all the fat — no need to cut or drain. Just be sure the beef you buy says both "grass-fed" and "grass-finished;" either one without the other means the cow likely wasn't exclusively fed grass.
- ✔ **Lamb:** All cuts are good; grass-fed is best.
- ✔ **Poultry:** All cuts of poultry are good. Organic, free-range, antibiotic- and hormone-free or pasture-raised are best.

✔ **Pork:** If you can't purchase pasture-raised pork or wild boar to avoid the toxins and omega-6 fatty acids of conventionally raised pork, choose another, cleaner protein source. If you buy organic bacon, make sure it's free of sugar, and eat it in moderation.

✔ **Game meats:** Game meats, such as elk, bison, duck, pheasant, and quail, are naturally low in fat and high in protein. When you can find them, they're great choices.

✔ **Organ meats:** Organic, antibiotic- and hormone-free organ meats, such as liver, kidney, and heart, are rich in nutrition. Just keep in mind that organic and pasture-raised is your best bet. Conventionally raised organ meats can be toxic, so pass on those options if you can't find a pasture-raised source.

✔ **Eggs:** Organic and pastured eggs provide the healthiest omega-6 to omega-3 ratios. You can tell the difference in the color of the yolk. A dark yellow yolk is the sign of a good egg.

Your healthiest choice for eggs is organic and pastured. You know the chickens were humanely and healthfully raised if the carton says "Certified Humane" or "Food Alliance Certified." Avoid "United Egg Producers Certified"; this certifier permits factory farm practices. When buying eggs, labels or cartons that read "vegetarian-fed" and "natural" have no impact on the quality of the eggs. Their titles sound like a breezy day at the farm but have no value.

✔ **Fish and seafood:** Wild-caught fish, seafood, and shellfish are healthier than farm-raised. Visit the Monterey Bay Aquarium Seafood Watch site (www.montereybayaquarium.org/cr/seafoodwatch.aspx) for recommendations from a trusted source.

✔ **Nitrite- and gluten-free deli meats and sausages:** Look on the label for added sugar, gluten, or other additives that can sabotage your healthy efforts. If you can't purchase quality deli meats and sausages, choose another protein; conventional choices can cause inflammation.

Grabbing Paleo-smart produce

Veggies provide you with tons of nutrients, reduce toxicity, increase fiber, and make you look better. They naturally reduce your chances of getting just about every disease — not to mention that they keep you healthy, young, and vibrant. Always try new and exciting vegetables in varying colors and fill your plate. The brighter and richer the color, the more good stuff you're giving your body. (*Tip:* Farmers' markets are great places to find veggies for experimenting.)

Fruits in moderation are an excellent antioxidant source. The healthier your body becomes, the more fruit you can tolerate without blood sugar swings.

One of the best qualities of fruit is its ability to naturally satisfy your taste for sweet while adding nutrition. However, just remember that eating some fruit is a good idea; eating gobs of it isn't. Fruit can satisfy sugar cravings, but it can also keep the sugar fits going. The fructose in fruit elevates blood sugar, so don't let the fruit displace vegetables. Vegetables first, fruit second.

Of course grabbing a piece of fruit is easier than steaming some vegetables, but you'll soon find ways to grab veggies just as quickly the more you get into your new habits and into the flow of things. Purchase a container of washed greens (like the prepared greens from Earthbound Farm), pop open the lid, drizzle on some olive oil, and add some Celtic sea salt and a squeeze of lemon if you like. Boom: instant salad. For a more elaborate touch, add few sliced strawberries. It takes less than two minutes, and it's really good. If you want to go a step further and add protein into your veggies, you have a full-fledged balanced meal.

Local, organic, and seasonal produce is best. Frozen organic is a good choice as well because the produce is flash frozen, locking in all the freshness and goodness.

The Environmental Working Group (EWG; www.ewg.org/foodnews/) tested various produce items and found which have high pesticide contamination and are therefore most beneficial to buy organic:

- ✔ **Buy organic:** Apples, cherries, grapes, nectarines, peaches, pears, lettuce, raspberries, strawberries, blueberries, bell peppers, celery, carrots, kale, mushrooms, spinach
- ✔ **Organic optional:** Bananas, mangos, papaya, kiwi, pineapples, asparagus, avocado, broccoli, cauliflower, onions

Check out Book I, Chapter 2, for lists of Paleo-approved veggies and fruits that you can stock in your kitchen.

Spicing things up

You can turn a mediocre dish into a hit with a splash of spice or a spice blend. You can purchase spices dried or fresh; just get your hands on spices that warm and ground you or make you come alive with energy, such as cayenne, cinnamon, curry, ginger, and peppermint.

Cayenne, chili powder, chipotle, red pepper flakes, and paprika are considered nightshades and may cause discomfort if you have joint pain, autoimmune conditions, multiple sclerosis, fibromyalgia, or chronic fatigue syndrome.

Allowing Paleo-smart fats

Putting healthy fats on your plate makes just about everything you do better! Fats nourish every structure and function of the body — including your very important brain. Fats also help you absorb nutrients more efficiently and keep you feeling full.

The key to choosing fats is to get the healthiest fats you possibly can. Fats are the second place on your shopping list (behind protein) where it's worth spending extra money. Here are some good options:

- **Avocadoes:** These fruits provide *monounsaturated fats,* which are incredibly healthy. Add some in a salad, mash and use as a dip for veggies, or just eat with a spoon.

- **Olives:** Olives also offer monounsaturated fats and are a great snack or salad addition.

- **Butter and ghee:** Butter from grass-fed, pasture-raised cows and organic, grass-fed ghee (also called *clarified butter*) are fantastic cooking oils because they're stable at a very high heat.

  Any butter, even grass-fed, contains milk proteins. If you're super-sensitive to milk proteins or have a condition you're trying to heal, you may want to stick to ghee, in which the milk proteins are boiled off.

- **Coconut fats:** Incorporate coconut through coconut butter, flakes, and milk and fresh coconut.

- **Nuts and nut butters:** Try those with almonds, Brazil nuts, cashews, chestnuts, hazelnuts, macadamia nuts, pecans, pistachios, and walnuts. ***Note:*** Due to their toxin level, peanuts and peanut butter are off the menu.

- **Oils:** Try macadamia oil, avocado oil, coconut oil, olive oil, and walnut oil.

- **Seeds:** Pumpkin, sesame, and sunflower seeds and pine nuts are great Paleo choices.

- **Animal fats:** Eating animal fats can be healthy when they come from pastured-raised, grass-fed sources, such as *tallow* (beef fat), lamb fat, duck fat, and *schmaltz* (chicken fat).

Packing a Paleo-smart pantry

Time to replenish your pantry with foods that are going to get you results. See, Paleo isn't so boring! With these pantry foods in your arsenal, you can get really creative:

- Shredded coconut (great as a snack or to add sweetness to dishes).
- Unsweetened coconut milk (full-fat canned), unsweetened almond milk, and flax milk (instead of dairy).
- Canned chilies.
- Salsa.
- Fish sauce. (Red Boat brand is good.)
- Gluten-free hot sauce.
- Gluten-free mustard.
- Vinegar: Red wine and apple cider.
- Unsweetened, sulfite-free pickles.
- Unsweetened applesauce.
- Canned fish: tuna, salmon sardines, crab, or mackerel. (Vital Choice [www.vitalchoice.com/shop/pc/home.asp] is a great brand for very clean, fresh fish.)
- Gluten- and soy-free beef jerky.
- Nuts and seeds.
- Unsweetened nut butters.
- Artichoke hearts.
- Olives (read the label for additives; should have olives, water, and salt as the only ingredients).
- Unsweetened, sulfite-free dried fruits.
- Arrowroot powder (used as a thickener; substitute for conventional flour and cornstarch).
- Coconut flour (instead of conventional flour).
- Almond flour (instead of conventional flour).
- Coconut aminos (instead of soy sauce).
- Broth: Chicken, beef, and vegetable.
- Raw honey.

✔ Pure maple syrup.

✔ Dark chocolate with at least 85 percent cacao.

✔ Unsweetened cocoa powder.

✔ Sun-dried tomatoes.

✔ Tomato sauce. (Rao's is a good brand: `www.raos.com/premium-sauces.aspx`.)

✔ Tomatoes in a jar or a carton.

Tomatoes are acidic and react with the metal in the cans. The interior coating of the cans contains Bisphenol A (BPA), a nasty, estrogen-mimicking chemical that can make you sick and fat and cause infertility problems. All the companies in the industry have BPA issues in their cans, so buying jarred tomatoes is best. BPA-free tetra paks like Pomi or Trader Joe's brand are safe. Look for jarred organic strained tomatoes and tomato paste from Bionaturæ (`www.bionaturae.com/tomatoes.html`) and conventional tomatoes in tetra pak cartons by Pomi (`http://pomi.us.com/home.php`) or Trader Joe's brand Italian Tomato Starter Sauce.

Any and all sweeteners, artificial sweeteners, and no-calorie sweeteners (including Paleo-approved ones) can open the floodgate for more carb and sugar cravings. You find some natural sweeteners on the pantry list, but don't let that mislead you into thinking that they're acceptable everyday indulgences. They're simply the best options for that once-in-a-while treat.

Sipping Paleo-smart drinks

The worst thing you can do is drink liquid (specifically sugary) carbohydrates. Even if the drink is made from fruit, it lacks the fiber and the other parts from fruit that help to buffer the glycemic response of sugary juice. Paleo-approved drinks don't contain any added or artificial sugars, toxic dyes, preservatives, or fake anything — including vitamins. You can enjoy the following options while enjoying your health:

✔ Tea (green, herbal, white).

✔ Water with fruit slices (lemon, lime, orange, berries, and so on). Add mint or spearmint leaves for extra flavor.

✔ Mineral water (Mountain Valley Spring Water is best: `www.mountainvalleyspring.com`).

✔ Coffee (organic is best).

Cooking Smart to Retain Flavor and Nutrition

Cooking can help move you either toward or away from health, depending on how you do it. Little cooking tweaks or pointers can make all the difference in the health of your meal. This section offers some valuable pointers to get you cooking in the know.

You certainly don't have to be a gourmet chef to use healthy cooking techniques. Anyone can use these simple methods to prepare foods; they lock in high-octane flavor and provide deep nutrition.

Paleo-smart cooking methods

Even the best intentions and the healthiest ingredients can be ruined by unhealthy cooking methods. For example, breading and deep-frying those grass-fed meats doesn't exactly support your health and weight goals. To get the most out of your Paleo kitchen, you need to prepare foods in a way that doesn't demean their nutritional value. The Paleo-approved cooking methods in this section help you do just that.

No matter what method you use to cook your food, using spices and herbs is one of the best ways to add color, flavor, and aroma to your meals. Try to choose fresh herbs that are bright, have a pungent color, and aren't wilted. Always add them toward the end of cooking. If you're using dried herbs, you can add them at the earlier stages of cooking. Go ahead and experiment!

Baking

You don't have to add anything extra to food when you bake. You can just place vegetables in a covered or uncovered pan or dish. The hot, dry air of your oven turns these foods into something special — without the extra calories or fat. Try baking some of the denser carbohydrates such as squash or sweet potatoes. The heat caramelizes the natural sugars, making for a delicious side dish.

Braising

When you *braise* meats, you first brown them on high heat to caramelize the outside and then slowly cook them at low heat in flavored liquid, such as water or broth, to make the meat tender and lock in all its flavors. Braise in the oven in a covered pan or on the stovetop in a heavy pot with a tight-fitting lid. Consider adding herbs, spices, and vegetables to the braising liquid and, when the meat is done, using the braising liquid to create a flavorful, nutrient-rich sauce.

Braising is a fantastic method to use for inexpensive, tougher cuts of meat because it tenderizes them the way other cooking methods can't. Cook times vary, but it's usually about 40 minutes per pound of meat.

Sautéing and stir-frying

Sautéing and stir-frying both involve quickly cooking foods in small amounts of fat over high, direct heat. *Sautéing* uses less fat than stir-frying does; you typically allow the food to brown before moving it around in the pan. *Stir-frying* uses more fat, and you move the food around in the pan more. They're both great methods for adding flavor to thinly, uniformly sliced meat and vegetables.

Roasting

Three words describe roasting: simple, healthy, and delicious. Just place a chicken or a beef roast in a pan, surround it with hearty vegetables, and put it in the oven for a few hours. The meat cooks in its natural juices, and you can simmer and strain the drippings in the bottom of the pan and turn them into a sauce.

Roasting and baking are similar methods of dry cooking, but you apply them to two different kinds of foods. You generally roast foods that have structure already, such as meat and vegetables. You typically bake foods that don't have much structure before going into the oven, such as casseroles or pies.

Slow cooking

Slow cooking just may be the most perfect way of cooking on the planet. Meats and vegetables cook on low temperatures over longer periods of time than with other cooking methods, so the meat gets tender and the flavors blend together. If you're busy and like warm, hearty meals, you'll love how the slow cooker can make just about anything while you're running around with kids, toiling at work, or just relaxing.

Steaming

Steaming is as basic at it gets: You bring a small amount of liquid to a simmer on the stove, place the food in a basket suspended above the liquid, and cover the pot. The hot steam circulates through the pot and cooks the food. This method is a great way to really lock the nutrition into your vegetables, brightening their colors and making them inviting to eat. You can even flavor the liquid by adding seasonings to the water, which brings out even more flavor as the food cooks.

Poaching

To *poach* foods, slowly simmer the ingredients in a liquid (such as water, stock, or broth) until they're tender and thoroughly cooked. The food retains its shape and texture without drying out, leaving it tender and delicious. Poaching is a great way to cook fish so it's tender and full of flavor.

Grilling

Grilling is a way to cook food over direct heat by placing the foods on a rack above a bed of charcoal or gas-heated rocks.

Although grilling is certainly a warm-weather favorite and the center of many fun gatherings of family and friends, don't make it your everyday cooking method. Grilling food damages its proteins, producing carcinogens. Good evidence indicates that *heterocyclic amines* (HCAs) produced in meat cooked at high temperatures are carcinogenic. This risk increases when the meat is cooked well-done.

You can minimize your carcinogen exposure by using the following grilling tips:

- ✔ **Don't use grilling as your go-to cooking method.** Incorporate some of the other cooking methods to your cooking repertoire.

- ✔ **Ditch the processed vegetable oils.** When using oils in marinades or directly on the grill, opt for saturated fats, which can withstand high heat without becoming rancid. Coconut oil and grass-fed butter are great options.

- ✔ **Incorporate lots of veggies.** When you eat grilled foods, pile on the vegetables. The antioxidants and phenols in them soften the impact of the mutations in the grilled meats.

- ✔ **Don't overheat.** Make sure you don't overcook or char the food, which greatly increases the carcinogens. Keep meat away from direct heat and don't let juices fall on the heat source. These juices cause flare-ups, which tend to char food.

Keeping healthy fats healthy: Smoke points

A *smoke point* refers to the temperature at which an oil is too hot to remain stable and starts breaking down and creating free radicals. When the oil starts to literally give off smoke, you've reached that point. You need to rinse the pan and add fresh oil. The more saturated the fat, the more stable it is and the higher temperature it can endure before becoming unhealthy.

Oils good for high-heat cooking include

- ✔ Butter and ghee
- ✔ Coconut oil
- ✔ Duck fat
- ✔ Lard (pork fat)
- ✔ Schmaltz (chicken fat)
- ✔ Tallow (beef fat)

Oils best to just drizzle over food or cook at very low temperatures include

- ✔ Avocado oil
- ✔ Flaxseed oil (occasional use only)
- ✔ Macadamia nut oil
- ✔ Olive oil
- ✔ Walnut oil

Chapter 4

Using Paleo Concepts in Your Fitness Routine

In This Chapter

▶ Realizing the importance of strength training

▶ Moving and breathing like you were designed to do

▶ Identifying what compels you to get fit and healthy

▶ Discovering the most effective and efficient exercise practices

▶ Monitoring your progress with health markers

*B*efore you get into the primal exercise routines and get to work in Book IV, we provide a few techniques in this chapter that will guarantee your success and, more important, your safety.

In Book I, Chapter 1, we talk about Paleo principles and values. In brief, we talk about *Paleo strategy* — the things you need to do to achieve vibrant health, a sexier physique, and peak performance. Here, we talk about *Paleo tactics* — the things you should do specifically. These tactics are the finer details. Some may even go so far as to call them minor details. But keep these words in mind: Big doors swing on little hinges. Often, the littlest tweaks produce the largest results.

In this chapter, we present nine simple techniques that everyone should do on a regular basis. For this set of guidelines, we've reverse-engineered the cave-man lifestyle.

All the techniques in this chapter are immediately applicable, and the quicker you put them into practice, the quicker you'll start dropping weight and building muscle, the quicker you'll start feeling vibrant and vivacious, and the quicker you can close this book! We'll even go so far as to say that anyone who practices these simple techniques 90 percent of the time will see 99 percent of his remediable health issues rapidly remedied.

Cultivating Strength

Many valuable physical attributes exist, from agility and balance to anaerobic/aerobic capacity, flexibility, and mobility, but before anything else, you should cultivate strength.

In this section, we explain what it means to cultivate strength by first defining what strength is and then showing you how strength helps you build a strong foundation for the other things you should do.

Knowing what strength really is

You can find many workable but somewhat lacking definitions for strength. For example, a haughty and somewhat respectable lifter once said that true strength is a 500-pound dead lift, a 400-pound squat, and a 300-pound bench press. On the other end of the spectrum, poet Judith Viorst says that strength is the ability to break a chocolate bar into four pieces with your bare hands.

Finally, one definition, both beautiful and correct, is stated simply as this: Strength is the ability to overcome resistance.

Resistance comes in many forms — mental, physical, internal, external; it's any force in opposition of what you're trying to do. The only way to gain strength is to work against resistance. For example, the push-up provides resistance of your own body weight. But by working against this resistance, you develop upper body strength.

Getting stronger to fix just about everything

Getting strong is the one simple, sweeping, and effective antidote to the general ailments of the masses. Here are just a few benefits of primal strength training:

- ✔ Decreased fat mass
- ✔ Improved focus/concentration
- ✔ Improved glucose tolerance (decreased risk of diabetes)
- ✔ Improved heart health

✔ Improved sleep quality

✔ Increased lean body mass

✔ Increased stamina

✔ Reduced risk of injury

✔ Stress relief

✔ Stronger bones (decreased risk of osteoporosis)

General bodily weakness inhibits everything, whereas the stronger you are (the more force you can produce), the easier everything else becomes. In other words, as you increase your strength capacity, you increase all capacities, including but not limited to the following:

✔ **Muscular endurance:** The ability to exert force over a prolonged period of time

✔ **Cardiovascular endurance:** The ability to sustain strenuous cardiovascular efforts for a prolonged period of time

✔ **Power:** How much force you can produce in a given amount of time

✔ **Coordination:** How well everything in your body plays together

So strength is the foundation on which everything else is built, and it's generally useless to train anything without training and building strength first. Consider this: Will the firefighter who trains for strength or the firefighter who trains for endurance be able to perform his tasks with greater efficiency? The answer is the one who trains for strength, because if the one who trains for endurance has no strength base — that is, if he's unable to lift the equipment or unable to drag an unresponsive person — then his general endurance is unusable. His endurance training has been for naught.

Endurance is possible only to the extent that you're stronger than the task at hand, meaning that lifting and carrying a 150-pound body will be an easy act of endurance for the person who can lift 300 pounds but an impossible task for the person who can lift only 75 pounds. To say it another way, the person who can lift 300 pounds even once will have no trouble lifting 100 pounds many times, but the person who can lift 100 pounds many times may not be able to lift 300 pounds even once. To understand this is to know that increasing strength increases endurance but not the other way around.

Endurance is simply a byproduct of strength. If you want to improve your endurance, get stronger!

Developing strength as a skill

The cave man was strong because strength was required for survival. But today, this whole business of strength often presents a dilemma. People think that strength is an attribute of the genetically gifted and that if they picked the wrong parents, they're out of luck.

Strength isn't hereditary; it's a skill, in the same vein that skiing, typing, and learning a new language are all skills. A skill is a habit of operation, something you acquire through observation and experience. You learn the rules, and then you operate according to the rules until you form a habit. In other words, you learn by doing.

So if you lack strength, it's not because you chose the wrong parents but because you chose the wrong habits. Therefore, if you're weak, you either aren't practicing effective habits or you're practicing ineffective habits.

Skills range in complexity. For example, learning a new language or how to play the piano are complex skills that take years to develop (at least to a level of significant proficiency). Strength, however, is a simple skill — one that anyone at any age can acquire rapidly. So just as a pianist acquires the skill of musicianship through diligent practice, you acquire strength in the same way. But instead of running scales, you lift weights.

Furthermore, skills also range in necessity. If you're unable to moonwalk, you need not offer any apologies. That's a hard skill to master and is relatively useless. Strength, however, is essential, and there's no excuse for not cultivating that skill. For strength — true strength — you need to follow only two simple rules:

- ✔ **Practice often.** No one has ever acquired a skill without practice. Strength is no exception. If you want to get strong at pull-ups, practice pull-ups. If you want to get strong at squats, practice squats.

- ✔ **Lift heavy some of the time.** If you want to get strong — really strong, that is — then you have to push your limits every so often. Not every day, but every couple of days you want to lift heavy and push yourself.

Realizing there's more to fitness than strength

Lifting heavy is all very well and primal. And torn sinew, from time to time, just *feels* good. But strength can be a little addicting. And as you probably know, too much of any one good thing can quickly turn it bad.

Although you want to train strength first, you don't want to do so exclusively or excessively. Strength is the capacity that lifts all other capacities, but it doesn't necessarily fill them. As your strength increases, so does the potential for endurance, flexibility, conditioning, and so on.

Prioritize strength, but don't neglect everything else. Many strong athletes stumble because they failed to give heed to their heart, and we've seen many strong lifters get injured because they paid no mind to the quality of their movement. Chasing strength and strength alone is a foolish and downright dangerous crusade.

So after this puzzling realization, you may be wondering, "What else am I to do?" This fundamental question deserves a fundamental answer. And that answer, of course, is everything else, covered conveniently in the rest of this chapter.

Moving Every Day

Life is movement. And the opposite of movement is motionlessness, which you could say is an apt definition of death. The cave man was constantly on the move in one way or another, so he suffered few of the problems that people do today, problems brought about largely from a lack of quality movement.

As people age and take on more responsibilities, they tend to slip into stillness. They sit too much, and they get rigid. They fail to move, so they start to creak like the Tin Man.

This pattern is unfortunate but highly preventable and, if it has already set in, easily remedied. A life rich in movement wards off the deleterious effects of aging. It keeps the cells fresh, the muscles toughened, and the joints well oiled. And if life is movement, then surely movement stimulates life — it rejuvenates muscle tissue, upsurges joint nutrition, and even spurs the growth of new brain cells.

You need to move every day, but that doesn't mean you have to work out with great intensity every day; just move. When you plan how to move every day, keep it easy, but do it often.

There's no such thing as a wrong movement. You can suffer only from a lack of movement.

For now, a few basic human movement patterns every day will suffice. Explore new positions, postures, and patterns, like the following:

✔ Bend	✔ March
✔ Carry	✔ Pull
✔ Crawl	✔ Push
✔ Flex	✔ Roll
✔ Hang	✔ Rotate
✔ Hinge	✔ Squat
✔ Jump	✔ Throw
✔ Lunge	✔ Twist

Don't confuse movement with exercise. Although exercise includes movement, the means and the ends aren't the same. Exercise induces stress and is often intense, such as five sets of five heavy reps on the back squat. Movement promotes rejuvenation and is usually lighthearted and playful, such as crawling around on the ground with a newborn.

Breathing the Way You Were Meant To

Through simple deductive reasoning — that is, you're alive, therefore, you're breathing — it's clear that you've met the simple act of breathing with a considerable amount of success. However, breathing is too complex and influential a task to be graded like finger painting or Lego blocks. And the type of breathing this section discusses isn't the involuntary act of breathing but the conscious type.

Human respiration — the seemingly simple act of breathing — is perhaps the most powerful regulatory agency in the body. The rate and depth of your breath has the power to arouse and depress the senses, and it has long been known that you can affect your mood simply and rapidly by changing your breathing.

Breathing affects everything from your mood to the quality of your sleep. Don't discount the benefits of taking a few minutes every day to practice deep, purposeful breathing.

Overbreathing — often referred to as *hyperventilation* — is where your breath is laborious and excessive. If you've ever had a panic attack, you've experienced hyperventilation and know it's frightening. Hyperventilating is paralyzing and sorely limits your ability to perform under stress.

Mostly, people just breathe too often. If you're taking more than 12 breaths a minute, you're overbreathing. Overbreathing, or hyperventilation, arouses anxiety (sometimes to the point of inducing panic), impairs cognition (sometimes to the point of memory loss), and promotes restlessness (sometimes to the point of insomnia).

Here are a few consequences of overbreathing:

✔ Anxiety

✔ Chronic fatigue

✔ Headaches

✔ Restlessness

✔ Stress

Abnormal breathing patterns, such as overbreathing, have been linked to a plethora of illnesses, from the annoying (gastritis) to the deadly (heart disease).

For best health and wellness, you need to *breathe consciously* every day — that is, you should practice slow, rhythmic, diaphragmatic breathing. Babies breathe this way, long and deep into the belly.

Conscious breathing is more about the exhalation than it is the inhalation. To practice conscious breathing, you breathe in for a count of four and breathe out for a count of eight. If you take the time to do this slow breathing every day, as often as possible, your efforts will be well rewarded. When you control your breath, you control your composure, your deliberation, and, to a certain degree, your aging.

Take five minutes now to try the following breathing exercise, known as *crocodile breathing:*

1. **Lie flat on your belly and rest your forehead on your hands.**

2. **Slowly draw in a breath as deep into your belly as possible for four counts.**

   Your belly should push out into the ground, and your sides should also have some outward visible movement. Your shoulders and chest, however, shouldn't rise.

3. **Hold the breath for a count of one, and then slowly exhale for a count of eight.**

Knowing What Compels You

People work out for two reasons: to move toward something, such as a heavier dead lift or a more chiseled midsection, and/or to move away from something, such as stiffness or poor self-esteem.

The following sections show you how to identify what compels you to work out and how to set goals for fitness that you can stick to.

Identifying your primal motivators

Some people choose to work out because they want to be something they're not, and some people choose to work out because they want to stop being something they are. Some people work out for vanity — they want to whittle their waistlines, tighten their butts, or carve out their abs to look like the sinewy superstar cover model — and there's nothing wrong with that. And then some people work out for glory — they want to be elite athletes, they want to crush the competition, and they want to do so mercilessly in front of thousands of raving fans — and there's nothing wrong with that, either.

These are just common examples of working out to move toward something. People want to get to somewhere new, and they want to be someone new. The promise of pleasure compels them.

The other reason is slightly less sexy but slightly more common. It's when people work out because they know they need to in order to be healthy or because the doctor said if they don't, they'll have a heart attack and die. They look into the mirror and see that their arms are soft and doughy, like a pair of breadsticks, and that their stomach has grown outward like The Blob. It's typically a revolting reality, and people will suddenly do anything to move away from such a poor self-image and poor health.

People reach a point, often a very painful point, where they're so disgusted and fed up with themselves and how they feel that they just can't take it any longer. Something needs to be done. They don't necessarily care where they go, as long as they get away from where they are right now. Most people have been there at one time or another.

Whatever the reason may be, you need to know why you're working out, and you need to remind yourself of that reason daily — because that's what compels you.

Everyone seeks fitness either to avoid pain or to gain pleasure (sometimes both). Identifying and understanding what compels you and reminding yourself daily of these reasons will help you stick to the program.

Setting goals that stick

When it comes to setting goals, it's best to aim high — higher even than you suspect you may be able to reach — and in many circumstances, it's best to forgo what's easily obtainable for something that's really going to challenge you. Even if you fail, chances are that you'll still land a lot higher than you would otherwise. Additionally, setting goals that are a bit lofty is enthralling. And goals that are enthralling tend to have a higher stick rate.

Set yourself a goal that excites you, regardless of how crazy it sounds. Boring goals rarely stick, because they're, well, boring! Get creative. Get a little rambunctious, even. Go for what you truly want.

Although losing two pounds may be a goal of yours, it's hard to get very excited about meeting that goal. So set a goal that's a bit more imaginative and loftier. For example, imagine that the editors of some glamorous publication want to feature you on the cover as the "best body of the year." All you have to do is get ready for the shoot. Now doesn't that sound like something worth working toward?

On the other hand, you want to be sure to set goals that are humanly possible and that you're actually able to achieve them in the amount of time you've given yourself. There's a difference between aiming high and being completely unrealistic.

To this end, you should set *S.M.A.R.T.* goals that meet the following criteria:

- ✔ **Specific:** "I want to lose weight" isn't a specific goal, but "I want to lose five pounds" is. Do your best to make your goals as specific as possible.

- ✔ **Measurable:** You should be able to measure your progress along the way. If you can't, then how will you ever know whether you're making any progress? Luckily, most fitness-related goals are measurable. Losing body fat is measurable (via body fat analysis) and so is gaining strength (via strength testing).

- ✔ **Attainable:** Although you want to set lofty goals, you don't want to set unrealistic goals. If you set goals that are entirely out of your current reach, you're only setting yourself up for failure and disappointment. You need to set goals that challenge you but that you can achieve so you get a feeling of accomplishment, which will motivate you to reach other goals.

- ✔ **Relevant:** For our purposes here, all your goals should be fitness related. Although being more fit and healthy may very well make you more productive at work, setting the goal of getting that promotion you've really wanted in three months is hardly relevant here.

- ✔ **Time-bound:** There's a saying that "a goal without a deadline is simply a dream." Without a clear-cut deadline, you have no reason not to procrastinate. So give yourself a deadline, one that's realistic but also pressing enough to give yourself the impetus you need to get to work!

Training the Primal Patterns Primarily

Conventional wisdom maintains that you can get most of the strength and fitness you'll ever need from a small fraction of all the exercises you've ever heard of and subtle variations therein. In other words, a handful of battlefield-tested exercises offers tremendous utility — far above and beyond that of most other exercises.

This proposition is a spin on the *Pareto principal,* or what's more commonly referred to as the *80/20 rule.* Simply put, the 80/20 rule states that 80 percent of all effects come from 20 percent of the causes. Commonly, a pea garden illustrates this phenomenon, demonstrating that 80 percent of the peas grown in any one garden are often the result of only 20 percent of the pea pods.

The 80/20 rule can be and has been applied to increase the efficiency of tasks in multiple domains. In business, the rule commonly reveals that 20 percent of customers contribute 80 percent of the income.

As you may suspect, the 80/20 rule can even be applied to fitness, although the ratio is probably a bit more skewed — more like 95 percent of all the results you could ever want come from 5 percent of all the possible things that you could ever do. And this 5 percent consists of the fundamental primal human movements, of which there are roughly six:

- ✔ Pushing
- ✔ Pulling
- ✔ Hinging
- ✔ Squatting
- ✔ Carrying
- ✔ Walking and sprinting (gait)

You get the details on these movements in the following sections.

Pushing

A *push* isn't an exercise per se but rather a category of movement. It includes the push-up (see Figure 4-1), the military press, and the bench press, all of which are big pushes.

Within each category of human movement, you want to do the movements that offer the highest return on investment. The push does that. And the

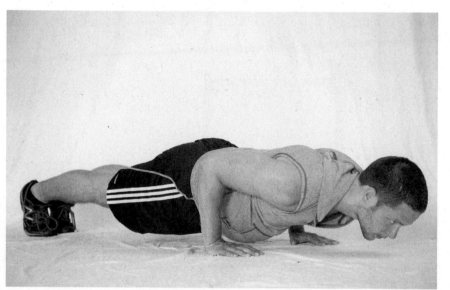

Figure 4-1:
The push-up
is the king of
pushes.

Photo courtesy of Rebekah Ulmer

push-up in particular is perhaps the perfect primal exercise, working trunk stability and upper-body pushing strength. This classic gym class exercise strengthens the chest, shoulders, triceps, and abs.

Pulling

There's nothing finer for a strong and muscular back than the pull-up (see Figure 4-2).

Don't fret if you're unable to perform even one rep of the pull-up, and certainly don't listen to the bunkum claiming that "females can't do pull-ups." Females most certainly *can* and most certainly *should* do pull-ups. Anyone who says otherwise has never had enough strength — or brains — to know better. Many women have progressed from zero to five pull-ups within two months' time. That's more than most males can do, and you can get there, too.

Hinging

Hinging — a movement horribly underpracticed — is a tremendously useful pattern, and throughout Book IV, you see it in what is perhaps the most marvelous fat-chopping device ever seen: the kettlebell swing. Hinging forges an

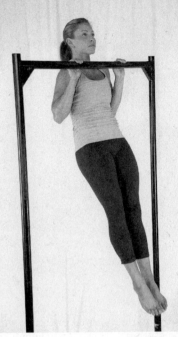

Figure 4-2:
The pull-up
is the
perfect
primal
complement
to the
push-up.

Photo courtesy of Rebekah Ulmer

iron posterior and is, or at least should be, the default movement pattern for picking stuff up off the ground.

As an athlete, you can produce a tremendous amount of force from a hinge — think of a lineman before the snap, a sprinter before the gun, or a broad jumper before the leap; these actions are all strong and all come out of a hinged position. Figure 4-3 shows the dead lift, which is perhaps the most common hinging pattern of all. The dead lift strengthens the hips and the back. When performing the dead lift, be sure to keep the back flat and the hips below the shoulders but above the knees. (See Book IV, Chapter 1, for full instructions on this movement.)

Squatting

In the category of the squat, you find a variety of options including the goblet squat, the pistol squat, and the front squat — all of which you find out about in great depth in Book IV, Chapter 1. The squat is an essential human movement

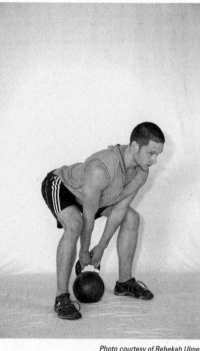

Figure 4-3:
The dead lift
is the best
movement
for picking
stuff up off
the ground.

Photo courtesy of Rebekah Ulmer

pattern. It keeps the hips supple and the knees strong. It's also a natural rest
position, meaning that you should be able to get down into a squat and sit there
comfortably for extended periods of time.

Figure 4-4 shows the primal or bodyweight squat. If you have the mobility,
it should feel almost effortless to sit in the bottom position of this squat.
You want to try to accumulate as much time as you can in the bottom of a
squat position throughout the day. Doing so will work wonders for your hips,
knees, and back.

Carrying

No single movement pattern is more primal — or more useful — than the
basic carrying of heavy objects. You do it every day, so it's quite important.

Carrying, as strength coach Dan John would say, "fills in the gaps." It's
something that everyone should do, but most people don't. Carrying helps

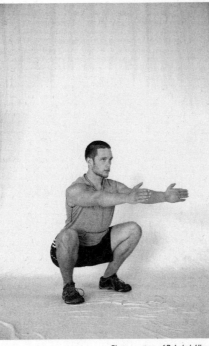

Figure 4-4:
The primal
squat, or
bodyweight
squat,
should
serve as a
natural rest
position.

Photo courtesy of Rebekah Ulmer

reinforce proper posture (which is often neglected) and strengthens the grip (finger and forearm strength is also paid very little attention). In Book IV, Chapter 3, you find out how to use the waiter's carry, the farmer's carry (see Figure 4-5), and the Turkish get-up to "fill in the gaps."

Walking and sprinting

Gait, or the manner of moving on foot, includes walking and sprinting. Jogging, especially for long distances, is not optimally effective for increasing your fitness. Instead, you should steep yourself primarily in the two ends of the force-velocity spectrum. You should move slowly very often and move very fast occasionally. There's little benefit to playing around in the middle (jogging).

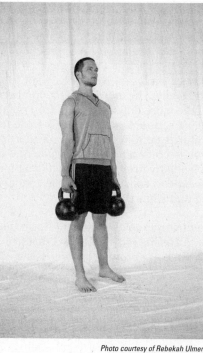

Figure 4-5:
Carries
truly earn
the title of
"functional"
exercise.

Photo courtesy of Rebekah Ulmer

Keeping Your Conditioning Inefficient

As with anything else, a heap of semantics surrounds the word *conditioning*. People argue that conditioning means a great many things, and they're right. Conditioning is a word with many definitions.

But for the purposes of this book, conditioning links to anything related to the strengthening of the heart muscle and, more thrillingly, fat loss. The sections to come explain in detail what conditioning is and how you should approach it.

Conditioning for strength or fat loss

Strength is efficiency. It's a finely tuned nervous system, if you will. For example, a more efficient person can produce more force with the same amount of muscle than a less efficient person; in other words, he uses his brawny resources more resourcefully.

The fewer moving parts, the more efficient a machine becomes. Although you're not a machine, this analogy still serves a useful purpose. Your movement, from the standpoint of strength, shouldn't consume any more than the bare minimum effort required. This, of course, takes practice.

But for conditioning — moreover, fat loss — you don't want to strive for efficiency. Quite the opposite, really. The more efficient you become, the less energy you expend, and the more difficult it is to drop pounds, which is another reason long, trudging runs are comparatively futile for fat loss. They may produce measly returns upfront, but those returns are quickly and severely diminished when you become an efficient jogger. And even if you're not an efficient jogger yet, jogging by itself is a more efficient means of travel than, say, sprinting is — you expend considerably more energy sprinting 50 yards than you do jogging that same distance.

So if you want to fight fat effectively, you need to fight it with inefficiency. You need to select movements and exercise protocols that are wasteful in terms of energy expenditure, such as sprinting and various metabolic conditioning routines.

Comparing efficiency and effectiveness

Naturally, to do something efficiently is to do something economically. Efficiency is easily measured by the ratio of input to output (how much you get for what you give). In the example of jogging versus sprinting, jogging is more efficient because you give less (energy) to get the same result (distance traveled).

Efficiency is also easily measured qualitatively by your perceived level of exertion. To wit: The more challenging or difficult an exercise or exercise regimen feels, the less efficient it probably is.

Effectiveness, on the other hand, has little to do with economy but more to do with ability — that is, the ability to produce a desired result. Effectiveness, unlike efficiency, isn't so easily quantified. In other words, effectiveness is *doing the right things,* whereas efficiency is *doing things right.* A chief distinction between the two is that just because something is efficient doesn't mean it's effective (and vice versa).

One example is step aerobics; another is Zumba. These exercises are efficient — as made clear by the relatively low level of exertion — but relatively useless weaponry for the battle against body fat.

Low-intensity aerobics, such as walking or hiking, are tremendously beneficial for overall health, and you should do them often. By themselves, however, they are ineffective for rapid changes in body composition.

So if your aim is to combat fat, effectively and unapologetically, then you need to downgrade to a more primitive arsenal. Do it in the way of the cave man, and really exert yourself. Sprint hard, lift heavy, and play often.

Doing the Least You Have to Do

The idea that a perpetually enlarging dose of exercise — that is, spending a lot of time in the gym — will continue to improve the body's function and appearance indefinitely is as unsound and nearly as dangerous as the notion that the complexion and health of the skin will improve in direct ratio to the number of hours spent basking in the sun. Exercise is to be practiced judiciously. You want to do just enough to get the job done and not a smidgeon more.

Too much exercise can lead to a chronic state of stress known as overtraining. Here are some of the symptoms to look out for:

- Amenorrhea (females)
- Anxiety
- Depression
- Constant pain or soreness
- Increased/abnormal heart rate
- Injury
- Insomnia
- Lack of enthusiasm for exercise
- Low energy/chronic fatigue
- Low libido
- Memory problems
- Poor concentration
- Weight gain

The chief aim of exercise is to impose a demand on the bodily systems — to inject stress and subsequently force an adaptation. The body requires time to recover from the stress, and to adapt, you must rest.

When you inject more stress than you can accommodate, recovery is inhibited, and you, at best, decelerate your progress and, at worst, die. Indeed, the latter is quite rare, but still, it can happen.

Intense exercise is a potent drug; a little does a lot of good, but a lot does very little good. In other words, if what you're doing is effective, the marginal returns are severely diminished after you've run the minimum dose. The minimum dose, or the *minimum effective dose* (MED) as Tim Ferriss refers to in his book *The 4-Hour Body* (Ebury), is "the smallest dose that will produce a desired outcome." Anything beyond the MED is simply wasteful. For example, if it takes only x number of reps to elicit the response you want, then don't do $x + 1$.

So how much is enough? The answer depends on what you want. But in any circumstance, it's probably less than you think.

The Big Seven: Tracking Your Progress with Health Markers

Professor Peter Drucker, a well-known management consultant, said, "What gets measured, gets managed." That's the philosophy behind the big seven health markers. Tracking your progress with these health markers gives you the actual data behind your success or shortcoming as you follow a Paleo lifestyle. It takes the guesswork out of the picture. The best part: If you're not on the right path, tracking data allows you to make a midcourse correction and correct a variable early on.

Body composition

If you took two people of the same height and weight and compared them, their bodies may look completely different due to their differing body composition. *Body composition* is the ratio between how much lean body mass you have and how much fat mass you have. It's your ratio of fat to muscle.

Body composition is the reason your clothes often fit differently after you start following a Paleo diet and fitness plan. Your ratio of lean body mass is going up, while your fat mass is going down. For many people, decreasing body fat is an important outcome of living Paleo, so knowing how to measure your body composition is essential.

You can measure body composition in several ways. The two most practical and assessable are *body fat calipers* and *bioelectrical impedance (BIA):*

✔ **Body fat calipers:** Calipers are used to measure skin folds. The calipers pinch several areas of the skin to measure the thickness of the fat layer under the skin. Measurements are then plugged into an equation to compute body fat. You see this method done at a lot of fitness centers. If you measure your body fat this way, make sure you get your before and after measurements done by the same person, using the same points and the same algorithm (formula to figure out body fat percentage).

A waistline of more than 40 inches in men and more than 35 inches in women can be an indication of heart disease.

✔ **BIA scale:** This scale is a useful way to check body composition from home. BIA works by sending an undetectable current through your body. Fluids within your body carry an electrical current; however, fat can't. The current measures the resistance to the electrical signal as it passes through water found in muscle and fat. The more fat in your body, the more resistant the current. It's safe and is accurate enough to get a good benchmark number. All you do is step on the scale, so it's very easy.

For the most accuracy with a BIA scale, wake up in the morning, drink a glass of water (the exact same amount and temperature each time you take the measurement), wait 30 minutes, go to the bathroom, and then measure. However, because the current is going through only your upper or lower body (depending on the scale), it's not 100 percent accurate, but it's the easiest way to get a number that's close enough. You're mainly going to use that number as a benchmark to see whether you're progressing. BIA scales with higher accuracy are the Tanita scales (www.tanita.com/en).

Strength

Strength comes from putting on more muscle. Having lean muscle mass makes your body run much more efficiently. In fact, the stronger you are, the longer you're likely to live because you decrease your chance of many diseases. Putting on muscle is like taking a pill against metabolic diseases. It's great for your bone density, and you'll stay healthier and look younger. What more incentive could there possibly be?

To see whether you're getting stronger, you need to see how much you can push or lift. A great strength test is the leg press machine. We love this exercise because you use many major muscle groups. Test your *three-rep max:* After warming up, lift as hard and as heavy as you can for three repetitions and rest, and then repeat this cycle for a total of three times. Jot down the absolute heaviest you can push. Repeat monthly to see your progression.

You can do this test with any strength exercise if you don't have access to a leg press. Just make sure you're lifting as much as you possibly can and you can't lift another pound by the end of the three reps.

If you don't want to test by lifting or pushing heavy weights, you can do a grip strength test, which requires a small hand-held device called a *dynamometer*. You grip the meter as hard as you can, and it records your strength.

Whichever strength test you choose, make sure you're seeing progress. When you begin a strength program, you'll be surprised how much you see your body start to sculpt. Adding muscle makes your body healthier, and you look better. Win-win!

Blood pressure

Your blood pressure is measured by the amount of blood your heart pumps and the amount of resistance to blood flow in your arteries. Your blood pressure will be high when your body is pumping blood through narrower arteries. You can think of it like this: It's easy for blood to go through a wide-open space, but it's harder to go through a narrow space, so your body has to work harder. That's when your blood pressure goes up.

You should check your blood pressure regularly for one clear-cut reason: Heart disease is a silent killer. You may have no indication whatsoever that you're facing a problem. The good news is many of the reasons we get high blood pressure are totally within our control to change. If you've been diagnosed with high blood pressure, you should invest in a home model meter. You can buy a good quality meter for about $50 to $100 in any drug store or major shopping outlet.

Here are blood pressure guidelines:

- **Normal blood pressure:** Less than 120/less than 80
- **Prehypertension:** 120–139/80–89
- **Hypertension stage 1:** 140–159/90–99
- **Hypertension stage 2:** 160 or more/100 or more

Blood sugar markers

Two simple blood tests tell you how your body handles sugar. They're called *fasting insulin* and *hemoglobin A1C*. These two tests together tell you how your body is processing sugar both long term and short term.

✔ **Fasting insulin:** If you've been eating processed foods over the years, your body may have developed resistance to insulin. Insulin resistance can also happen naturally as you age. The fasting insulin test is a predictor of insulin resistance and other metabolic diseases that have become such a problem with so many people. It's a quick blood draw, but as the name indicates, you must fast the night before the test.

When you eat the wrong kind of carbohydrates, blood sugar increases dramatically. Insulin gets pumped out constantly until, finally, your body stops listening to the messages. This excess insulin can cause your body's signals to get confused, causing a resistance to insulin, which can lead to all kinds of problems, like diabetes and obesity. So you can see the value in the fasting insulin test!

✔ **Hemoglobin A1C:** This test is more of a trend analysis of what's happening to blood glucose over a period of four to six weeks' time. This test has great stability because the variability of test levels isn't affected by stress or illness because it's not just a snapshot in time.

Another reliable and inexpensive way to test for blood sugar if you want to test in your own home is to use a glucometer, which you can purchase from your local pharmacy. This test is called a *postprandial* (post-meal) *blood sugar test,* meaning you test your blood after eating. The American Association of Clinical Endocrinologists recommends that your post-meal blood sugar goes no higher than 140mg/dl.

The consequences of high blood sugar are pretty severe; you can experience diabetic complications, such as nerve damage, visual problems, or stroke. These tests are easy, so take the time to check your numbers as a base line. If you're concerned about the results you get, see your doctor.

When you start eating the foods you were designed to have, you're going to love seeing how your numbers improve a great deal. It really does give you the certainty to know that you're on the right track.

C-reactive protein

C-reactive protein is protein found in the blood that, when elevated, is an indicator of inflammation in the body. This inflammation may be a predictor of heart disease. Inflammation can damage the inner lining of the arteries and make a heart attack more likely.

When your body continues to stimulate proinflammatory immune cells that may not be needed, you can get chronic inflammation. The following are some of the signs and symptoms:

- Allergies and sensitivities
- Body aches and pain
- Skin problems
- Stiffness
- Swelling
- Weight gain

Checking for C-reactive protein is a great idea when you consider some of the problems that chronic inflammation can cause:

- Alzheimer's disease
- Arteriosclerosis
- Cancer
- Diabetes
- Heart disease
- High blood pressure
- Osteoporosis
- Parkinson's disease

The great news is the Paleo eating plan and recipes are completely non-inflammatory foods. So if you do have chronic inflammation, the Paleo plan is a great place to start! Paleo-approved foods are also natural inflammation busters, so eating Paleo is a great preventive lifestyle as well.

Cholesterol and triglycerides

Fats and their related compounds are called *cholesterol.* Liquid fats are *oils,* and solid fats are simply *fat.* Fats in food are called *dietary fats.* Fats aren't bad for you. In fact, they're an important part of feeling and looking your best. Getting fats in the right balance is the key.

Triglycerides are the most common kind of fat that comes from food. You make this fat to burn for energy. When you eat more calories than you need, extra calories change into triglycerides and are stored in fat cells for when your body needs energy. Lifestyle is one of the most common causes of high triglycerides, and sugary carbohydrates are a major player.

The following sections go into detail about both cholesterol and triglycerides and how to keep the right levels in your system.

Checking out your cholesterol

Despite common belief, cholesterol is actually a good thing! You need this fatty substance for your brain, the production of hormones, and *cellular membranes* (the stuff that lines your cells). Dietary cholesterol doesn't significantly affect cholesterol levels in the blood or risk for heart disease.

Your body needs cholesterol to be healthy. Cholesterol is found in the walls of your cells, in your fatty tissues, in your organs, in your brain, and in your glands. Here's what cholesterol does for you:

- ✔ Protects your cells
- ✔ Helps your nerve cells get information from one place to another
- ✔ Provides the building block for vitamin D
- ✔ Enables your gallbladder to make the digestive juice bile
- ✔ Gives you the raw material on which you build hormones

You make cholesterol in your liver. You also get cholesterol from foods that come from animals: meat, poultry, fish, and eggs.

The fear of cholesterol stems from the potential for fatty deposits to cause a restriction of blood flow. Your heart needs oxygenated blood flow; without it, you're susceptible to a heart attack. And if you don't have enough blood flow to the brain, you can get a stroke. However, you can combat these fears by eating the right foods (such as all the foods on the Paleo-approved list in Book I, Chapter 2) and strengthening your blood vessels.

The best way to prevent fatty deposits from lining your vessels is to eat foods that are nutrient dense so you maintain your immune function and strengthen the integrity of your blood vessels. Eating Paleo-approved foods, which include foods like grass-fed meats with a favorable omega-6 to omega-3 ratio, makes it easy. These foods are non-inflammatory and naturally raise your good cholesterol.

Your good cholesterol is called HDL. Think of it as "happy" and your bad cholesterol, LDL, as "lacking." The goal is to eat foods that increase the good stuff and reduce the bad. Paleo, grass-fed proteins and healthy fats do just that. Paleo fruit and vegetables are great for strengthening your vessels.

Getting the skinny on triglycerides

Triglycerides are the fats that are constantly circulating in your bloodstream. When your triglycerides are elevated, it's an indication that some kind of metabolic problem, such as Type 2 diabetes, coronary heart disease, or obesity, may be occurring.

Here's the kicker: Eating too much of the wrong type of carbohydrates (grains, potatoes, sugary drinks, and so on) causes elevated triglycerides, which happens because the liver converts excess carbohydrates into triglycerides for storage. If you're producing too much triglyceride, your body stores more.

Elevated triglycerides are a lifestyle issue that's well within your reach to remedy. When you start living Paleo, lifestyle health issues usually start to melt away.

Finding out your levels

Finding out your cholesterol and triglyceride levels is simply a matter of getting a blood test from your physician. If levels are high, blood vessels can become clogged by plaque deposits, leading to coronary heart disease. The best defense? Living Paleo foods and exercise; the perfectly balanced fats in Paleo foods and the functional Paleo movements keep your coronary artery disease risk low.

For a more advanced cholesterol screening, find a physician in your area who uses Genova Diagnostics. This advanced testing, called CV Health, will not only give you all the valuable numbers you need for cholesterol and triglycerides but will also give you the size of the cholesterol particles in your blood, which is imperative. Ask your doctor whether he works with this lab. If not, you can call Genova Diagnostics (check out www.gdx.net) to find a doctor in your zip code who works with their lab.

pH (acid-base balance)

Testing for your body's pH is easy, inexpensive, and very telling of your body's state of health. When your acid-base balance is healthy, you look and feel much younger. That's why living Paleo is such a brilliant life plan to follow.

Most people are on the acidic side of the acid-base spectrum. When you consume processed foods and sugary drinks and experience all the stress that an inverted way of eating, living, and thinking brings, you get acidic. Negative emotions (like anger and resentment) and negative lifestyle habits (too much screen time, smoking, or alcohol) play a role in your body's acidity as well — it's not just about food; it's about the way you live day to day.

Chapter 5

Making Paleo Practical in a Modern World

In This Chapter

▶ Tackling common roadblocks associated with switching to Paleo

▶ Traveling and eating out without sacrificing your good habits

▶ Celebrating holidays and special occasions the Paleo way

▶ Bringing your family onboard the Paleo train

Getting started on any new lifestyle can be a challenge, and the best way to smooth out the rough spots is to be ready for them. When you understand what's coming, you can better equip yourself to stay on course, whether the obstacles come at you from your friends, family, or right inside your own mind.

When you've made the commitment to follow a Paleo lifestyle, eating the Paleo Big Three becomes second nature, especially when you're cooking and eating at home. But if you're like most humans, you're a social creature who likes to get out and see the rest of the world once a while.

This chapter shows you how to get past common points of resistance and make a Paleo lifestyle work when it's most challenging, like when you're away from home or celebrating a holiday. It also shows you how to navigate a restaurant menu and model good habits for your family.

Dealing with Potential Pitfalls

Long-term success is where Paleo really shines. When you address your roadblocks and jump over hurdles, you begin to embrace the power of what eating Paleo can add to your life. Find out here about common setbacks so you're ready to remove doubts or excuses and can succeed with your Paleo transition.

Clearing diet-related hurdles

How and what you eat has a direct relationship to how you feel. The foods you eat elicit a chemical response in your body, and you feel those effects, whether good or bad. The following sections explain what your body may be experiencing during a change in diet, what diet-related hurdles may get in your way, and how you can get back on track.

The carb flu

The degree to which your body experiences the *carb flu* — the unpleasant, flulike symptoms you may experience when you begin your journey of cutting out sugar and sugary carbohydrates — is purely individual. Some people snap out of this phase in a couple of days; for others, it takes closer to three weeks. Here are the symptoms commonly associated with the carb flu:

- Mental fuzziness
- Headaches
- Moodiness
- Shakiness
- Fatigue × 10
- Achy joints

Experiencing these symptoms as you begin the Paleo diet means nothing more than your body is transitioning. Think of your body pushing the compost button and trying to start over with cleaner, more efficient fuel. Your body is going through a good detox and flipping the switch to the more efficient fat-burning system of using fats (dietary and body fat) and proteins to create the energy it needs, rather than the sugary carbs it was accustomed to using.

If you feel a little shaky during a workout, give your body time to adjust and try eating some protein and fat before you train. A piece of protein and a handful of nuts work well for most, but adjust to what works best for you.

This transition is part of the process and a small price of admission to what you'll get in the end, so hang in there! Try to ease off any intense training when you're dealing with the carb flu and let your body recalibrate.

Cravings

Your cravings in the beginning can be intense. You may even *dream* about foods when you're making the transition to Paleo. These cravings are easy to confuse with hunger. Your brain causes these cravings as it adjusts to going without the sugary stuff that it's used to.

You've removed all the carbohydrate-dense, nutrition-poor foods, such as packaged, processed, sugary carbs, grains, and legumes. Often, being hungry is your body recalibrating to a new system, and these carbs may have been the source of most of your calories. Replacing these calories with healthy fats from grass-fed animal fats, coconut, or avocado fuels your body efficiently and sustains you so your hunger diminishes with healthy raw material.

Be sure to drink enough water. Your body can often confuse the low signal for water as a low signal for food. Drink at least half your body weight in ounces of water each day.

Make sure you're getting enough protein and fat, which can help sustain you. Building your plate with proteins, fats, and non-starchy vegetables is critical. You want to give your body the rest and the right raw material to start this process of change and to curb cravings.

Accelerating through common roadblocks to living Paleo

Most people encounter roadblocks at some point in their life. These roadblocks are the frustrations you may go through when you know what you have to do but are apprehensive about accelerating. They're the fears you have when you know change is closing in. They're the stories you tell yourself that make eating Paleo difficult to endure.

The Paleo lifestyle is about you. It's about changing your life for the better and saying good-bye to illness, weight gain, and fatigue. If there was ever a time when you needed to be in charge of what you allow yourself to buy into, it's now.

"It's just too hard"

Have you ever had to recover from surgery? Heal from a disease? Been through the treatment or recovery process with someone with cancer? Or tried to deal with a progressive disease that no one can diagnose, and you feel hopeless that you'll ever return to "the real you" again? Now that's hard. Real hard.

Don't think of living Paleo as being hard but rather liberating! Finally, you're getting a road map to a healthy you that actually works. For many, it means thinking differently, behaving differently, and changing a lot of patterns. It's new; it's scary; and it takes guts. But don't let yourself think it's too hard. Without question, you're capable of living Paleo.

"I'm too busy; I don't have time for this"

Preparing whole foods from scratch definitely takes some time. But when you face this roadblock, you have to be honest about your time and time management. Do you have time sucks throughout the day? You know, things you do that you can give up or do less of. TV and social media are big ones for most.

When you get down to the nitty-gritty of the matter, the issue is more about your *organization* than your *time*. Organize your time and your meals so eating Paleo isn't a big deal. When you organize, you get in and out of the grocery store faster, make your meals faster, and don't spend time fumbling around aimlessly. When you're not clear or organized, it costs you time.

The more access you have to real foods, the better you'll feel and the more you'll get done regardless of time crunches. Also, the more you practice Paleo meal planning, shopping, and food prep, the easier it will become.

"I'm not losing any weight"

If you're eating a true Paleo diet, it's nearly impossible for your weight not to shift. You're introducing so many benefits to your health that your weight should naturally normalize. If you're not getting results, it may be attributed to one of these causes:

- ✔ Eating too much fruit, which contains fructose and creates an insulin response that causes your body to lay down fat.

- ✔ Not getting enough sleep.

- ✔ Not getting organized, which can lead to grabbing convenience foods or other non-Paleo options.

- ✔ Expecting results too quickly.

- ✔ Eating too many nuts or seeds. (A handful is plenty.)

- ✔ Indulging too often in Paleo treats.

- ✔ Skipping the fat; having the right quantities of fat (not too much, not too little!) actually helps you lose fat.

- ✔ Not measuring your food properly. Make sure you know what a portion is and how it looks on your plate.

- ✔ Falling into old eating habits.

- ✔ Not managing stress.

"I feel like I can't eat anything on this diet"

For almost every SAD (Standard American Diet) food, some kind of Paleo conversion exists, maybe not spot-on but close. Mourning pasta is normal, but the Paleo "yes" list is more giving and more delicious than you think. The Paleo diet includes enough meats, vegetables, fruits, fats, nuts, and spices to make thousands of meals. Investigate your produce aisles and talk to your butcher or fishmonger. Get creative with pantry items. Consult cookbooks, websites, and chefs. Loads of resources and options are available within the Paleo framework.

Be patient, use this book as a reference, step outside your comfort zone, get creative, and acquaint yourself with as many spices as you can to put some zing in your meals.

"My friends and family think I've gone mad"

Everyone wants support from family and friends. Some people will support you unconditionally. Others will give their support after they see you transform. But some people may despise your enthusiasm, efforts, or transformation and won't give you an inch of support. Just be prepared for the different ways people may react and let yourself be okay with it. It's about you and your health, anyway.

"I can't afford to eat Paleo"

You can do Paleo on a budget. Having said that, if you're used to buying nutritionally void, supersized junk foods and eating fast food a couple times a week, eating Paleo will cost a little more. In the long run, though, you end up spending money on the health care you will most certainly need in the future. Eating Paleo can be done on a budget and keep your engine going far longer and stronger than supersized French fries.

"I can't find healthy meats or vegetables where I live"

You don't have to have a gourmet grocer or Whole Foods nearby to eat Paleo. Eating Paleo doesn't require following hyper-specific rules. You just need to find meat, vegetables, fruits, nuts, seeds, and some good oil. If you don't have a Whole Foods, Trader Joe's, or a gourmet grocer nearby, no big deal whatsoever.

In fact, the large national grocery chains, like Sam's Club, Costco, and Wal-Mart, and any of your local grocery chains, farmers' markets, CSAs, and local butcher shops have most of what you need. For some of the pantry items, like coconut oil or almond flour, you may have to seek out a natural foods store or an online source, but every year, conventional stores are expanding their stock to healthier, more natural foods.

Book I

Getting
Started
with
Paleo

"I don't know how to cook"

Cooking Paleo is about the easiest way to prepare meals that you can possibly imagine. You're working with basic foods, and you can access an overwhelming number of amazing resources to get started. The best part is you can create super nutritious, wonderfully easy dishes in a snap. Books II and III are chock-full of recipes that require little kitchen experience but are big on flavor and interest.

Incorporating Paleo into vegetarian and vegan lifestyles

Eating Paleo does recommend the inclusion of animal protein. However, you can enjoy eating Paleo and gain considerable health benefits without making animal protein a part of your Paleo plan.

Getting enough protein

If you eat some eggs and fish, try to build your plate with these foods as your protein and use the plant-based proteins only as the exception, not the rule. Eating plenty of eggs and fish along with veggies, fruits, and nuts ensures that you get the protein you need.

On the other hand, if you choose not to eat any meat, fish, or eggs, you have to look to other vegetarian protein to get your nutrition. The most optimal choices are organic, dense protein sources, like non-GMO plant-based foods, including the following:

- Beans: Lentils, black beans, pinto beans, and red beans
- Edamame
- Full-fat pasture-raised yogurt and kefir
- High-quality protein powders, hemp, or pea protein
- Natto
- Tempeh
- Tofu

Don't look to string cheese, cottage cheese, or conventional yogurt or dairy products as your protein sources. These foods may cause congestion or inflammation in the body. In fact, a lot of people are finding that they're intolerant to dairy. If your body shows signs of a dairy sensitivity, such as feeling tired after eating any dairy products, constant sniffles, coughing, or acne or skin rashes, then making dairy your protein source is definitely not going to move you toward health.

Avoiding frankenfoods

Whether you decide to eat a little meat, eggs, or fish or stick with plant-based proteins, avoiding *frankenfoods* is of utmost importance. *Frankenfoods* are made to look like real foods but are nothing more than fake foods from head to toe. They include processed soy and meat alternatives. Unlike soy foods, such as edamame, tempeh, and traditional miso, which are closer to their natural state, these foods are a far cry from anything real.

You have to get your protein somewhere, but look past these food products for your options. This stuff just isn't healthy for anyone. Period. In fact, these options aren't even foods. They're *food products,* usually a mixture of a wheat protein with a subpar oil. Frankenfoods to avoid include the following:

- Soy milk
- Tofu hot dogs
- Veggie bacon
- Veggie burgers
- Veggie chicken
- Veggie chicken wings
- Veggie loafs
- Veggie "sausage" links

Make sure your protein sources are as healthy and as natural as can be. Also, make sure you're getting plenty of healthy fats and loads of fruits and veggies. People who take the vegetarian approach tend to have intestinal, inflammatory, and autoimmune types of problems; healthy fats help reduce that inflammation.

Dining Out and Traveling

Eating out is an inevitable and pleasurable part of our culture. But when you're committed to a Paleo diet, it becomes something of a challenge — although one you can meet with a little forethought and information. Similarly, vacations can often be detrimental to good nutrition. Preparation goes a long way when you travel away from home.

Choosing the right restaurant

Research and preparation are the first steps to enjoying a successful restaurant experience. Review restaurant menus in advance to ensure that you can find food that fits into your eating plan. By deciding in advance what to order, you can prevent temptation or confusion from derailing your good intentions.

Whenever possible, choose restaurants that serve locally sourced ingredients, like meat and organic produce from nearby farms. The phrase *farm to table* is usually a reliable indicator that the quality of the ingredients is top-notch, and restaurants concerned with serving only the best ingredients are also interested in responding to diners' requests, so you have free rein to be a "picky eater."

Living Paleo doesn't require you to be perfect but is meant to encourage you to make intentional food choices that make you feel good physically and emotionally. You may choose to indulge in a non-Paleo treat occasionally. Choose only the most delicious options, and then savor every bite.

Making informed choices

Here are some tips to help you win over your server and get the information you need to make Paleo-friendly choices:

- ✔ **Call ahead.** Don't be afraid to ask for what you need; people are often happy to accommodate you, especially if it means repeat business.

- ✔ **Ask about gluten.** Although gluten-free options may still involve grains, a gluten-free menu is a good starting point for asking questions and finding meals that don't include glutinous grains.

- ✔ **Say "no" to the pre-meal freebies.** When the server delivers snacks like bread or chips with your menu, smile and say, "No, thank you."

- ✔ **Ask about oils.** Most restaurants use canola oil for their griddles, pan frying, deep frying, and salads. If you know you're sensitive to oils high in omega-6 fatty acids, skip any foods cooked in canola oil.

- ✔ **Make substitutions.** You can always swap side dishes — request a side of fruit instead of potatoes at breakfast, for example — or ask for a double order of good things like vegetables.

- ✔ **Get creative.** Request that sauces be served on top of vegetables instead of pasta, or ask for sandwich fillings on a bed of lettuce instead of between bread.

✔ **Check the dressing.** Factory-made salad dressings are notorious for including hidden sugars, soy, and corn, so ask your server about the salad dressing. If it's commercially made, opt instead for vinegar or lemon juice and extra-virgin olive oil for your salad. Order whatever dressing you choose on the side so you can control your portion.

Managing the restaurant menu

If you're diligent and ask lots of questions, eating in a restaurant can be a fun, pleasurable experience. *Remember:* You're not aiming for perfection. Just do your best, and then relax and savor your food.

Forget *battered* and *crispy* and look for these cooking methods and descriptions to find the most Paleo-friendly choices on the menu — and remember to ask clarifying questions of your server to verify ingredients and cooking methods.

✔ Braised	✔ Sautéed
✔ Broiled	✔ Smoked
✔ Grilled	✔ Sous vide
✔ Poached	✔ Steamed
✔ Roasted	

Beware of soups and stews. They can be a satisfying one-stop source of quality protein and vegetables, unless the chef thickens them with a flour-based roux or adds cream for a smooth texture. Ask lots of questions about soups and stews, including whether they contain soy, flour, other grains, or dairy.

Be inquisitive! Terms like *salsa* and *relish* usually indicate fresh vegetables diced and tossed together with seasonings to add zing to meats and vegetables, which means they can be Paleo friendly. But these condiments can also include added sugar, soy, and wheat, so ask plenty of questions before you dig in.

Planning for Paleo on the road

Finding high-quality, Paleo-friendly food while traveling can be difficult. The situation is further complicated when you're tired or stressed by the challenges of traveling. Here are some guidelines to ensure that a few special treats don't ruin your entire vacation with gastrointestinal distress, lethargy, or moodiness:

✔ **Eat very clean before you go.** In preparation for your trip, follow the Paleo eating guidelines extra closely.

✔ **Choose only the best.** Set your standards high and treat yourself with only the best version of the special foods you choose, whether bread in France or barbecue in North Carolina.

✔ **Set parameters.** Will you allow yourself one treat per day? One treat per meal? Maybe you'll eat clean at breakfast and lunch, but make dinner a special meal. Decide in advance how you want to manage your meals so you're not caught off guard or overtaken by cravings during your trip.

✔ **Savor every bite.** When you've selected a treat, eat it slowly and experience every bite with all your senses.

✔ **Refocus when you get home.** Enjoy your memories of your special dining experiences and get right back into your Paleo groove.

Finding or bringing airport-friendly snacks

Let's face it: The food options at most airports are pretty terrible, and airplane food is not only junky, but it's also not very tasty (when it's even offered). Arm yourself with a small, insulated bag to carry foods that need to be kept cool, and stuff nonperishables into your carry-on for snacks any time.

What follows are some foods that won't send the TSA into a panic and will travel well without refrigeration:

✔ Sugar-free, high-quality deli meats

✔ Smoked salmon

✔ Hard-boiled eggs

✔ Cooked chicken, cut into easily managed pieces

✔ Cooked meatballs or burger patties

✔ Cooked sweet potatoes

✔ Raw veggies, cut into easily managed pieces

✔ Fresh fruit, cut into easily managed pieces

✔ Avocado or guacamole

✔ Olives

Take these items in your carry-on bag:

- ✔ Sugar-free beef jerky
- ✔ Coconut flakes
- ✔ Nuts
- ✔ Dried fruit
- ✔ Canned sardines, tuna, or salmon
- ✔ Snack bars that contain only dried fruit and nuts
- ✔ Squeeze packs of nut butter and/or coconut butter

Snacking while driving: The "emergency" car cooler

A road trip (or train travel) lets you take your good Paleo habits with you. With some advance cooking and a well-stocked cooler, you're all set for Paleo eating wherever your wanderlust takes you. Put together the following items in your toolkit to keep with you while on the road:

- ✔ Small cutting board
- ✔ Paring knife
- ✔ Can opener
- ✔ Empty BPA-free storage containers
- ✔ Ziploc bags in a variety of sizes
- ✔ Salt, pepper, and other spices in travel-sized jars
- ✔ A small sponge and dish soap
- ✔ Toothpicks

For perishable items, pack the following in your cooler:

- ✔ Sugar-free, high-quality deli meats
- ✔ Smoked salmon
- ✔ Hard-boiled eggs
- ✔ Cooked chicken, cut into easily managed pieces
- ✔ Cooked meatballs or burger patties
- ✔ Cooked sweet potatoes
- ✔ Whole raw veggies
- ✔ Whole fresh fruit

- Salsa
- Baba ghanoush
- Homemade salad dressing (see recipes in Book III, Chapter 2)

These items are great for the road; keep them in your dry-goods bag:

- Sugar-free beef jerky
- Coconut flakes
- Nuts
- Dried fruit
- Canned sardines, tuna, or salmon
- Snack bars that contain only dried fruit and nuts
- Jars of nut butter and/or coconut butter

Enjoying Special Occasions

Especially on holidays or special occasions, like a wedding, food is more than just nourishment for the body; it's a way to bring people together in celebration. The good news is that you can balance treats with your Paleo commitment so you have the best of both worlds.

Planning ahead for social events

Following your Paleo guidelines will eventually feel like second nature in the comfort of your house, but socializing can present a new world of challenges. Here are some suggestions to help you carry your Paleo habits with you wherever your social life takes you:

- **Do your research.** A quick review of a restaurant's menu in advance can mean the difference between a relaxing, enjoyable meal and a gluten-infused nightmare. Read all the options on the menu and decide what you're going to order before you go.

- **Bring your own food.** This trick isn't always applicable or appropriate, but in many cases, it works like a charm. Are you going to a casual event, like a picnic? There's no harm in packing your own food in a cooler bag. And believe it or not, you can even pack your own food for a wedding, if you do it with class and care. Between the ceremony and the reception, there's usually a lull of at least an hour. That's the perfect opportunity to eat a Paleo-friendly snack or mini meal to nourish your body.

✔ **Eat before you go.** A party at a friend's house, an afternoon of window shopping, or a movie night doesn't need to derail your good habits. Eat a solid Paleo meal before you go and bring Paleo-friendly snacks with you to sustain you if you get hungry or to give you something to eat when your companions indulge in a snack along the way.

✔ **Enlist help.** Tell your family and friends that you're sticking to your new Paleo habits to explain why you're not gulping beer, noshing on Grandma's sugar cookies, or diving face first into the plate of nachos you usually order while watching the playoffs. Don't be shy about creating an army of support to help you get over challenging humps.

✔ **Be firm.** If someone gives you a hard time — a waiter, a co-worker, a friend — simply look him in the eye and say with as much steel (and patience) in your voice as possible, "Eating this way is important to me. I'm sure you understand my desire to be as healthy as possible." It's virtually impossible for anyone to argue with that.

When spending time with friends and family, you want your focus to be on the conversation, laughter, and camaraderie of your favorite people. Don't fall into the trap of thinking that a party is *primarily* about the food and the cocktails; it's really about enjoying social interaction with people you like. If you take the focus off the food and drink and redirect your attention to the people you're with, you'll enjoy the occasion, and following your Paleo guidelines will feel effortless.

Eating Paleo during celebrations and holidays

Living Paleo doesn't mean that you'll never eat your mom's legendary coffee cake or a piece of comforting lasagna ever again. But choosing food indulgences carefully and intentionally is essential for optimal mental and physical health.

Food traditions are some of the most cherished, and Thanksgiving may not seem like Thanksgiving without the green bean casserole you eat every year. But new traditions can be just as rewarding as old ones — and sometimes the old ones can be updated without anyone being the wiser. As you find out in this section, starting new traditions that make your family and friends healthier is easy and fun, and bringing old traditions into your Paleo lifestyle keeps that traditional feeling but in a new and improved way.

Planning a Paleo party menu

To truly celebrate holidays, create menus that feature Paleo foods that nourish your body and taste great, and then on very special occasions, select a treat that's worth the compromise. Here are some suggestions to help with holiday menu planning when you're the host:

- ✔ **Make it fun.** If you make the food fun and engaging, chances are no one will notice how healthy it is. For a party, try setting up a burger bar with all the fixings and invite guests to build their own burgers. Put out colorful bowls of raw vegetables, guacamole, Tangy BBQ Sauce and Olive Oil Mayo (see the recipes in Book III), pickles, jalapeños, and shakers of spices and seasoned salts. Or set out a build-your-own taco bar with chicken and ground beef taco meat, salsas, avocado, and a variety of lettuce leaves for wrapping. By encouraging everyone to play with their food, you amp up the fun as well as the nutrition.

- ✔ **Satisfy with side dishes.** For more formal dinners and holidays like Thanksgiving, Christmas, and Easter, serving some kind of roast meat or poultry is often tradition. That's perfect for a Paleo lifestyle! And the sides are where you can enjoy some special ingredients to make the meal memorable. Go-alongs, like roasted sweet potatoes with clarified butter and Mashed Cauliflower or Cauliflower Rice (find the recipes in Book II) studded with dried fruit, are Paleo-friendly options that will delight your guests' taste buds.

- ✔ **Go with grain-free goodies.** There's no denying that the attachments to cookies on Christmas and a cake to celebrate a birthday are pretty strong. You can satisfy those yearnings with grain-free, gluten-free baked goods. These special occasion foods can be part of a healthy, balanced Paleo lifestyle, but remember to keep them to a minimum. You can find excellent grain-free recipes in cookbooks and online; just be sure to verify that the ingredients conform to your Paleo guidelines. Book III gives you dessert recipes.

- ✔ **Mix it up with finger foods.** Nothing says party food like fancy appetizers, and turning Paleo ingredients into finger foods that your friends and family won't be able to resist is easy. Raw vegetables become something special when they're cut into unusual shapes and dipped in homemade sauces, like Ranch Dressing or Cashew Butter Satay Sauce (see the recipes in Book III). Tuna salad turns into party food when you add apples and pecans and then serve it on thin apple slices or cucumber rounds. Tuck a smoked almond inside a dried date for a salty-sweet treat. Simple, fresh ingredients can become memorable when you dress up their presentation and focus on bold flavors.

✔ **Don't forget the eye candy.** It's been said that we eat first with our eyes, and Paleo ingredients are beautiful: brightly colored fresh fruits and vegetables, toasty brown nuts, jewel-toned dried fruits. Take a little extra time to create enticing presentations of Paleo foods, and even the most devoted junk-food junkie at your gathering won't be able to resist.

✔ **Indulge in really good dark chocolate.** High-quality, organic, dark chocolate is a not-too-sweet treat that satisfies the desire for something sweet without derailing all your hard work. Look for bars that are at least 70 percent cacao, and then break them into bite-size pieces, place on a beautiful serving dish with a few dry-roasted nuts and unsweetened coconut flakes, and relish how no one complains that they're denied a gloppy, over-the-top dessert.

Having the occasional drink

Drinking alcohol on a regular basis isn't part of the Paleo lifestyle, but enjoying a cocktail on occasion is okay, whether it's raising Champagne in celebration, sipping a glass of red wine to relax, or cooling off at a hot fiesta with an icy margarita. The key to successfully imbibing alcohol while living Paleo is choosing the right adult beverages and consuming them in a responsible, intentional way.

One way to manage social situations when you're not going to drink alcohol is to get a glass into your hand immediately upon entering the room. Simply walk up to the bartender and request a large club soda with two slices of lime or a few olives. With that glass in your hand, you look like everyone else in the room!

But what do you do if you want to enjoy a cocktail once in a while? Some choices for alcohol fit better into the Paleo lifestyle than others. Here are the smartest options for when you want to indulge:

✔ **Wine and Champagne:** Wine, especially red wine, may have some heart health benefits, and some evidence suggests that it even helps ward off infectious cold viruses. Wine includes antioxidants that help fight cancer and reduce the signs of aging.

✔ **Vodka, gin, rum, and tequila:** Distilled spirits don't offer the health benefits of wine, but they don't include carbohydrates or gluten, either, so they're acceptable choices. They're best enjoyed chilled on their own or mixed with club soda and garnished with lemon and lime wedges or olives.

Adapting your favorite recipes

Many standard recipes can be updated with Paleo ingredients to make them comply with your new habits. It may take some experimentation, but you'll gain more confidence as you practice in your Paleo kitchen. Table 5-1 lists some common substitutions to help you rework your favorite recipes.

Table 5-1	Paleo-Friendly Ingredient Substitutions
Original Ingredient	*Paleo Substitution*
White flour	Almond flour, coconut flour
White or brown sugar	Honey
Milk, cream, or yogurt	Coconut milk
Red wine	Balsamic vinegar
White wine	Chicken broth
Soy sauce	Coconut aminos
White potatoes	Sweet potatoes, turnips, rutabagas, cauliflower
Pasta	Zucchini noodles, spaghetti squash, shredded cabbage
Rice	Cauliflower rice
Shortening, vegetable oil, seed oils (canola, sunflower, rapeseed)	Coconut oil, clarified grass-fed butter
Butter	Clarified grass-fed butter

Indulging with pleasure

One of the most important aspects of living Paleo is developing the ability to balance the times when you comply completely with the Paleo rules and when you loosen your standards to enjoy a special treat. Your ability to stray from the strict Paleo path is dependent on your goals and health concerns, like whether you have a disease that requires you to avoid certain foods.

Here are some questions you can ask yourself to help you decide when is a good time for a treat and whether that treat is worth the indulgence:

✔ Do you have a medical concern, such as a gluten sensitivity, allergy, celiac disease, or diabetes, that requires you to avoid this food?

✔ Will eating this food trigger a domino effect of overeating?

✔ Will this food satisfy your craving, or will it merely be a momentary distraction?

✔ Are you eating this food for the pleasurable taste, to satisfy true hunger, to comfort an unpleasant emotion, or as entertainment?

✔ Will eating this food cause you any discomfort, such as gastrointestinal distress, bloating, interrupted sleep, or moodiness, after you eat it? If so, is it worth it?

✔ Is this version of the food the best you can find?

✔ How will you feel after eating this food? For example, will you be satisfied, happy, remorseful, ashamed, or hungrier?

Transitioning the Family

Leading by example, or being a strong, silent leader, is the most effective way to influence kids. You simply can't bully your way into transformation. When someone pursues change with no heart, it's not lasting change. That's where the theory "they'll come to you when they're ready" holds. If you want other members of your household to embrace change, be a great role model. Have healthy foods available and have *your* food values in order. That's how you can affect change.

The following sections cover some basic strategies for being the example who leads toward a healthier home.

Teaching kids the "why" behind the "what"

Have you ever gone through the motions of doing something just because? Maybe someone said to do it, maybe it was a role you had to take on for work, or maybe it was just something you got in the habit of doing? Something is usually missing when you do something just because, and that something is heart. When you do things with heart, the passion to succeed follows.

No matter what age or stage your kids are in, explain some simple facts. You don't have to make a big deal about it; it can even be in passing. As long as you do, teach them the *why*. Here are some examples:

- You should be able to pronounce the ingredients on a food label; otherwise, they're probably chemicals that you don't want in your body.

- If too many ingredients are on the label, the foods are too processed and won't give you the nutrients your body needs to grow and be healthy. You'll get some energy but no nutrition.

- Fruits and vegetables have antioxidants, which keep you healthy and protect you against getting sick.

- Fruits and vegetables have vitamins and minerals, which make every structure and function of your body work. When you get too low on these vitamins, you get sick more easily, and performing in all areas of life as well as you can is difficult.

- Fruits and vegetables have fiber, which helps move things along your intestines so your body stays cleansed and not clogged.

- You need healthy proteins to build and repair everything in your body, like strong muscles.

- Healthy fats make your brain and all your cells work better so you can do everything better.

- If you want your cells to flow really nicely, you have to be hydrated. Your cells need water so they don't stick together, which causes you to get tired and worn out.

Keep your explanations simple — no big words or lengthy lectures — just some simple facts so your children understand why eating healthy foods is important. Explaining the *why* behind the choices you make helps them feel ownership and helps them *want* to have a healthier lifestyle. That's a sure-fire prescription for success!

Providing tasty, nutritious treats

Kids love treats. In fact, many of them would trade you in for a banana split! You can manage these cravings in the following ways:

- The only way you can completely avoid sugar in your kids' diet is to not have any sweeteners or sweet stuff in your household so there's no begging or battles. Remember the rule: What you do, the kids follow. But don't expect your kids to appreciate you removing the sugar from their lives. Your best strategy is to always give a clear explanation as to why you're making your kitchen healthier in terms that they'll clearly understand.

✔ If you do decide on a treat, such as ice cream, go out and get it instead of stocking it at home. That way when you're home, the temptation isn't present.

✔ Redefine desserts by making Paleo treats with wholesome ingredients, like fruit and almond and coconut flours. Many of them are simple to put together and really delicious. (Check out the recipes in Book III, Chapter 4.)

✔ Don't fall into the circus animal pattern of rewarding kids with sweets. Don't confuse the fact that food is there to nourish, not to show love or reward.

✔ Let your kids know that some sweets, such as birthday cake at parties or holiday cookies that you bake together, are okay *some of the time*. Make sure they understand the difference between special occasion treats and everyday real foods.

✔ Pull the plug on sweet drinks in your home. Don't buy soda or sweet drinks. No sports drinks (unless you need them). Sugary drinks have become a huge problem for kids, and this rule should be an absolute deal breaker with no wiggle room. No liquid sugar! Get your kids used to water and iced herbal teas if they want something else. Just a pitcher of water with some oranges and lemons is usually enough to keep them happy. Hold strong on this one. Explain why; they'll get it.

These off-limit, toxic sweeteners aren't good for a growing neurological system (or any system for that matter):

✔ Acesulfame-K (Sweet One)

✔ Aspartame (Equal, NutraSweet)

✔ High-fructose corn syrup

✔ Saccharin (Sweet'N Low)

✔ Sucralose (Splenda)

The top choices (by a landslide) in sweeteners for your kiddos include the following:

✔ Dates (you'd be surprised how well these work)

✔ Fresh fruit juice (great for baking and dressings)

✔ Organic maple syrup

✔ Raw honey (although not under the age of 2, due to the risk of botulism, a very serious illness)

✔ Ripe bananas

Paleo treats are made with these ingredients, and they taste so good that your kids won't feel like they're missing a thing.

Here's an easy-peasy treat to try: Take some berries and drizzle some honey on top — kids love this. Or just a bowl of berries and coconut milk can do the trick! By the way, you can easily transform fruit into wonderful ice creams and mousses.

Managing mealtimes

Mealtimes are an important part of any family. Although eating together as a family every day isn't always possible, even if you manage it on the weekends, you'll reap the rewards. When you do get to have meals together, your family starts seeing mealtimes as an enjoyable family experience, not a chore or a war zone.

Avoid distractions, include the kids in the conversation, and focus on any positive interactions. Doing so makes your mealtime a good opportunity to touch on appropriate mealtime behaviors and making smart food choices. The more you manage mealtimes, the healthier the entire family will eat.

Pick a meal, any meal

Start your family on the path to putting real foods back in their diet with one meal and work your way toward more. Pick whatever meal works best with the rhythm of your home. The point is to start somewhere. Breakfast is one of the best meals to start with because it's when your family's the hungriest and willing to try different foods.

Always keep hard-boiled eggs on hand. You can eat them on their own or chop them into sausage or bacon for a quick and easy breakfast.

The 2-plus-1 dinner rule

The 2-plus-1 rule goes like this: At every dinner, have *two* cooked vegetables and *one* raw vegetable on the table. Make it a rule, something your family can expect. If you make a dish that includes a vegetable, that counts; if you make spaghetti squash for dinner, that's one vegetable. Just make sure you include a raw vegetable as well, such as snow peas, sugar snap peas, kohlrabi, jicama, cucumbers, carrots, and crisp bell peppers.

What this 2-plus-1 rule does is anchor into a child's mind that vegetables at mealtimes are standard. Therefore, having vegetables becomes normal to them. You can use this time to talk about the different kinds of vegetables (or seasonal vegetables) and encourage them to try new ones.

Try to prepare fruits and vegetables just before cooking or serving, because nutrient levels begin to diminish as soon as you cut the produce.

The "no biggie" rule

Don't let food create stress in your household. What stress creates in your body is worse than what eating a cupcake does. The key is to have a positive influence without creating stress.

What you focus on grows. So don't focus on the food issues your kiddo may be having. Don't allow mealtimes to be battlegrounds. Control what you can, and let the rest go.

You influence your family by being a strong leader and keeping a healthy and positive home. Your job is to walk the talk and not give negative actions/reactions too much energy. Approach healthy eating like it's a part of who you are and carry that certainty with you. It will rub off.

The non-negotiable bite

Here's a great rule to help your family try new flavors: They have to try one bite. That's it — one itty-bitty bite. Your kids can scrunch up their noses and stick out their tongues all they want, but they've gotta give it a try. If they try it and discover they don't like it, let them know that's okay with you. At least they tried.

Keep in mind that a rejection is often not a true indication of dislike. Reintroduce them to the food at another point, and the results may be different.

The point in the non-negotiable bite rule is to get your family's taste buds (and brain) used to real foods. Every time they try a vegetable, their body creates neurological pathways. These pathways create habits, making eating healthy second nature. Think of it this way: With every tiny bite, you take a small chunk out of their veggie resistance and move one step closer to balanced mealtimes. But it may take 15 to 20 tries before your child gets to acceptance. Don't give up!

Building a kid-friendly plate

Knowing how to build a healthy plate is the cornerstone of healthy eating. Understanding that a healthy plate includes vegetables, some fruit, a little protein, good-for-you fats, and healthy starches sets the stage for a lifetime of health.

Don't *ever* talk calories with your kids. If your child needs to eat more, the messages from the brain determine hunger. When your children experience a true physiological need for calories and when they're truly hungry, they'll eat. If they need to lose weight, talk to them about eating better for health. Health should *always* be the focus. Don't focus on bad foods or make a big deal about it. Control what you can, and do your best to teach your kids how to make choices outside of the home.

The end goal is to have your kids eating real foods that are rich in every nutrient under the sun, including lean proteins, healthy fats and oils, low-starch vegetables, healthy carb-dense vegetables, fruits, nuts, and seeds and their butters.

Fruits and vegetables

A portion size of fruits and vegetables for kids differs from an adult's portion size and is smaller than you may think. A portion size is the amount a child can hold in one hand, and as her hand grows, so should the size of the portion. For school-age kids, a portion is about half a cup. Try to incorporate the following amounts in your kids' diet:

- Three to five servings (kid-sized handfuls) of vegetables a day
- Two to four servings (kid-sized handfuls) of fruit a day

Healthy carbs

Be sure to include some dense sources of healthy carbohydrates for your kids. Kids are active and usually need more of a refuel than adults. Here are some healthy carb suggestions:

- Beets
- Butternut squash
- Carrots
- Kohlrabi
- Parsnips
- Pumpkin
- Raw cassava
- Raw jicama
- Spaghetti squash
- Sweet potatoes
- Taro root
- Winter squash
- Yams

Healthy fats

Kids older than 2 years of age should get about 30 percent of their daily calories from fat. Here are some great healthy fats for your kids:

- Bacon
- Coconut milk or shredded coconut
- Eggs
- Fatty fish (salmon, trout, or mackerel)
- Flax milk
- Grass-fed butter
- Guacamole dips
- Healthy oils
- Nut butters
- Nuts
- Olives
- Seeds

Make up a trail mix of shredded coconut, nuts, and seeds, and throw in some dark chocolate, which has some valuable nutrients as well.

Protein

Kids need about 10 to 15 percent (about three servings per day) of their diet to come from protein. The more they're growing (growth spurts) and the more active they are, the more building blocks they need. Animal proteins are better tailored to meet the needs of infants and growing children than are plant proteins, which is why nature provides human milk for babies.

Convincing your significant other

The best thing you can do to get your partner involved is to show — don't tell — how amazing and delicious living Paleo can be. Doing so requires you to be a strong leader and lead by example above and beyond all else. First, give your absolute best, most compelling pitch as to why trying Paleo for 30 days is so important. If your partner accepts your pitch, do what you can to support him or her. Be enthusiastic to help during the transition, because you know that after 30 days, your partner will be on board.

If your significant other doesn't want to try Paleo, your only course of action is to be a strong leader. Show by example how much energy you have and how much better you feel. Prepare some Paleo recipes and let your partner see how simple it is to stay on board. Show him or her that Paleo meals are simple and delicious and won't make you heavy, bloated, constipated, or get your blood sugar all out of whack. Eating can actually make you feel better, not worse.

Let your significant other see how your body, mind, and spirit transform for the positive. If, after you do all of this, your significant other still decides that trying to live Paleo is just not something he or she is willing to do, accept your partner for who he or she is — crappy food and all. Don't get resentful or frustrated; the stress hormones counterbalance your great strides and efforts. It simply isn't worth what it does to you internally.

The best thing you can do is keep on keeping on. Create the best life you can and keep the best attitude you can. That's what's in your control.

Book II
Recipes for Every Occasion and Meal

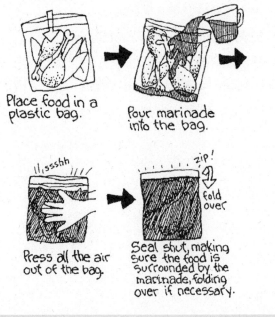

Using a Plastic Bag to Marinate Food

Place food in a plastic bag.

Pour marinade into the bag.

ll,ssshh

Press all the air out of the bag.

zip!
fold over

Seal shut, making sure the food is surrounded by the marinade, folding over if necessary.

Illustration by Elizabeth Kurtzman

web
extras

Find kid-approved ways to fill a lunch box and keep young tummies happy at
www.dummies.com/extras/paleoaio.

Contents at a Glance

Chapter 1: Crafting Paleo Breakfasts **139**
  Expanding Your Breakfast Options 139
  Enjoying Paleo-Friendly, Grain-Free Goodies 140

Chapter 2: Packing Nutrition into Soups and Salads **157**
  Making Your Own Savory Soups, and Buying Wisely When You Can't 158
  Seizing the Versatility of the Salad 160

**Chapter 3: The Meat (and More) of the Matter:
Paleo Main Dishes** **189**
  Building Paleo Meals from Top-Quality Meats 189
  Buying Fresh Fish for Fab Dishes 191

Chapter 4: Paleo Life in the Slow (Cooker) Lane **209**
  Getting the Scoop on Slow Cooking 209

Chapter 5: Vegetable Dishes That Satisfy **227**
  Evolving Past Starches: Paleo-Friendly Hot Side Dishes 228

Chapter 6: Paleo for Kids: Recipes Your Littles Will Love **245**
  Packing Kid-Friendly Paleo Lunches 245

Chapter 1

Crafting Paleo Breakfasts

Recipes in This Chapter

▶ Pizza Frittata
↻ Huevos Rancheros
▶ Breakfast Sausage Scramble
▶ Thai Rolled Omelet
▶ Eggs in Spicy Tomato Sauce
▶ Grilled Eggs with Homemade Chorizo
▶ Machacado and Eggs
↻ Mini Cinnamon Pancakes
↻ Almond Banana Pancakes
↻ Morning Honey Muffins
↻ Anytime Waffles
↻ Lime-Blueberry Poppy Seed Coffee Cake
↻ Frozen Blueberry Breakfast Bars

In This Chapter

▶ Finding new (very old) ways to start your day

▶ Building breakfasts savory and sweet

How you start the day sets the tone for your entire day. Breakfast is a big piece of that puzzle. Your breakfast can either fuel you or make you feel like diving into the nearest coffeepot head-first. If your breakfast doesn't get you in your zone, then you're probably not fueling right.

One of the most important Paleo principles is to dial into how food makes you feel. More than any other barometer, the mind-body connection keeps you in check. The Paleo Big Three (protein, healthy carbs, and fats) will never let you down. When you create meals by using these foods, you're golden.

Expanding Your Breakfast Options

Labels kind of box you in, and the same goes for the notion of breakfast, lunch, or dinner. So-called breakfast foods really are just food. They don't have to be granola, cereal, bagels, or anything in a brightly colored box. A good breakfast is defined by foods that accomplish three things:

✔ Taste good while satisfying you

✔ Create a healthy blood sugar balance to prevent energy crashes

✔ Fortify you with nutrients to fuel your mind and body

Eating real foods produces these results. If you warm up a bowl of soup for breakfast, you're not breaking any rules, and you're not weird. As long as what you're eating satiates you, creates a favorable blood sugar balance, and fortifies your body and mind, you're good to go. You're going to get a better workout, take better care of your kids, and crush it at work or whatever you do the rest of the day. When you're fueling a healthy body, good stuff happens. Ditch the label "breakfast foods" and just focus on real foods for breakfast. You'll get used to it before you know it.

If you pass on most desserts because you don't want the extra sugar, you may feel duped to know that traditional breakfast cereals often have more sugar than most desserts. The Environmental Working Group's review of 84 popular cereals showed that most of them were loaded with sugar. In fact, one of the most popular kids' cereals is a staggering 56 percent sugar by weight.

Enjoying Paleo-Friendly, Grain-Free Goodies

The grain-free treats in this chapter (pancakes, waffles, and coffee cake) are technically Paleo but are higher in natural sugars and fats than standard meals of protein, vegetables, and fat. These recipes are much healthier options than traditional pancakes, waffles, and coffee cake, but they're still treats, which means they're meant for occasional indulgences, special occasions, and celebrations. Why not designate one Sunday a month as "Waffle Brunch Day" or plan a "Breakfast for Dinner" night once a week to turn an ordinary day into something special!

To make the most of your grain-free goodies, always eat them with high-quality protein, savor every bite, and throughout the rest of the day, try to minimize your intake of nuts and fruit.

Pizza Frittata

Prep time: 15 min • **Cook time:** 20 min • **Yield:** 4 servings

Ingredients	Directions
12 large eggs	**1** Preheat the oven to 400 degrees.
1 teaspoon Italian Seasoning (see recipe in Book III, Chapter 3)	**2** In a large bowl, beat the eggs, Italian Seasoning, salt, and pepper until blended.
¾ teaspoon salt	
½ teaspoon ground black pepper	**3** Heat a large oven-safe skillet over medium-high heat and add the coconut oil. When it's melted, add the onion and sauté until translucent, about 5 minutes. Add the bell pepper and tomatoes; cook until tender, about 5 minutes.
2 tablespoons coconut oil	
1 medium onion, diced	
1 cup diced green bell pepper	**4** Pour the beaten eggs into the pan and add the basil. Using a spatula to stir, gently scrape the bottom of the skillet to form large curds, about 2 minutes. Shake the pan to evenly distribute the ingredients and allow to cook undisturbed so the bottom sets, about 30 seconds.
1 cup grape tomatoes, halved	
8 large fresh basil leaves, coarsely chopped	
One 5-ounce package Applegate Farms Natural Pepperoni	**5** Arrange the pepperoni slices on top of the frittata. Place the pan in the oven and bake until the top is puffed and beginning to brown, about 13 to 15 minutes. Remove the skillet from the oven and allow to set for 5 minutes, and then cut into wedges to serve.

Per serving: Calories 412 (From Fat 277); Fat 31 g (Saturated 14 g); Cholesterol 583 mg; Sodium 956 mg; Carbohydrate 9 g (Dietary Fiber 2 g); Protein 25 g.

Tip: This dish is wonderful hot, straight out of the oven. It's also good at room temperature for a quick snack or lunch.

Vary It! Replace pepperoni with cooked ground beef, turkey, or pork. Add variety with your other favorite pizza topping vegetables, like zucchini or eggplant slices, mushrooms, or artichoke hearts. Serve the frittata at lunch or dinner with a quick topping of arugula salad. Just toss fresh arugula with a little red wine vinegar, extra-virgin olive oil, salt, and pepper, and pile the greens on top of the hot or room temperature frittata.

Huevos Rancheros

Prep time: 10 min • **Cook time:** 20 min • **Yield:** 4 servings

Ingredients	Directions

Ingredients

½ tablespoon coconut oil

1 medium onion, diced

2 cloves garlic, minced

1 teaspoon ground cumin

1 teaspoon unsweetened cocoa

¼ teaspoon cayenne pepper

Two 14.5-ounce cans diced fire-roasted tomatoes

One 6-ounce can diced green Anaheim chiles

1 canned chipotle chile in adobo sauce, chopped

Salt and pepper to taste

8 fresh eggs

Garnishes: minced fresh cilantro, diced avocado, fresh lime juice (optional)

Directions

1 Heat a large skillet over medium-high heat and add the coconut oil. When it's melted, add the onion and sauté until translucent, about 5 minutes. Add the garlic, cumin, cocoa, and cayenne pepper; cook until fragrant, about 30 seconds.

2 To the pan, add the tomatoes, green chiles, and chipotle chile. Stir to combine, taste, and season with salt and black pepper. Bring to a boil, and then reduce heat to simmer and cook until slightly thickened, about 15 minutes.

3 Working in batches, if necessary, carefully purée the cooled sauce in a food processor or blender. Return to the skillet.

4 With the back of a large spoon, make eight shallow wells in the sauce. Break an egg into a cup, and then carefully pour the egg into the well in the sauce; repeat with the rest of the eggs. Sprinkle each egg with salt and pepper, and then cover the pan and cook over medium-low heat until the eggs are cooked: 4 to 5 minutes for runny yolks, 6 to 7 minutes for set yolks.

5 Serve immediately, dividing the sauce and eggs among four plates. Sprinkle with cilantro, avocado, and a squeeze of lime juice (if desired).

Per serving: Calories 235 (From Fat 108); Fat 12 g (Saturated 5 g); Cholesterol 372 mg; Sodium 837 mg; Carbohydrate 15 g (Dietary Fiber 3 g); Protein 15 g.

Vary It! If you prefer fried eggs to poached, fry the eggs separately in a little coconut oil and then top them with the ranchero sauce.

Note: The sauce can be made ahead of time and frozen or stored in the refrigerator for a quick weekday breakfast.

Breakfast Sausage Scramble

Prep time: 10 min • **Cook time:** 20 min • **Yield:** 6 servings

Ingredients	Directions
1 pound ground pork	*1* Place the pork in a large mixing bowl and add the applesauce, marjoram, thyme, nutmeg, ginger, cayenne pepper, salt, black pepper, and allspice. Knead with your hands until combined.
½ cup unsweetened applesauce	
¼ teaspoon ground marjoram	
½ teaspoon dried thyme leaves	*2* Heat a large skillet over medium-high heat and add the coconut oil. When it's melted, crumble the pork into the pan, using a wooden spoon to break up large clumps. Sauté the pork until it's browned and cooked through, about 10 minutes. Remove the pork to a bowl with a slotted spoon; set aside.
¼ teaspoon ground nutmeg	
¼ teaspoon ground ginger	
¼ teaspoon cayenne pepper	
¼ teaspoon salt	*3* Drain all but 1 tablespoon of fat from the pan. Add the onion and sauté until translucent, about 5 minutes. Add the bell pepper and cook until tender, about 5 minutes.
¼ teaspoon ground black pepper	
⅛ teaspoon allspice	
1 tablespoon coconut oil	*4* Add the pork back to the pan and stir to combine. Pour in the eggs and cook, stirring frequently, until set. Season with salt and pepper to taste. Serve immediately.
1 medium onion, diced	
1 large red bell pepper, diced	
10 large eggs, scrambled	
Salt and pepper to taste	

Per serving: Calories 301 (From Fat 182); Fat 20 g (Saturated 8 g); Cholesterol 299 mg; Sodium 319 mg; Carbohydrate 6 g (Dietary Fiber 1 g); Protein 23 g.

Vary It! Substitute ground turkey or chicken for the pork.

Tip: Leave out the eggs, and this sausage works great as patties, too. Just form 2-inch patties with the pork and cook in a hot skillet until evenly browned. They're an excellent accompaniment for Anytime Waffles, coming up in this chapter.

Thai Rolled Omelet

Prep time: 5 min • **Cook time:** 10 min • **Yield:** 1 serving

Ingredients	Directions
2 eggs	*1* Crack the eggs into a medium bowl and add the fish sauce, cilantro, scallions, and a squeeze of lime juice. Whisk together until frothy.
½ teaspoon fish sauce	
1 tablespoon chopped fresh cilantro	*2* Heat the ghee in a seasoned 8-inch cast-iron skillet or a regular 8-inch skillet with sloped sides over high heat. Swirl the melted fat to cover the sides of the pan. When the ghee is shimmering, add the egg mixture.
1 tablespoon chopped scallions	
Lime wedge (¼ lime)	*3* Let the eggs sit undisturbed for 10 to 15 seconds.
1 tablespoon ghee	*4* Tip the pan back toward you at a slight angle so the omelet begins to bunch up at the far edge of the pan and then roll over itself. (You can help it roll with a spatula if needed.)
	5 When the omelet is mostly cooked through, tip it out of the pan. Serve immediately.

Per serving: Calories 211 (From Fat 135); Fat 15 g (Saturated 5 g); Cholesterol 372 mg; Sodium 484 mg; Carbohydrate 4.5 g (Dietary Fiber 0.5 g); Protein 14 g.

Recipe courtesy Michelle Tam, author of Nom Nom Paleo (http://nomnompaleo.com)

This recipe has been vetted by the team at Whole9 (http://whole9life.com) and is considered acceptable for a cleansing 30-day Paleo launch.

Eggs in Spicy Tomato Sauce

Prep time: 10 min • **Cook time:** 20–25 min • **Yield:** 3 servings

Ingredients	Directions
¼ cup olive oil	**1** Preheat the oven to 400 degrees.
3 jalapeño peppers, seeded and minced	**2** Heat the olive oil in a deep ovenproof skillet over medium heat. Add the peppers and onion and sauté until the onion is slightly browned, about 5 minutes.
1 green bell pepper, diced	
1 white or yellow onion, diced	
4 cloves garlic, minced	**3** Add the garlic, cumin, and paprika and sauté 2 minutes.
½ teaspoon ground cumin	
2 teaspoons paprika	**4** Add the tomatoes. Reduce the heat and simmer 15 to 20 minutes (longer if you're using fresh tomatoes), stirring occasionally, until the sauce is thickened and most of the liquid is gone. Add salt to taste.
28 ounces diced tomatoes in their juice, or 2 pounds fresh tomatoes, chopped	
Salt to taste	**5** Make 6 indentations in the veggie mixture: 5 in a circle around the skillet and one in the center. Place the skillet on the oven rack.
6 eggs	
¼ cup chopped parsley	
	6 Crack an egg into a small dish and carefully pour it into one of the indentations. Repeat with the remaining eggs. Close the oven and bake for about 20 minutes. Garnish with the parsley and serve warm.

Per serving: *Calories 465 (From Fat 296); Fat 33 g (Saturated 7 g); Cholesterol 369 mg; Sodium 249 mg; Carbohydrate 25 g (Dietary Fiber 6 g); Protein 19 g.*

Note: Also known as shakshuka, this dish is loved around the world for its comforting flavor and simple preparation. (It's especially popular in Israel.) Although the sauce is often sopped up with pita bread, it's thick enough that you can skip the bread and eat it with a spoon (or spread extra sauce over leftover meat for a really fantastic meal).

Tip: The three jalapeños make this dish pretty spicy. If you prefer less heat, use one or two instead.

Recipe courtesy Mark Sisson, author of Primal Blueprint and Mark's Daily Apple (www.marksdailyapple.com)

This recipe has been vetted by the team at Whole9 (http://whole9life.com) and is considered acceptable for a cleansing 30-day Paleo launch.

Grilled Eggs with Homemade Chorizo

Prep time: 5 min • **Cook time:** 30 min • **Yield:** 4 servings

Ingredients	Directions
2 dried ancho or guajillo chilies, stems and seeds removed	**1** In a dry pot heated on high, toast the chilies on each side for about 25 seconds so they start to blister. Add 2½ cups of water, bring to a boil, and then turn off the heat.
¼ cup apple cider vinegar	
1 pound ground pork	**2** Cover the pot and let the chilies soak until soft, about 30 minutes. Drain the water and blend the chilies and vinegar in a blender until a smooth paste forms.
1 teaspoon chili powder	
1 teaspoon paprika	
1 teaspoon dried oregano	**3** In a large bowl, mix the chili paste, pork, chili powder, paprika, oregano, cumin, cinnamon, salt, and garlic with your hands until well combined. This mixture is your chorizo sausage.
½ teaspoon ground cumin	
⅛ teaspoon ground cinnamon	
½ teaspoon salt	**4** Brown the chorizo in a skillet over medium heat, breaking the meat into small pieces, until it's cooked through and slightly browned on the outside, about 8 to 10 minutes.
2 cloves garlic, minced	
2 large bell peppers	**5** Cut the bell peppers in half through the stem. Scrape out the seeds and cut out the white membrane. Place the pepper halves on an unheated grill.
4 eggs	
Celtic sea salt	**6** Crack an egg into each pepper half and sprinkle with a handful of chorizo. Heat the grill and place the filled pepper over the hottest part of the grill to char the skin and give it a smoky flavor.

7   Close the grill and cook for 8 to 10 minutes for a soft yolk. Check on the progress of the eggs once or twice as they cook, until they reach desired doneness.

8   Sprinkle with Celtic sea salt and serve with extra chorizo on the side.

Per serving: Calories 337 (From Fat 132); Fat 15 g (Saturated 4.5 g); Cholesterol 280 mg; Sodium 502 mg; Carbohydrate 8 g (Dietary Fiber 3 g); Protein 44 g.

Note: Chorizo is a delicious spicy Spanish pork sausage. The most important seasoning in homemade chorizo is dried chiles (ancho and guajillo are most common). Many grocery stores sell dried chiles, and you can also buy them at Hispanic markets or from online spice stores.

Tip: To help keep the bell peppers from tipping over on the grill, mold some rings out of aluminum foil to hold them upright. Place the foil rings and peppers on the cold grill, add the filling, and then turn the grill on.

*Recipe courtesy Mark Sisson, author of Primal Blueprint and Mark's Daily Apple (*www.marksdailyapple.com*)*

*This recipe has been vetted by the team at Whole9 (*http://whole9life.com*) and is considered acceptable for a cleansing 30-day Paleo launch.*

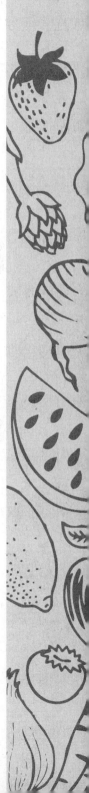

Machacado and Eggs

Prep time: 5 min • **Cook time:** 10 min • **Yield:** 3 servings

Ingredients	Directions
6 eggs	*1* Crack the eggs into a medium bowl, sprinkle with the salt and pepper, and then lightly beat with a fork or whisk. Set aside.
Pinch of salt	
Pinch of pepper	
2 tablespoons coconut oil, divided	*2* Heat a skillet over medium-high heat and add 1 tablespoon of the coconut oil. When the pan is hot, add the remaining ingredients except the eggs.
¼ cup carne seca (also called machacado) or dried beef	
¼ cup diced onion	*3* Sauté, stirring with a wooden spoon, until the onions are tender, about 7 to 10 minutes.
1 clove garlic, minced	
½ a jalapeño, ribs and seeds removed, minced	*4* Push the vegetables and beef to the side of the pan and add the remaining coconut oil. Add the eggs to the pan and push the meat into the eggs.
½ a medium tomato, seeded and diced	
¼ teaspoon chili powder	*5* Allow the egg to begin to set, and then stir with a wooden spoon. Continue to gently scramble until the eggs are cooked to your desired doneness. Taste and adjust the seasonings.

Per serving: Calories 365 (From Fat 216); Fat 24 g (Saturated 12 g); Cholesterol 369 mg; Sodium 1,180 mg; Carbohydrate 6 g (Dietary Fiber 1 g); Protein 31 g.

This recipe has been vetted by the team at Whole9 (http://whole9life.com) and is considered acceptable for a cleansing 30-day Paleo launch.

Mini Cinnamon Pancakes

Prep time: 5 min • **Cook time:** 10 min • **Yield:** 12 pancakes

Ingredients	Directions
2 eggs	*1* Whisk the eggs, coconut milk, banana, vinegar, and vanilla in a medium bowl until combined.
3 tablespoons coconut milk	
3 tablespoons mashed ripe banana	*2* In a separate bowl, mix together the dry ingredients.
½ teaspoon apple cider vinegar	*3* Combine the wet and dry ingredients and mix well. The batter should be fairly thin.
½ teaspoon vanilla extract	
1½ tablespoons coconut flour	*4* Heat a tablespoon of ghee over medium heat in a small frying pan or griddle. When the fat starts sizzling, add a tablespoon of batter to the pan for each pancake. You should be able to fit three or four pancakes in the pan.
½ teaspoon ground cinnamon	
¼ teaspoon baking soda	
⅛ teaspoon kosher salt	*5* Flip each pancake over when bubbles form on the surface and the edges are golden (about 1½ minutes). Cook for an additional 30 to 60 seconds on the other side.
2 tablespoons ghee for frying	
	6 Repeat Steps 4 and 5 until you've used all the batter. (You may not need to add as much ghee each time.) Serve immediately.

Per serving: *Calories 32 (From Fat 20); Fat 2.5 g (Saturated 1 g); Cholesterol 31 mg; Sodium 63 mg; Carbohydrate 2 g (Dietary Fiber 0.5 g); Protein 1 g.*

Tip: Top with fresh fruit or pureed berries for a sweet treat.

Recipe courtesy Michelle Tam, author of Nom Nom Paleo (http://nomnompaleo.com)

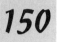

Almond Banana Pancakes

Prep time: 3 min • **Cook time:** 5 min • **Yield:** 2 servings

Ingredients	Directions
1 egg	**1** Beat the egg and mix well with the bananas.
2 ripe bananas, mashed	
1 heaping tablespoon almond butter	**2** Stir in the almond butter, adding more than a tablespoon if you want a more pancake-like texture.
1 tablespoon grass-fed butter	**3** In a large skillet, melt the butter over low heat and then pour the batter into small cakes, about 4 inches across.
	4 Brown on each side (keeping at low temperature) and serve warm.

Per serving: Calories 275 (From Fat 146); Fat 16 g (Saturated 5 g); Cholesterol 107 mg; Sodium 50 mg; Carbohydrate 29 g (Dietary Fiber 4.5 g); Protein 7 g.

Tip: Top pancakes with grass-fed butter, fresh berries, or a touch of raw honey. Add vanilla and/or cinnamon for a delicious accent.

Note: This dish is a good option for a quick breakfast and an alternative to pancakes made with almond or coconut flour, which may be a little heavier.

Recipe courtesy Mark Sisson, author of Primal Blueprint and Mark's Daily Apple (www.marksdailyapple.com)

Morning Honey Muffins

Prep time: 10 min • **Cook time:** 15 min • **Yield:** 6 servings

Ingredients	Directions
3 eggs	**1** Preheat the oven to 400 degrees. Prepare a muffin tin by placing paper liners in 6 cups.
3 tablespoons honey	
2 tablespoons coconut oil, melted	**2** Combine the eggs, honey, coconut oil, coconut milk, salt, and vanilla.
2 tablespoons canned coconut milk	
¼ teaspoon salt	**3** Sift together the baking powder and coconut flour and then combine with the wet ingredients. Mix well and then fold in the mashed banana and chopped pecans (if desired).
¼ teaspoon vanilla extract	
¼ teaspoon baking powder	
¼ cup coconut flour	**4** Divide your batter into the lined muffin cups and bake for 15 minutes.
1 mashed ripe banana	
½ cup chopped pecans (optional)	

Per serving: Calories 160 (From Fat 86); Fat 10 g (Saturated 6 g); Cholesterol 92 mg; Sodium 146 mg; Carbohydrate 17 g (Dietary Fiber 2.5 g); Protein 4 g.

Tip: These muffins are great with eggs or just eaten on their own. You can freeze a bunch of these for breakfast on the run.

Recipe courtesy George Bryant, CEO and author of Civilized Caveman Cooking Creations (http://civilizedcavemancooking.com)

Anytime Waffles

Prep time: 15 min • **Cook time:** 5 min • **Yield:** 4 servings

Ingredients	Directions
⅓ **cup unsweetened shredded coconut**	*1* Preheat the oven to 350 degrees. Spread the coconut on a baking sheet in a single layer and toast until golden, about 4 minutes. Remove from the oven and set aside to cool.
1½ **cups almond flour or almond meal**	
½ **teaspoon baking soda**	*2* In a medium bowl, mix the almond flour, baking soda, salt, and cinnamon with a fork. Set aside.
½ **teaspoon salt**	
½ **teaspoon ground cinnamon**	*3* In a large bowl, whisk together the eggs, coconut milk, sweet potato, and vanilla until smooth. Add the toasted coconut and dry ingredients to the wet ingredients and whisk until combined.
5 **large eggs**	
¼ **cup coconut milk**	
¾ **cup cooked sweet potato, mashed**	*4* Allow the batter to rest for 10 minutes. Meanwhile, pre-heat the waffle iron.
1 **teaspoon pure vanilla extract**	*5* Pour ½ to 1 cup of batter onto the waffle iron, depending on the size of your model. If you're not sure, use the smaller amount. Close the lid and allow the batter to cook, about 2 to 3 minutes.
	6 Remove the waffle to a baking sheet and place in the warm oven while you prepare the rest of the waffles. Serve the waffles hot with eggs or other protein and a small amount of honey or pure maple syrup.

Per serving: Calories 450 (From Fat 321); Fat 36 g (Saturated 11 g); Cholesterol 233 mg; Sodium 258 mg; Carbohydrate 10 g (Dietary Fiber 7 g); Protein 18 g.

Note: You may substitute unsweetened, canned sweet potatoes for fresh sweet potatoes.

Tip: Almond meal and almond flour are simply very finely ground almonds. You can find almond flour in the baking aisle of most grocery or health food stores; you can also purchase it online.

Vary It! Substitute a ripe, mashed banana for the sweet potato and add ¼ cup chopped pecans for banana-nut waffles.

Lime-Blueberry Poppy Seed Coffee Cake

Prep time: 10 min • **Cook time:** 40 min • **Yield:** 12 servings

Ingredients	Directions
½ cup coconut flour	**1** Preheat the oven to 350 degrees.
½ teaspoon salt	
¼ teaspoon baking soda	**2** In a small bowl, mix coconut flour, salt, and baking soda with a fork. Set aside.
6 eggs	
½ cup coconut oil, melted	**3** In a large bowl, whisk eggs, coconut oil, honey, vanilla, lime zest, and lime juice until smooth. Stir in the flour mixture, poppy seeds, and blueberries until just combined.
¼ cup honey	
½ tablespoon pure vanilla extract	
Zest of 1 lime	**4** Grease an 8-x-8-inch square pan with coconut oil, and then dust with coconut flour. Pour the batter into the pan and spread into the corners with a rubber scraper. Bake until lightly golden and a toothpick inserted in the center comes out clean, about 35 to 40 minutes.
2 tablespoons lime juice	
1½ tablespoons poppy seeds	
1¼ cup fresh blueberries (or frozen, defrosted)	**5** Cool the cake in the pan, and then cut into 12 squares. Store covered in the refrigerator or at room temperature.

Per serving: Calories 170 (From Fat 115); Fat 13 g (Saturated 9 g); Cholesterol 106 mg; Sodium 165 mg; Carbohydrate 11 g (Dietary Fiber 3 g); Protein 4 g.

Vary It! Substitute raspberries or strawberries for the blueberries — or replace the lime juice and zest with lemon.

Frozen Blueberry Breakfast Bars

Prep time: 20 min, plus freezing time • **Cook time:** 15–20 min • **Yield:** 10 servings

Ingredients	Directions
Blueberry Topping (see the following recipe)	**1** Preheat the oven to 350 degrees and line an 8-x-8-inch baking pan with parchment paper, making sure the paper covers all four sides of the pan.
½ **cup almonds**	
1 cup pecans	**2** In a food processor, chop the almonds, pecans, and macadamia nuts until they're coarse ground.
½ **cup macadamia nuts**	
½ **cup coconut flour**	**3** Add the coconut flour, arrowroot powder, baking soda, and salt, and then pulse to combine. Add the coconut oil, coconut milk, honey, and vanilla and process until the ingredients clump together and form the dough.
2 teaspoons arrowroot powder	
1 teaspoon baking soda	
⅛ **teaspoon salt**	
½ **cup coconut oil, melted**	**4** Press the dough evenly on the bottom of the prepared pan and bake until the edges and top start to turn golden brown, about 15 to 20 minutes. Set the pan to cool on a wire rack.
2 tablespoons full-fat coconut milk	
2 tablespoons raw honey	**5** Pour the Blueberry Topping evenly over the cooled crust and freeze until firm. Cut into bars and sprinkle the top with blueberries.
1 teaspoon vanilla extract	
Blueberries for garnish	**6** Allow the bars to sit at room temperature for about 10 minutes before serving. Store leftovers in the freezer.

Blueberry Topping

2 cups frozen blueberries, thawed

⅓ cup chopped bananas

1 tablespoon coconut oil, melted

1 teaspoon lime juice

Cream from one 13.5-ounce can full-fat coconut milk

1 Puree the blueberries, bananas, coconut oil, and lime juice in a food processor.

2 Using a stand mixer or hand mixer, mix the blueberry mixture and the coconut milk cream until fluffy and fully combined.

Per serving: Calories 342 (From Fat 270); Fat 31 (Saturated 14 g); Cholesterol 0 mg; Sodium 171 mg; Carbohydrate 18 g (Dietary Fiber 5 g); Protein 4 g.

Note: The cream from a can of coconut milk is what you get when you refrigerate a can of full-fat coconut milk overnight and scoop out what forms at the top of the can, discarding the water.

Chapter 2

Packing Nutrition into Soups and Salads

In This Chapter

▶ Warmth and satisfaction from stove to spoon

▶ Flavor-packed salads for maximizing meals

Recipes in This Chapter

▶ Deep Healing Chicken Broth

↻ Immune-Building Vegetable Broth

▶ Coconut Curry Chowder

▶ Turkey Spinach Soup

▶ Curried Cream of Broccoli Soup

▶ Chicken Fennel Soup

▶ Bacon Butternut Squash Soup

↻ Provençal Veggie Soup

↻ Tomato Fennel Soup

▶ Teriyaki-Turkey Meatball Soup

▶ Thai Butternut Squash Soup

▶ Hearty Chili

↻ Watermelon Soup

▶ Kale with a Kick Salad

▶ Avocado and Egg Salad

↻ Tuscan Spinach Salad

▶ Curried Chicken Salad

▶ Mango and Fennel Chicken Salad

▶ Simple Crab Salad

↻ Turkish Chopped Salad

▶ Waldorf Tuna Salad

↻ Chopped Salad with Tahini Dressing

↻ Vietnamese Cucumber Salad

▶ Chinese Chicken Salad

↻ Classic Cole Slaw

🍴🥄🍲🌶🥕

Soups and salads are fantastic for their *nutritional density,* meaning they have tons of nutrition packed into their calories. Nutritionally dense foods are ideal to get a lean, strong body.

Soups are so comforting, grounding, and healing — and if you get a good bowl, you leave the table feeling as if you've had an experience. Salads bring crunch and flavor that's as appealing as it is valuable: the nutrients, water content, and fiber leave your skin glowing, your hair shiny, your eyes bright, and your body clean.

The soups and salads you find here are filled with flavor, easy to prepare, and easy on the wallet.

If you have digestive problems like irritable bowel syndrome (IBS), inflammatory bowel disease (IBD), celiac disease, Crohn's disease, leaky gut, colitis, diverticulitis, diverticulosis, or ulcerative colitis, raw vegetables can irritate your gut. Well-cooked vegetables are a better choice for you until your gut begins to heal — and it will.

Making Your Own Savory Soups, and Buying Wisely When You Can't

You're giving yourself more of what you need if you use the recipes in this chapter instead of buying ready-to-eat soups or broths at the grocery store. But if you find yourself in a situation where you have to buy ready-made soup or broth, you can still ensure that you're getting the best ingredients and none of the bad stuff.

Most canned soups contain gluten, preservatives, monosodium glutamate (MSG), and high sodium levels. Be extra careful to check labels and watch for sneaky names for wheat/gluten or MSG that often find their way into the broths:

✔ **Sneaky names for wheat and gluten:** If the following ingredients appear on a label, the food may contain wheat and/or gluten:

- Artificial flavoring

- Bleached flour

- Caramel color

- Dextrin

- Flavorings

- Hydrolyzed plant protein (HPP)

- Hydrolyzed vegetable protein (HVP)

- Hydrolyzed wheat protein

- Hydrolyzed wheat starch

- Malt

- Maltodextrin

- Modified food starch

- Natural flavoring

- Seasonings

- Soy sauce

- Vegetable protein

- Vegetable starch

- Wheat germ oil

- Wheat grass

- Wheat protein

- Wheat starch

✔ **Sneaky names for MSG:** If the following ingredients appear on a label, the food contains MSG:

- Any "flavors" or "flavoring"

- Any hydrolyzed protein

- Anything hydrolyzed

- Anything ultra-pasteurized

- Autolyzed yeast

- Barley malt

- Calcium caseinate

- Calcium glutamate

- Carrageenan

- Citrate

- Citric acid

- Gelatin

- Glutamate

- Glutamic acid

- Magnesium glutamate

- Malt extract

- Maltodextrin

- Monoammonium glutamate

- Monopotassium glutamate

- Monosodium glutamate

- Natrium glutamate

- Pectin

- Protease

- Sodium caseinate

- Soy protein

- Soy protein concentrate

- Soy protein isolate
- Soy sauce
- Soy sauce extract
- Textured protein
- Whey protein
- Whey protein concentrate
- Whey protein isolate
- Yeast extract
- Yeast food
- Yeast nutrient

Seizing the Versatility of the Salad

Salads are one of those foods that just have to be redefined. They're far from being a boring, tasteless sidekick to a main meal. You can experiment with all different kinds of lettuce bases, like romaine, mesclun, spinach, or kale. You can spice up salads with exotic, fiery, or sweet spices and add any protein from meat to fish to eggs.

Salads are also the perfect food to tote along to a picnic or potluck. You can make a bright, beautiful display with a special dressing. (For Paleo-friendly dressing options, check out Book III, Chapter 2.)

You can find more great Paleo salad recipes online at www.dummies.com/extras/paleocookbook.

Deep Healing Chicken Broth

Prep time: 5 min • **Cook time:** 11 hr • **Yield:** Six 1-cup servings

Ingredients	*Directions*
4-pound roasting chicken	**1** Rinse and pat the chicken dry. Place it in the slow cooker, season with the salt and pepper, and cook for 3 hours on high.
½ teaspoon salt	
¼ teaspoon ground black pepper	
¼ cup roughly chopped onions	**2** Remove the chicken from the slow cooker and let it cool enough that you can handle it. Take all the chicken off the bones; refrigerate or freeze the chicken for future use.
¼ cup roughly chopped celery	
¼ cup roughly chopped carrots	**3** Return the bones and skin to the slow cooker and add the onions, celery, carrots, and rosemary.
½ teaspoon dried rosemary	
	4 Fill the slow cooker about two-thirds full with water (just enough to cover the carcass and bones, about 6 cups).
	5 Cook on low for 8 hours. Before using, strain the broth and discard the bones, skin, cooked vegetables, and rosemary.

Per serving: Calories 20 (From Fat 9); Fat 1 g (Saturated 0 g); Cholesterol 0 mg; Sodium 574 mg; Carbohydrate 1 g (Dietary Fiber 0 g); Protein 2.5 g.

Tip: If you buy a precooked roasted chicken, you can skip Step 1 and prepare this recipe before going to bed to wake up to a beautiful, delicious broth.

This recipe has been vetted by the team at Whole9 (http://whole9life.com) and is considered acceptable for a cleansing 30-day Paleo launch.

Immune-Building Vegetable Broth

Prep time: 15 min • **Cook time:** 2 hr, 15 min • **Yield:** 6 servings

Ingredients	*Directions*
6 unpeeled carrots, scrubbed and roughly chopped	*1* Put the vegetables and the garlic in a large stockpot, and add enough water to cover everything by 1 inch (about 10 cups). Cover the pot and bring to a boil.
8 stalks celery, including leafy part, roughly chopped	
2 unpeeled onions, roughly chopped	*2* Remove the lid, turn the heat to low, and simmer uncovered for about 2 hours. If the veggies start to show above the water line, add more water. Carefully skim any foam off the top as the broth simmers.
2 unpeeled large sweet potatoes, scrubbed and quartered	
1 unpeeled garnet sweet potato, scrubbed and quartered	
8 cloves garlic	
1 bunch cilantro, including stems, chopped	
½ cup chopped fresh flat-leaf parsley	
One 8-inch piece of kombu (seaweed)	
14 peppercorns	
4 dried allspice berries	
2 dried bay leaves	
Sea salt to taste	
Fresh lemon juice to taste	

3 Add the cilantro, parsley, kombu, peppercorns, allspice berries, and bay leaves during the last 10 minutes of cooking. Strain the broth through cheesecloth in a large bowl.

4 When the broth is cool, check the seasoning; add the salt and lemon juice as needed. Completely cool the broth before refrigerating or freezing.

Per serving: Calories 98 (From Fat 9); Fat 1 g (Saturated 0 g); Cholesterol 0 mg; Sodium 115 mg; Carbohydrate 23 g (Dietary Fiber 5 g); Protein 2.5 g.

Note: This broth is for healing. It's loaded with minerals and healing agents — perfect for when you have a cold or feel one coming on. You can use it as your base for all your soups to keep your immune system humming. Make a big batch and keep some in containers in your freezer; you never know when you'll need some!

Tip: Garnet sweet potatoes have darker flesh than regular sweet potatoes.

Vary It! Instead of the allspice berries and bay leaf, you can make this broth with some ginger or turmeric for a nice healing tonic. Rosemary and oregano are nice too.

This recipe has been vetted by the team at Whole9 (http://whole9life.com) and is considered acceptable for a cleansing 30-day Paleo launch.

Coconut Curry Chowder

Prep time: 15 min • **Cook time:** 25 min • **Yield:** 6 servings

Ingredients	Directions
1 onion	*1* Preheat the oven to 400 degrees.
3 small sweet potatoes	
4 tablespoons coconut oil, divided	*2* Peel and slice the onion into thin slices about 1 inch long. Chop the sweet potatoes into ½-inch cubes. Set aside.
1 teaspoon garlic powder	
1 teaspoon ground ginger	*3* Place 2 tablespoons of the coconut oil into a 9-x-9-inch baking pan and melt in the oven until the coconut oil is liquid, about 2 minutes.
1 teaspoon salt	
1 pound haddock filets	*4* Remove the pan from the oven; add the garlic powder, ginger, and salt, stirring to combine. Dip the haddock in the oil mixture so all sides are evenly coated and bake the fish in the pan for 15 minutes.
2 tablespoons green curry paste	
2 strips bacon, cooked and chopped	*5* While the fish is baking, add the remaining coconut oil to a medium stockpot over high heat. Add the onions and stir continuously until caramelized and translucent, about 2 minutes.
One 14.5-ounce can coconut milk	
4 cups chicken broth	*6* Stir in the green curry paste and add the sweet potatoes, bacon, coconut milk, and broth. Reduce the heat to medium and simmer for 20 minutes.

7 Remove the fish from the oven and test for doneness by flaking the flesh with a fork. If it flakes easily, flake all the fish into bite-sized pieces and add them and the oil into the soup pot.

8 Stir gently for about 5 minutes and taste.

Per serving: *Calories 431 (From Fat 270); Fat 30 g (Saturated 24 g); Cholesterol 43 mg; Sodium 1,346 mg; Carbohydrate 24 g (Dietary Fiber 4 g); Protein 20 g.*

Tip: You can substitute another mild white fish for the haddock. We recommend the Thai Kitchen brand of green curry paste.

Recipe courtesy Audrey Olson, author of Primal Kitchen: A Family Grokumentary (`www.primalkitchen.blogspot.com`)

This recipe has been vetted by the team at Whole9 (`http://whole9life.com`) and is considered acceptable for a cleansing 30-day Paleo launch.

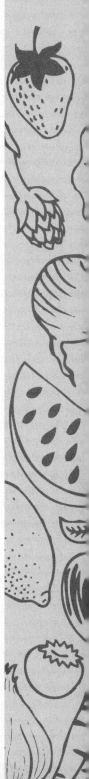

Turkey Spinach Soup

Prep time: 10 min • **Cook time:** 25 min • **Yield:** 4 servings

Ingredients	Directions
2 tablespoons coconut oil 1 medium onion, diced 2 cloves garlic, minced 1 pound ground turkey 1 tablespoon coconut aminos 10 cups chicken broth ¼ teaspoon salt ¼ teaspoon ground black pepper 4 cups fresh spinach leaves, coarsely chopped Fresh rosemary (optional)	*1* Heat the coconut oil in a large stockpot over high heat. Add the onion and garlic and sauté for 2 minutes. Add the ground turkey and sauté for an additional 7 minutes. *2* Add the coconut aminos. Stir frequently for 2 minutes. *3* Add the chicken broth, salt, and pepper. Simmer for about 20 minutes. *4* Add the spinach and rosemary (if desired) and sauté for 2 minutes. Serve.

Per serving: Calories 347 (From Fat 126); Fat 14 g (Saturated 8 g); Cholesterol 81 mg; Sodium 650 mg; Carbohydrate 6 g (Dietary Fiber 1.5 g); Protein 50 g.

Recipe courtesy Audrey Olson, author of Primal Kitchen: A Family Grokumentary (www.primalkitchen.blogspot.com)

This recipe has been vetted by the team at Whole9 (http://whole9life.com) and is considered acceptable for a cleansing 30-day Paleo launch.

Curried Cream of Broccoli Soup

Prep time: 20 min • **Cook time:** 40 min • **Yield:** 6 servings

Ingredients	Directions
2 tablespoons coconut oil or ghee	*1* Melt the coconut oil or ghee over medium heat in a large stockpot. Add the leeks, onions, and shallots and sauté until softened, stirring frequently.
4 leeks, white and light green parts, washed and thinly sliced	
1 large onion, diced	*2* Add the broccoli, apple, and broth, topping off with water if the vegetables aren't fully submerged. Crank the heat to high, bring the soup to a boil, and then lower the heat and simmer for 20 minutes or until the vegetables are soft.
3 medium shallots, diced	
2 pounds broccoli florets	
¼ medium apple, diced	*3* Stir in the curry powder and season with salt and pepper to taste.
1 quart Deep Healing Chicken Broth (see recipe earlier in this chapter)	
1 tablespoon curry powder	*4* Turn off the heat and let the soup cool slightly. Use an immersion blender to puree the ingredients into a smooth broth.
Kosher salt to taste	
Ground black pepper to taste	*5* Stir the coconut milk into the soup until incorporated. Bring the soup back to a boil over high heat and ladle into serving bowls.
1 cup coconut milk	

Per serving: Calories 265 (From Fat 158); Fat 18 g (Saturated 12 g); Cholesterol 14 mg; Sodium 104 mg; Carbohydrate 23 g (Dietary Fiber 7 g); Protein 9 g.

*Recipe courtesy Michelle Tam, author of Nom Nom Paleo (*http://nomnompaleo.com*)*

*This recipe has been vetted by the team at Whole9 (*http://whole9life.com*) and is considered acceptable for a cleansing 30-day Paleo launch.*

Chicken Fennel Soup

Prep time: 15 min • **Cook time:** 30 min • **Yield:** 4 servings

Ingredients	Directions
2 tablespoons ghee or grass-fed butter	**1** In a large stockpot, heat the ghee or butter over medium heat. Add the onions and chicken and sauté until the onions are translucent, about 3 minutes.
1 white onion, diced	
1 pound boneless, skinless chicken thighs or chicken breasts, chopped	**2** Add the fennel and sauté until it's softened and the chicken is partly cooked through, about 4 minutes. Add the celery, garlic, and carrots and sauté for a few minutes until fragrant.
1 fennel bulb, diced	
3 stalks celery, chopped	
3 cloves garlic, crushed	**3** Add the salt, pepper, basil, dried parsley, and stock. Bring to a boil and then simmer for 25 minutes.
2 carrots, chopped	
1 teaspoon salt	**4** Top with the fresh parsley and serve.
1 teaspoon ground black pepper	
1 teaspoon dried basil	
1 teaspoon dried parsley	
4 cups Deep Healing Chicken Broth (see recipe earlier in this chapter)	
Fresh parsley for garnish	

Per serving: Calories 420 (From Fat 279); Fat 31 g (Saturated 7 g); Cholesterol 138 mg; Sodium 630 mg; Carbohydrate 6 g (Dietary Fiber 2 g); Protein 33 g.

Recipe courtesy Arsy Vartanian, author of Rubies & Radishes (www.rubiesandradishes.com)

This recipe has been vetted by the team at Whole9 (http://whole9life.com) and is considered acceptable for a cleansing 30-day Paleo launch.

Bacon Butternut Squash Soup

Prep time: 15 min • **Cook time:** 1 hr • **Yield:** 6 servings

Ingredients	*Directions*
1 large butternut squash, peeled and cut into large chunks	*1* Preheat the oven to 350 degrees.
3 carrots, peeled and cut into large chunks	*2* Toss the squash and carrots with the coconut oil. Arrange the mixture in a baking dish and roast uncovered for 35 minutes or until tender.
1½ tablespoons coconut oil, melted	
½ pound bacon	*3* In a large stockpot or Dutch oven, cook the bacon over medium heat until crisp. Drain on paper towels and set aside. Sauté the onion and apple in the bacon fat until tender, about 5 minutes.
1 small onion, chopped	
1 small apple, peeled and chopped	
3 cups chicken stock	*4* Add the squash, carrots, chicken stock, and coconut milk and bring to a boil, stirring often.
1 cup coconut milk	
1 teaspoon salt	*5* Remove the pot from the heat and use an immersion blender to blend your soup until smooth. (Alternately, you can blend the soup in a food processor or blender in several small batches and return it to the pot.)
1 to 2 tablespoons ground cinnamon to taste	
1 tablespoon ground nutmeg	
	6 Bring the blended soup to a simmer and season with the salt, cinnamon, and nutmeg. Serve in large bowls garnished with crumbled bacon or freeze and save for later.

Per serving: Calories 396 (From Fat 248); Fat 28 g (Saturated 15 g); Cholesterol 42 mg; Sodium 1,574 mg; Carbohydrate 21 g (Dietary Fiber 2.5 g); Protein 19 g.

Recipe courtesy George Bryant, CEO and author of Civilized Caveman Cooking Creations (http://civilizedcavemancooking.com)

This recipe has been vetted by the team at Whole9 (http://whole9life.com) and is considered acceptable for a cleansing 30-day Paleo launch.

Provençal Veggie Soup

Prep time: 20 min • **Cook time:** 30 min • **Yield:** 4 servings

Ingredients	Directions
1 tablespoon ghee	**1** Heat the ghee in a large stockpot. Add the leeks and sauté until soft, about 7 to 8 minutes.
2 medium leeks, white and light green parts, washed and chopped	
4 medium carrots, peeled and chopped	**2** Add the carrots, celery, and garlic and sauté until fragrant, about 5 minutes.
2 stalks celery, chopped	
4 cloves garlic, crushed	**3** Add the remaining vegetables, the vegetable stock, and the herbs. Bring to a boil and then simmer uncovered for 30 minutes or until the vegetables are tender.
2 medium zucchini, chopped	
2 medium summer squash, chopped	**4** Add salt and pepper to taste before serving.
6 ripe tomatoes, peeled, seeded, and chopped	
6 cups vegetable broth	
3 sprigs fresh thyme	
¼ cup chopped fresh basil	
2 tablespoons chopped fresh parsley	
Salt and pepper to taste	

Per serving: Calories 196 (From Fat 42); Fat 4.5 g (Saturated 2.5 g); Cholesterol 9 mg; Sodium 686 mg; Carbohydrate 30 g (Dietary Fiber 6 g); Protein 4 g.

Tip: If you can't get your hands on any fresh tomatoes, substitute jarred diced tomatoes.

Recipe courtesy Arsy Vartanian, author of Rubies & Radishes (www.rubiesandradishes.com)

This recipe has been vetted by the team at Whole9 (http://whole9life.com) and is considered acceptable for a cleansing 30-day Paleo launch.

Tomato Fennel Soup

Prep time: 20 min • **Cook time:** 30 min • **Yield:** 4 servings

Ingredients	Directions
1 tablespoon ghee 3 shallots, chopped	*1* Heat the ghee in a large stockpot. Add the shallots and sauté until softened, about 5 minutes.
3 cloves garlic, crushed 2 bulbs fennel, chopped	*2* Add the garlic and fennel; cook another 3 to 5 minutes until the garlic is fragrant.
8 cups chopped fresh tomatoes Juice of 1 lemon ½ teaspoon dried basil 4 cups vegetable broth	*3* Add the rest of the ingredients and bring to a boil. Lower to a simmer and cook uncovered for 30 minutes.
Salt and pepper to taste	*4* Add salt and pepper to taste before serving.

Per serving: Calories 258 (From Fat 51); Fat 6 g (Saturated 2 g); Cholesterol 9 mg; Sodium 1,283 mg; Carbohydrate 44 g (Dietary Fiber 8 g); Protein 6 g.

Tip: If fresh tomatoes aren't in season, substitute jarred diced tomatoes.

Recipe courtesy Arsy Vartanian, author of Rubies & Radishes (www.rubiesandradishes.com)

This recipe has been vetted by the team at Whole9 (http://whole9life.com) and is considered acceptable for a cleansing 30-day Paleo launch.

Teriyaki-Turkey Meatball Soup

Prep time: 10 min • **Cook time:** 15 min • **Yield:** 4 servings

Ingredients	Directions
1 pound ground turkey	*1* In a large bowl, mix the turkey with the cayenne pepper, salt, pineapple, coconut aminos, dried ginger, garlic, and egg. Measure a level tablespoon of turkey and roll into a meatball shape. If the meat sticks to your hands, wet your hands with water between rolling. Set meatballs aside.
½ teaspoon ground cayenne pepper	
¼ teaspoon salt	
½ cup canned crushed pineapple (sugar-free, packed in its own juice), drained well	
1 tablespoon coconut aminos	*2* With the bottom of a glass or the handle of a heavy knife, smash the ginger slices to release their flavor. Place them in a large pot and add the broth; bring to a boil over medium-high heat.
½ teaspoon dried ginger	
1 clove garlic, minced	
1 large egg, lightly beaten	
2-inch piece fresh ginger, cut into ½-inch slices	*3* Reduce the heat to simmer and add the meatballs. Simmer, covered, until the meatballs are cooked through, about 8 minutes. Season with salt and pepper to taste and add the spinach. Cook uncovered until the spinach is just wilted, about 2 minutes.
8 to 10 cups chicken broth	
8 cups fresh spinach leaves, coarsely chopped	
Salt and pepper to taste	*4* Serve in deep bowls and sprinkle with scallions and sesame seeds (if desired).
3 to 4 scallions, white and green, very thinly sliced	
1 tablespoon sesame seeds, toasted (optional)	

Per serving: Calories 333 (From Fat 182); Fat 20 g (Saturated 5 g); Cholesterol 139 mg; Sodium 2,469 mg; Carbohydrate 10 g; (Dietary Fiber 2 g); Protein 28 g.

Vary It! Substitute ground pork for the ground turkey. You may also substitute other greens for the spinach. Collard greens, Swiss chard, kale, and escarole are all good choices.

Thai Butternut Squash Soup

Prep time: 10 min • **Cook time:** 40 min • **Yield:** 4 servings

Ingredients	Directions
One 14.5-ounce can coconut milk, divided	**1** Open the can of coconut milk and scoop out about 2 tablespoons of the coconut cream that has risen to the top. Place in a small bowl and mix with the red curry paste until combined. Cover and set aside. Reserve remaining coconut milk in can.
One 4-ounce jar Thai Kitchen red curry paste	
1 tablespoon coconut oil	
2 medium onions, finely chopped	**2** Heat a large, deep pot over medium-high heat, and add the coconut oil. When the oil is melted, stir in the onions with a wooden spoon and cook until they're translucent, about 7 minutes.
4 cloves garlic, minced	
2 tablespoons minced fresh ginger	
1 teaspoon peppercorns	**3** Add the garlic, fresh ginger, peppercorns, lemongrass, and cumin. Cook, stirring, for 30 seconds, and then add the squash, chicken broth, coconut milk, and chicken to the pot. Bring to a boil.
2 stalks lemongrass, trimmed, smashed, and cut in half crosswise	
1 tablespoon ground cumin	**4** Reduce the heat to simmer and cook, covered, until the squash is tender and the chicken is cooked through, about 30 minutes. Remove the lemongrass and chicken from the pot. Place the chicken in a bowl to cool; when cool enough to handle, shred with two forks and set aside.
1 large butternut squash, seeds removed and cut into 2-inch cubes	
6 cups chicken broth	
1 pound boneless, skinless chicken breasts	**5** Add the curry paste to the soup pot, along with the lime zest and lime juice. Stir to combine. Then, working in batches, carefully puree the soup in a food processor or blender and return to the pot until heated through.
Zest of 1 lime	
Juice of 1 lime	
1 cup fresh cilantro leaves, coarsely chopped	**6** Ladle the soup into bowls and sprinkle with the shredded chicken, chopped cilantro, and additional fresh lime juice.

Per serving: Calories 515 (From Fat 311); Fat 35 g (Saturated 25 g); Cholesterol 70 mg; Sodium 2,088 mg; Carbohydrate 26 g (Dietary Fiber 7 g); Protein 29 g.

Note: You can find Thai red curry paste in most grocery stores and online retailers. The Thai Kitchen brand is sugar-free and Paleo friendly.

Hearty Chili

Prep time: 20 min • **Cook time:** 2 hr • **Yield:** 8 servings

Ingredients	Directions
2 tablespoons coconut oil	**1** Heat a large, deep pot over medium-high heat, and add the coconut oil. When the oil is melted, add the onions, bell peppers, and jalapeño. Stir with a wooden spoon and cook until the vegetables are tender, about 7 minutes.
2 medium onions, diced	
2 green bell peppers, diced	
1 fresh jalapeño, diced	
4 cloves garlic, minced (about 4 teaspoons)	**2** Add the garlic, and as soon as it's fragrant (about 30 seconds), crumble the ground meat into the pan with your hands, mixing with the wooden spoon to combine. Continue to cook the meat, stirring often, until it's no longer pink.
1 pound ground beef	
1 pound ground pork	
1 teaspoon dried oregano leaves	**3** In a small bowl, crush the oregano between your palms to release its flavor, and add the chili powder, cumin, and salt. Combine with a fork and then add to the pot, along with the tomato paste. Stir until combined, about 2 minutes.
3 tablespoons chili powder	
2 tablespoons ground cumin	
1 teaspoon salt	
One 6-ounce can tomato paste	**4** Add the chopped tomatoes with their juice, beef broth, and water to the pot. Stir well. Bring to a boil; reduce the heat and simmer, uncovered, for 2 hours.
One 14.5-ounce can chopped tomatoes	
One 14.5-ounce can beef broth	**5** Serve in deep bowls and top with garnishes.
1 cup water	
Garnishes: diced red onion and avocado; minced fresh cilantro leaves	

Per serving: Calories 387 (From Fat 176); Fat 20 g (Saturated 9 g); Cholesterol 73 mg; Sodium 670 mg; Carbohydrate 12 g (Dietary Fiber 4 g); Protein 25 g.

Note: This dish freezes well, so make a double batch for chili any time.

Watermelon Soup

Prep time: 10 min, plus chilling time • **Yield:** 6 servings

Ingredients	*Directions*
5 cups seeded and cubed watermelon, divided	*1* Blend 3 cups of the watermelon and 1 cup of the mango in a food processor or blender until smooth.
2 cups peeled and diced mango, divided	*2* Dice the remaining watermelon and mango into smaller pieces and stir into the puree. The soup should be chunky.
¼ cup lime juice	
3 tablespoons chopped fresh mint	*3* In a separate bowl, combine the lime juice, mint, ginger, honey, and cardamom. Add to the watermelon mixture and stir well.
1 tablespoon fresh ginger, minced	
1 tablespoon honey	*4* Chill for at least 2 hours and serve.
¼ teaspoon ground	
⅛ cardamom	

Per serving: *Calories 85 (From Fat 4.5); Fat 0.5 g (Saturated 0 g); Cholesterol 0 mg; Sodium 2.5 mg; Carbohydrate 22 g (Dietary Fiber 1.5 g); Protein 1.5 g.*

Recipe courtesy Alissa Cohen, chef and author of Living on Live Food (www.alissacohen.com)

Kale with a Kick Salad

Prep time: 10 min • **Cook time:** 4 min • **Yield:** 6 servings

Ingredients	*Directions*
2 strips bacon	*1* In a medium skillet, fry the bacon until crispy (about 4 minutes). Transfer it to several layers of paper towels to drain, blotting slightly. Chop the bacon into small pieces.
1 cup diced avocado	
½ cup diced red onion	
1 cup diced tomato	
One 8-ounce bunch kale, ribs removed and leaves chopped	*2* In a mixing bowl, toss all the ingredients together, squeezing and massaging the kale as you mix to wilt the kale and cream the avocado.
2½ teaspoons olive oil	
1½ teaspoons fresh lemon juice	*3* If possible, let the mixture sit for 30 minutes for the best flavor. Otherwise, go ahead and indulge right away!
½ teaspoon cayenne pepper	
1 teaspoon Celtic sea salt	

Per serving: Calories 118 (From Fat 36); Fat 7 g (Saturated 1.5 g); Cholesterol 3 mg; Sodium 309 mg; Carbohydrate 12 g (Dietary Fiber 4 g); Protein 4.5 g.

Note: Kale provides a rich supply of disease-fighting nutrients. It also makes your skin glow and your eyes shine! Red kale is our favorite for this recipe.

Note: Celtic sea salt is a highly nutritious salt because it's unrefined and full of minerals. You can purchase it at Whole Foods or from online retailers such as Amazon or www.celticseasalt.com. Otherwise, any unrefined sea salt will do just fine!

This recipe has been vetted by the team at Whole9 (http://whole9life.com) and is considered acceptable for a cleansing 30-day Paleo launch.

Avocado and Egg Salad

Prep time: 10 min • **Cook time:** 8–10 min • **Yield:** 6 servings

Ingredients	Directions
10 eggs	**1** Place the eggs in a large pot and cover with cold water. Bring to a gentle boil and then turn off the heat and cover the pot with a lid. Let the eggs sit for 15 minutes.
2 ripe avocadoes, peeled, pitted, and diced	
1 tablespoon stone-ground mustard	**2** Drain the eggs and place in a bowl of ice water until they're cool enough to handle. Shell and dice the eggs and place them in a large bowl with the avocado. Mix together, mashing the avocado slightly.
3 tablespoons fresh lemon juice	
1 tablespoon minced fresh dill	
2 tablespoons minced fresh parsley	**3** Combine the remaining ingredients with the egg mixture until mixed through. Add salt and pepper to taste.
1 teaspoon paprika	
Salt and pepper to taste	
Chopped tomatoes for garnish (optional)	**4** Top with the chopped tomatoes, if desired, and serve.

Per serving: Calories 212 (From Fat 144); Fat 16 g (Saturated 4 g); Cholesterol 310 mg; Sodium 108 mg; Carbohydrate 6 g (Dietary Fiber 3.5 g); Protein 12 g.

Tip: This avocado/egg salad is a perfect recipe for an on-the-go-breakfast, wrapped in lettuce for lunch, or as a quick snack.

Tip: We recommend the Organicville brand mustard.

Recipe courtesy Arsy Vartanian, author of Rubies & Radishes (www.rubiesandradishes.com)

This recipe has been vetted by the team at Whole9 (http://whole9life.com) and is considered acceptable for a cleansing 30-day Paleo launch.

Tuscan Spinach Salad

Prep time: 10 min • **Cook time:** 10 min • **Yield:** 4 servings

Ingredients	*Directions*
2 eggs	*1* Place the eggs in a saucepan and cover with cold water. Bring to a gentle boil and then turn off the heat and cover the pot with a lid. Let the eggs sit for 10 minutes.
2 cups baby spinach	
1 cup chopped fresh basil	
3 tablespoons olive oil	*2* Drain the eggs and place in a bowl of ice water until they're cool enough to handle. Remove the shells and roughly chop the eggs.
1 red onion, chopped	
1 tablespoon chopped fresh oregano	
⅓ cup lemon juice	*3* Combine the eggs and the remaining ingredients in a large bowl and serve.
2 tablespoons chopped black olives	
1 avocado, peeled, pitted, and diced	

Per serving: Calories 211 (From Fat 166); Fat 19 g (Saturated 3 g); Cholesterol 93 mg; Sodium 87 mg; Carbohydrate 8 g (Dietary Fiber 3.5 g); Protein 5 g.

Vary It! You can substitute any protein you love for the hard-boiled eggs.

This recipe has been vetted by the team at Whole9 (`http://whole9life.com`) and is considered acceptable for a cleansing 30-day Paleo launch.

Curried Chicken Salad

Prep time: 25 min • **Yield:** 4 servings

Ingredients	Directions
1 pound boneless, skinless chicken breast halves, cooked and diced	**1** In a large bowl, combine everything but the avocado. Add salt and pepper to taste.
½ cup Paleo mayonnaise (see recipe in Book III, Chapter 2)	**2** Cut each avocado in half, remove the pit, and top each half with the chicken salad.
¼ cup dried apricots, minced	
⅛ cup dried cranberries, minced	
½ small Gala apple, diced	
2 tablespoons chives, minced	
½ stalk celery, diced	
1 tablespoon minced scallion, white part only	
2 tablespoons minced red onion	
1 teaspoon mild curry powder	
Salt and pepper to taste	
2 avocadoes	

Per serving: Calories 581 (From Fat 339); Fat 38 g (Saturated 6 g); Cholesterol 114 mg; Sodium 263 mg; Carbohydrate 22 g (Dietary Fiber 7 g); Protein 40 g.

Recipe courtesy Arsy Vartanian, author of Rubies & Radishes (www.rubiesandradishes.com)

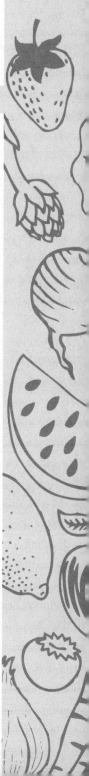

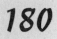

Mango and Fennel Chicken Salad

Prep time: 20 min • **Yield:** 4 servings

Ingredients	Directions
2 boneless, skinless grilled chicken breasts, chopped	*1* In a large bowl, combine the chicken, fennel, scallion, and parsley.
1 small fennel bulb, finely chopped	
2 scallions, chopped	*2* Divide the spinach into 4 servings and top each with the chicken mixture, mango, and avocado.
1 tablespoon minced fresh parsley	
2 cups baby spinach	*3* Drizzle with the vinaigrette.
1 mango, chopped	
1 avocado, peeled, pitted, and diced	
Sweet and Spicy Vinaigrette (see recipe in Book III, Chapter 2)	

Per serving (salad without the dressing): Calories 177 (From Fat 36); Fat 4 g (Saturated 1 g); Cholesterol 52 mg; Sodium 100 mg; Carbohydrate 15 g (Dietary Fiber 4 g); Protein 21 g.

Note: Spinach is a great source of vitamins and minerals, which keeps you in a state of nutrient sufficiency. When you're nutrient sufficient, it's like you have a protective barrier against disease and aging.

Tip: When selecting fresh spinach in the store, look for crisp, evenly colored leaves. If the leaves are still on the stalk, they shouldn't be wilted and should be free of slime and spots.

Recipe courtesy Arsy Vartanian, author of Rubies & Radishes (www.rubiesandradishes.com)

This recipe has been vetted by the team at Whole9 (http://whole9life.com) and is considered acceptable for a cleansing 30-day Paleo launch.

Simple Crab Salad

Prep time: 5 min • **Cook time:** 10 min • **Yield:** 4 servings

Ingredients	Directions
1 pound lump crab meat, drained and picked through	*1* Combine the crab, scallions, parsley, lemon juice, and mayonnaise in a medium bowl. Mix well.
2 scallions, thinly sliced	
2 tablespoons minced fresh Italian parsley	*2* Season with salt and pepper to taste.
1 tablespoon fresh lemon juice	
2 tablespoons Paleo mayonnaise (see recipe in Book III, Chapter 2)	
Kosher salt to taste	
Ground black pepper to taste	

Per serving: Calories 134 (From Fat 41); Fat 8 g (Saturated 1 g); Cholesterol 103 mg; Sodium 642 mg; Carbohydrate 1 g (Dietary Fiber 0 g); Protein 16 g.

Note: Make sure you use real crab for this recipe; imitation crab meats contain gluten.

Tip: You can assemble this quick and easy salad in no time at all; just make sure your fridge is always stocked with Paleo mayonnaise and canned crab. Serve it over salad greens or make a quick appetizer by spooning it into endive spears.

Recipe courtesy Michelle Tam, author of Nom Nom Paleo (http://nomnompaleo.com)

This recipe has been vetted by the team at Whole9 (http://whole9life.com) and is considered acceptable for a cleansing 30-day Paleo launch.

Turkish Chopped Salad

Prep time: 15 min • **Yield:** 6–8 servings

Ingredients	Directions
¼ cup minced fresh parsley leaves	*1* In a medium bowl, combine the parsley, lemon juice, garlic, cumin, paprika, oregano, and sumac (if desired). Whisk until blended and then slowly drizzle in the olive oil. Season with salt and pepper to taste.
Juice of 2 lemons	
1 clove garlic, minced	
¼ teaspoon ground cumin	
¼ teaspoon paprika	*2* Dice all the vegetables to roughly the same size — a ¼-inch dice is nice — and place in a large mixing bowl. Slice the olives and add to the bowl.
¼ teaspoon dried oregano	
¼ teaspoon sumac (optional)	
¼ cup extra-virgin olive oil	*3* Pour the dressing over the salad and toss until the vegetables are coated. Taste and adjust seasonings.
Salt and pepper to taste	
2 medium cucumbers, peeled	
2 medium green peppers, seeded	
3 medium tomatoes	
½ medium red onion	
1 bunch radishes, tops removed	
6 ounces brined ripe black olives, drained	

Per serving: Calories 125 (From Fat 103); Fat 12 g (Saturated 1.5 g); Cholesterol 0 mg; Sodium 166 mg; Carbohydrate 6 g (Dietary Fiber 1.5 g); Protein 1 g.

This recipe has been vetted by the team at Whole9 (http://whole9life.com) and is considered acceptable for a cleansing 30-day Paleo launch.

Waldorf Tuna Salad

Prep time: 5 min, plus standing time • **Yield:** 2 servings

Ingredients	Directions
1 small Gala or Fuji apple, diced	**1** Mix the apple, scallions, nuts, and parsley with a fork in a medium bowl.
2 scallions, dark green tops only, thinly sliced	
2 tablespoons coarsely chopped pecans	**2** Add the tuna, mashing with the fork to break up the tuna until no big chunks remain.
1 tablespoon minced fresh parsley	
Two 5-ounce cans wild-caught tuna in water, drained	**3** Add the mustard powder and mayo to the bowl and mix with a rubber spatula until blended. Allow the tuna salad sit for 15 minutes so the flavors meld, and then taste and adjust the seasonings.
½ teaspoon mustard powder	
3–4 tablespoons Olive Oil Mayo (see recipe in Book III, Chapter 2)	
Salt and pepper to taste	

Per serving: Calories 337 (From Fat 126); Fat 14 g (Saturated 1.5 g); Cholesterol 50 mg; Sodium 665 mg; Carbohydrate 13 g (Dietary Fiber 3 g); Protein 38 g.

Tip: Use wild-caught tuna whenever possible. Vital Choice brand is a good one: www.vitalchoice.com/shop/pc/home.asp.

This recipe has been vetted by the team at Whole9 (http://whole9life.com) and is considered acceptable for a cleansing 30-day Paleo launch.

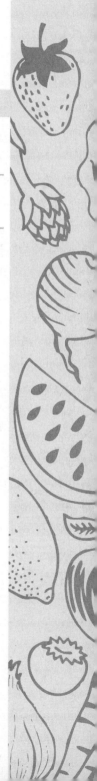

Chopped Salad with Tahini Dressing

Prep time: 15 min • **Yield:** 6–8 servings

Ingredients	Directions
⅓ cup tahini sauce	*1* Place the tahini sauce, lemon juice, water, and garlic in a food processor. Blend until smooth, taste, and season with salt and pepper. Set aside.
⅓ cup lemon juice	
⅓ cup water	
1 garlic clove, crushed	*2* Place the minced parsley in a large bowl. Dice all the vegetables into ¼-inch cubes and add to the parsley. Slice the olives and add to the bowl. Drizzle olive oil over the vegetables, season with salt and pepper, and toss until coated.
Salt and pepper to taste	
1 cup fresh parsley leaves, minced (about ¼ cup)	
2 medium cucumbers, peeled	
1 medium red bell pepper, seeded	*3* Pile the vegetables on individual salad plates and drizzle with 2 tablespoons of the tahini dressing. Store leftover salad and tahini dressing in the refrigerator, covered, for up to three days.
1 medium green bell pepper, seeded	
3 medium tomatoes	
½ medium red onion	
1 bunch radishes	
One 6-ounce can large black pitted olives	
½ tablespoon extra-virgin olive oil	

Per serving: Calories 166 (From Fat 103); Fat 11 g (Saturated 1 g); Cholesterol 0 mg; Sodium 267 mg; Carbohydrate 15 g (Dietary Fiber 3 g); Protein 4 g.

Note: You can find tahini sauce (ground sesame seeds) in the international section of most grocery and health food stores.

Vary It! Just about any raw vegetable works great in this salad. Try adding slivered red cabbage, fresh fennel, or a few hot peppers.

Tip: This salad is a big hit at potluck dinners — just double the recipe and serve the dressing on the side. No one will even notice that it's Paleo.

185

Vietnamese Cucumber Salad

Prep time: 10 min, plus standing time • **Yield:** 4–6 servings

Ingredients	Directions
2 English (seedless) cucumbers	**1** Cut the cucumbers in half lengthwise, and slice into very thin half-moons. Place in a large bowl.
2 medium carrots	
4 medium radishes	**2** Finely dice the carrots, radishes, and jalapeño; add to the cucumbers and toss until combined.
1 small jalapeño	
1 clove garlic, minced	**3** In a medium bowl, place the garlic, cashews, basil, mint, lime juice, rice vinegar, olive oil, and coconut aminos. Whisk until combined.
2 tablespoons dry roasted cashews, finely chopped	
6 to 8 large basil leaves, finely chopped (about 2 tablespoons)	**4** Pour the dressing over the vegetables and toss until evenly coated, about 2 minutes. Taste and season with salt and pepper. Allow flavors to meld for 10 minutes and serve.
10 fresh mint leaves, finely chopped (about 1½ tablespoons)	
1 tablespoon lime juice	
1 tablespoon rice vinegar	
½ teaspoon olive oil	
1 tablespoon coconut aminos	
Salt and pepper to taste	

Per serving: Calories 109 (From Fat 23); Fat 3 g (Saturated 1 g); Cholesterol 0 mg; Sodium 255 mg; Carbohydrate 18 g (Dietary Fiber 3 g); Protein 3 g.

Tip: Add cooked chicken, pork, or shrimp to make this salad a complete meal.

Vary It! Make spring rolls by spreading a butter lettuce leaf with ½ teaspoon Olive Oil Mayonnaise (Book III, Chapter 2). Place a large spoonful of cucumber salad in the leaf and roll to form a spring roll shape.

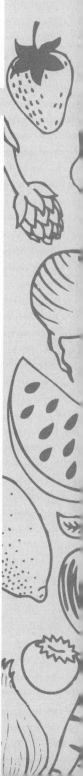

Chinese Chicken Salad

Prep time: 2 hr • **Cook time:** 20 min • **Yield:** 4 servings

Ingredients	Directions
6 cups water, divided	**1** Place a 1-gallon zipper storage bag inside a large bowl. Pour in 4 cups water; add the salt, peppercorns, 3 cloves smashed garlic, and jalapeño. Stir to dissolve salt and add the chicken. Seal the bag and refrigerate for 2 hours.
2 tablespoons salt	
1 teaspoon whole peppercorns	
3 cloves garlic, lightly smashed, plus 1 clove garlic, minced	**2** Rinse the chicken well under running water and place in a single layer in a large pot. Add 2 cups water, bring to a boil, and then reduce the heat to a gentle simmer. Cover and cook for 10 minutes.
1 fresh jalapeño, cut into rings	
1 pound boneless, skinless chicken breast	**3** Turn off the heat, allowing the chicken to sit, covered, another 15 to 20 minutes. When the chicken is cooked, place the chicken in a large bowl and use two forks to shred it.
¼ cup coconut aminos	
¼ cup rice vinegar	
1 tablespoon sesame oil	
1 teaspoon mustard powder	
½ teaspoon ground black pepper	
½ teaspoon crushed red pepper flakes	
¼ teaspoon dried ginger	
¼ cup light-tasting olive oil (not extra-virgin)	
1 pound Napa cabbage, cored and very thinly sliced	

½ pound snow peas, cut into slivers

1 red bell pepper, thinly sliced

3 to 4 scallions, green and white, thinly sliced

2 carrots, grated

½ cup loosely packed cilantro leaves, chopped

¼ cup sliced almonds, toasted (optional)

2 tablespoons sesame seeds, toasted (optional)

4 In a small bowl, whisk the coconut aminos, rice vinegar, sesame oil, 1 clove minced garlic, mustard powder, ground black pepper, red pepper flakes, and ginger until combined. Continue whisking and add oil in a slow, steady stream until combined.

5 Place the cabbage, snow peas, bell pepper, scallions, carrots, cilantro, and chicken in a large bowl. Toss to combine, and then add the dressing and toss well for 2 to 3 minutes until evenly coated. Allow the flavors to meld for 10 minutes before eating. Sprinkle with almonds and sesame seeds, if desired; serve immediately.

Per serving: Calories 463 (From Fat 72); Fat 8 g (Saturated 2 g); Cholesterol 96 mg; Sodium 811 mg; Carbohydrate 49 g (Dietary Fiber 5 g); Protein 40 g.

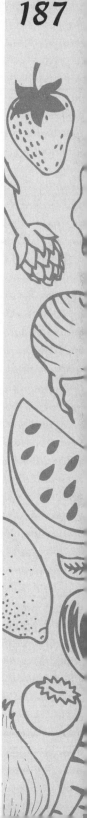

Classic Cole Slaw

Prep time: 15 min, plus standing time • **Yield:** 4 servings

Ingredients	Directions
⅔ cup Olive Oil Mayo (see recipe in Book III, Chapter 2)	**1** In a small bowl, whisk together the Olive Oil Mayo, red onion, lemon juice, vinegar, honey (if desired), salt, and pepper. Set aside.
2 tablespoons grated red onion	
1 tablespoon lemon juice	**2** In a large bowl, toss the cabbage, carrots, and parsley with two wooden spoons. Add the dressing and toss vigorously for 2 minutes to ensure that the vegetables are evenly coated. Cover and refrigerate for at least 1 hour before serving.
1 tablespoon white wine vinegar	
½ tablespoon honey (optional)	
½ teaspoon salt	
¼ teaspoon ground black pepper	
1 head green cabbage, very thinly sliced	
3 large carrots, shredded	
½ cup loosely packed parsley leaves, roughly chopped	

Per serving: Calories 392 (From Fat 287); Fat 32 g (Saturated 2 g); Cholesterol 21 mg; Sodium 513 mg; Carbohydrate 23 g (Dietary Fiber 8 g); Protein 5 g.

Note: To cut the cabbage, slice in half through the stem end. Remove and discard the tough inner core, and then thinly slice the cabbage into long, thin shreds.

Vary It! Add 1 to 2 teaspoons of caraway seeds for a traditional German touch, or make it a little sweeter by adding 1 cup shredded canned pineapple (unsweetened, packed in its own juice) or ⅓ cup raisins. You can also replace the whole head of green cabbage with half a head of green and half a head of red for colorful variety.

Tip: This recipe is easy to double for a potluck or cut in half for a dinner-for-two serving. This slaw tastes better the second day, so make it in advance if time permits.

Chapter 3

The Meat (and More) of the Matter: Paleo Main Dishes

Recipes in This Chapter

▶ Leafy Tacos
▶ Chicken Fingers
▶ Orange Shrimp and Beef with Broccoli
▶ Club Sandwich Salad
▶ Winter Squash and Sausage Hash
▶ Citrus Carnitas
▶ Thai Green Curry Chicken
▶ Tandoori Chicken Thighs
▶ Slow-Roasted Rack of Lamb
▶ Spicy Stuffed Eggplant
▶ Grilled Buffalo Shrimp
▶ Coconut Shrimp with Sweet and Spicy Sauce
▶ Creamy Baked Scallops
▶ Roasted Oysters
▶ Macadamia Nut Crusted Mahi-Mahi
▶ Olive-Oil Braised Albacore
▶ Salmon a L'Afrique du Nord

᎐╏◖∮⌇⤳

In This Chapter

▶ Making great meals from pork, chicken, lamb, beef, and more
▶ Working fish and seafood into the Paleo dinner menu

*P*aleo protein has a certain punch. It's a nutritionally dense food that provides you with what you need to build a healthy body. To keep yourself healthy and satisfied, you can enjoy any protein dish any time of day and for any meal of the day.

This chapter is loaded with a variety of protein recipes that feature pork, chicken, lamb, beef, fish, and seafood. All the proteins in this chapter are snuggled up with other yummy ingredients — like broccoli, bell peppers, olives, tomatoes, and sweet potatoes — that make them really pop.

Building Paleo Meals from Top-Quality Meats

Health is contagious. The healthier the food, the more health it brings to your body. Of course, the opposite is true as well. You may have heard some of the debate over grass-fed and grain-fed meats; the animals' diet is one factor that makes a big difference in the meat you eat. One of the biggest differences between grass-fed and grain-fed animals is the overall fat content. Take beef, for example. Grass-fed beef is lower in total fat and omega-6 fatty acids. The opposite is true of grain-fed animals. A healthy diet has an omega-6 fatty acid to omega-3 fatty acid ratio of about 4:1. The ratio of omega-6s to omega-3s in grass-fed animals is about 3:1. Grain-fed beef ratios exceed 20:1 omega-6s to omega-3s.

When you're deciding where to spend your money at the grocery store, keep the following facts in mind to help you make the best choice in regard to meat quality:

- ✔ Animals that are pasture raised and forage on a natural diet of grass have less stress and live healthier lives. There's little or no need to treat them with antibiotics or drugs.

- ✔ Grass-fed meat is a great source of conjugated linoleic acid (CLA), which is a good component in fat found primarily in the meat and dairy products from *ruminant* (cud-chewing) animals. It reduces the risk of heart disease, cancer, obesity, and diabetes and boosts immunity. Grain-fed animals tend to be lower in CLA than their grass-eating relatives.

- ✔ Grass-fed meat is higher in B vitamins, calcium, magnesium, and potassium than meat from grain-fed animals.

- ✔ Meat from grass-fed cattle typically has a much lower risk of E. coli because the cows are cleaner at the time of slaughter and are typically processed by a skilled local butcher or farmer who ensures the meat doesn't come in contact with feces.

- ✔ Grass-fed beef has ten times the amount of vitamin A and three times more vitamin E than grain-fed beef. It's also safe from mad cow disease (MCD).

- ✔ Pasture-raised, locally sourced poultry is the cleanest source of chicken and turkey you can purchase. The birds are able to roam freely in their environment, where they eat bugs, nutritious grasses, and other plants that are part of their natural diet. Organic, free-range poultry is also a good choice. Birds consume organic feed and have access to the outdoors. They are not given antibiotics unless they are ill.

If you're going to eat pork, make sure it comes from an organic, pasture-raised source. Otherwise, it's just too unhealthy; you're simply better off choosing another protein source. When selecting deli meats, make sure they're organic, gluten-free, sugar-free, and nitrite-free.

Buying Fresh Fish for Fab Dishes

Some people buy only frozen fish and seafood or avoid these versatile and nutritious protein sources altogether because they aren't sure how to buy quality fresh items. Here are some tips to help you enjoy the healthiest, freshest fish and seafood possible:

- Go to only the best fishmongers or to a reputable store and ask for the catch of the day. The fish store or counter should never smell fishy or like you're standing in the middle of a low tide.

- Fish should have a salty air scent, not a fishy smell.

- Fish should be firm and shiny, and the fillet should bounce back when you touch it.

- Fish fillets should be moist, and the flesh shouldn't separate or be discolored. Gaps in the meat as well as brown or yellow edges are signs of aging.

- Fish shouldn't have liquid on the meat. That milky look on fish means the fish is aging.

- Whole fish should have bright, clear (not cloudy) eyes and bright red gills.

- Shrimp should be firm and moist with translucent shells.

- Clams, mussels, and oysters should have tightly closed shells. If the shells gape slightly, tap them with a knife. If they don't close, discard them.

- Shucked clams, mussels, and oysters should be plump. Make sure their liquid is clear and slightly opalescent.

You don't want *frankenfish* — fish loaded with bad stuff like toxins such as mercury, PCBs, and hormones or antibiotics that you ingest when you eat the fish. Two great resources that can help guide you to the best choices in your area are www.montereybayaquarium.org/cr/seafoodwatch.aspx and www.cleanfish.com. Wild-caught, fresh fish is always best!

Fish is filled with omega-3 fatty acids, which are critical to the function of every cell in your body. Unfortunately, most people are deficient in these crucial fatty acids, so finding a clean source of fish or taking purified fish oil or a fish oil tablet to help bump up your levels is worthwhile.

Book II

Recipes for Every Occasion and Meal

Leafy Tacos

Prep time: 2 min • **Cook time:** 20 min • **Yield:** 4 servings

Ingredients	Directions

Ingredients

2 teaspoons coconut oil

1 small onion, minced

3 cloves garlic, minced

2 tablespoons chili powder

1 teaspoon ground cumin

1 teaspoon ground coriander

½ teaspoon dried oregano leaves

¼ teaspoon ground cayenne pepper

½ teaspoon salt

1 pound ground beef

2 tablespoons tomato paste

½ cup chicken broth

2 teaspoons cider vinegar

Salt and pepper to taste

1 large head lettuce (butter, romaine, or leaf)

Garnishes: diced avocado, onion, tomato, jalapeño, minced cilantro

Directions

1 Heat the coconut oil in a skillet over medium heat until hot, about 2 minutes; add the onion and cook until softened, about 4 minutes.

2 Add the garlic, chili powder, cumin, coriander, oregano, cayenne, and salt. Stir until fragrant, about 30 seconds.

3 Add the ground beef to the pan and cook, breaking up the meat with a wooden spoon until no longer pink, about 5 minutes.

4 Add the tomato paste, chicken broth, and vinegar. Stir to combine and bring to a simmer. Reduce heat to medium-low and cook uncovered for 10 minutes, until the liquid has reduced and thickened. Taste and adjust the seasonings with salt and pepper.

5 Spoon the taco meat into individual lettuce leaves and top with garnishes.

Per serving: Calories 304 (From Fat 159); Fat 18 g (Saturated 8 g); Cholesterol 80 mg; Sodium 548 mg; Carbohydrate 10 g (Dietary Fiber 5 g); Protein 27 g.

Note: Commercial taco seasonings often contain hidden sugars, gluten, and soy. Why eat processed seasonings when making your own is so easy — and flavorful? You can also top your tacos with your favorite tomato salsa; just be sure to check the label for non-Paleo ingredients.

Tip: This recipe is easy to double. Use leftovers tossed in a taco salad, spooned into a baked sweet potato, or scrambled into eggs.

Chicken Fingers

Prep time: 10 min • **Cook time:** 20 min • **Yield:** 4 servings

Ingredients	Directions
⅔ cup almond meal	**1** Preheat the oven to 425 degrees. Line a large baking sheet with parchment paper and place a wire baking rack on top.
1 teaspoon paprika	
1 teaspoon coarse (granulated) garlic powder	**2** In a shallow bowl or plate, combine the almond meal, paprika, garlic powder, salt, pepper, thyme, and all-spice. Mix with a fork to combine. In another shallow bowl, beat the egg white until frothy.
1 teaspoon salt	
½ teaspoon ground black pepper	
½ teaspoon dried thyme	**3** Pat the chicken dry with paper towels and then dip a piece into the egg white, shaking to remove any excess. Roll in almond meal and place on the pre-pared baking sheet. The chicken tenders should not touch. Repeat until all pieces are coated.
¼ teaspoon allspice	
1 large egg white	
1 pound chicken tenders (or boneless, skinless chicken breast, sliced into strips)	**4** Bake 15 to 20 minutes, turning once halfway through baking.

Per serving: Calories 240 (From Fat 110); Fat 12 g (Saturated 1 g); Cholesterol 63 mg; Sodium 669 mg; Carbohydrate 6 g (Dietary Fiber 3 g); Protein 28 g.

Note: You can make these chicken fingers without the almond meal if you're trying to minimize your nut intake. Just roll the chicken tenders in the spice blend and follow the baking instructions.

Vary It! To make spicy chicken fingers, add ¼ to ½ teaspoon ground cayenne pepper to the almond meal or give them a smoky spin with smoked paprika. You can also substitute pieces of firm, white fish for the chicken to make fish sticks or use beef strips for chicken-fried steak.

Tip: Serve with Paleo Ranch Dressing (Book III, Chapter 2) for dipping along with Mashed Cauliflower, Classic Cole Slaw, or Sweet Potato Shoestring Fries (Book II, Chapter 5).

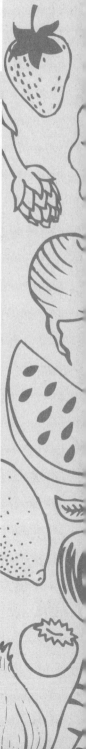

Orange Shrimp and Beef with Broccoli

Prep time: 15 min • **Cook time:** 10 min • **Yield:** 4 servings

Ingredients	Directions
1 tablespoon sesame seeds, optional	**1** Heat a large sauté pan or wok over medium-high heat. When the pan is hot, add the sesame seeds and stir constantly until they're lightly toasted, about 3 to 5 minutes. Remove from the pan and reserve for later.
3 oranges	
3 tablespoons coconut aminos	
1 tablespoon rice vinegar	**2** With a vegetable peeler, peel wide strips of zest from half of one of the oranges. Cut the zest into 1-inch pieces and set aside.
2 tablespoons arrowroot powder (optional)	
3 teaspoons coconut oil, divided	**3** Squeeze the juice from all the oranges into a small bowl; you should have about ¾ cup. Add the coconut aminos and rice vinegar; stir to combine.
¾ pound beef sirloin, trimmed and sliced against the grain into ⅛-inch-thick slices	**4** In another small bowl, mix the arrowroot powder with 2 tablespoons of water to form a paste; whisk into the orange juice and set aside.
½ pound shrimp, peeled, deveined, and halved	
1 large onion, thinly sliced	**5** Heat 1 teaspoon of coconut oil in the pan over high heat until very hot, about 2 minutes. Add the beef, shrimp, and onion. Stir-fry until the beef is no longer pink on the outside, about 1 minute. Transfer to a plate and cover loosely with foil.
8 cloves garlic, minced	
¼ teaspoon dried ginger	
¼ teaspoon ground cayenne pepper	**6** Add the remaining 2 teaspoons of coconut oil to the pan and heat until very hot. Add the garlic, ginger, cayenne, and reserved orange zest. Stir-fry until fragrant, about 30 seconds. Add the broccoli, red pepper, and water. Cover and steam, stirring occasionally, until the water has evaporated and the broccoli is tender, about 3 to 4 minutes.
2 pounds broccoli, cut into small florets	
2 red bell peppers, seeded and thinly sliced	
⅓ cup water	**7** Whisk the stir-fry sauce and pour into the pan. Bring to a boil and cook until the sauce is slightly thickened, about 1 to 2 minutes. Add the beef and shrimp, stirring to coat with the sauce. Remove from heat and sprinkle with scallions and toasted sesame seeds.
½ cup scallions, green parts only, thinly sliced	

Per serving: *Calories 551 (From Fat 164); Fat 18 g (Saturated 8 g); Cholesterol 146 mg; Sodium 462 mg; Carbohydrate 62 g (Dietary Fiber 14 g); Protein 36 g.*

Club Sandwich Salad

Prep time: 10 min • **Cook time:** 4 min • **Yield:** 4 servings

Ingredients	*Directions*
4 strips high-quality, nitrate-free bacon	*1* Cut the bacon crosswise into ¼-inch-wide pieces and place in a large, cold skillet; turn the heat to medium-high and fry the bacon until it's crisp, about 3 to 4 minutes. Remove the bacon from the pan with a wooden spoon and drain on a paper towel.
1 head green or red leaf lettuce, torn	
2 large cucumbers, peeled and thinly sliced	
12 ounces cooked boneless, skinless chicken breast, diced	*2* Divide the lettuce among four plates and line the rim with cucumber slices.
2 ripe tomatoes, diced	*3* In a large bowl, gently toss the chicken, tomatoes, avocado, red onion, and parsley. Divide on top of the lettuce-cucumber bed.
1 ripe avocado, diced	
½ medium red onion, thinly sliced	
½ cup fresh parsley leaves, coarsely chopped	*4* Drizzle each serving with Ranch Dressing, sprinkle with bacon, and serve immediately.
⅓ cup Ranch Dressing (see recipe in Book III, Chapter 2)	

Per serving: Calories 309 (From Fat 120); Fat 13 g (Saturated 3 g); Cholesterol 78 mg; Sodium 972 mg; Carbohydrate 17 g (Dietary Fiber 8 g); Protein 33 g.

Tip: This dish travels well for packed lunches. Package the chicken and dressing separately from the vegetables and assemble just before eating.

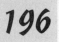

Winter Squash and Sausage Hash

Prep time: 15 min • **Cook time:** 25 min • **Yield:** 2 servings

Ingredients	*Directions*
2 cups ½-inch-diced winter squash	*1* Preheat the oven to 375 degrees.
1 cup diced mushrooms	*2* In a medium bowl, toss the squash, mushrooms, garlic, and sausage together.
2 cloves garlic, crushed	
½ pound spicy sausage (no sugar added), casing removed and meat diced into 1-inch cubes	*3* Spread the vegetable mixture into a baking dish, making sure not to overcrowd, and bake for 25 minutes or until the veggies are tender and the sausage is browned.
1 tablespoon coconut oil	
4 eggs	*4* While the veggie mixture is baking, heat a medium skillet over medium heat. Starting with half the oil and adding more as needed, fry the eggs, two at a time, to your desired doneness.
Fresh parsley for garnish	
Salt and pepper to taste	
	5 Remove the vegetable mixture from the oven and top with the fried eggs. Garnish with parsley and salt and pepper to taste.

Per serving: Calories 476 (From Fat 272); Fat 30 g (Saturated 13 g); Cholesterol 455 mg; Sodium 1,167 mg; Carbohydrate 18 g (Dietary Fiber 4 g); Protein 35 g.

Recipe courtesy Arsy Vartanian, author of Rubies & Radishes (www.rubiesandradishes.com)

This recipe has been vetted by the team at Whole9 (http://whole9life.com) and is considered acceptable for a cleansing 30-day Paleo launch.

Citrus Carnitas

Prep time: 5 min • **Cook time:** 2–3 hr • **Yield:** 8 servings

Ingredients	Directions
1 tablespoon ground cumin	*1* In a large zip-top bag, combine the cumin, garlic powder, salt, coriander, black pepper, and cayenne; shake to mix well.
1 tablespoon garlic powder	
½ tablespoon salt	
1 teaspoon ground coriander	*2* With a sharp knife, trim the excess fat off the pork shoulder and cut the pork into large chunks. Place the pork in the bag and shake until it's coated with the spices.
1 teaspoon ground black pepper	
¼–1 teaspoon ground cayenne pepper to taste	*3* Transfer the pork to a large stockpot. Add the lime and lemon juices and then add enough water to just cover the meat.
3 pounds boneless pork shoulder	
½ cup lime juice	*4* Bring the pot to a rapid boil over high heat; reduce the heat to keep a steady, strong simmer with the pot uncovered. (Turn on the exhaust fan over your stovetop for this step.)
½ cup lemon juice	
1 tablespoon coconut oil	*5* After 2 hours, check the pot. The water level should be much lower and maybe even almost gone.
	6 Heat a large skillet with the coconut oil over medium-high heat and carefully transfer the pork to the skillet. Brown the pork on all sides.
	7 Transfer the pork to a plate and let it rest for 5 minutes before serving.

Per serving: Calories 283 (From Fat 135); Fat 15 g (Saturated 4.5 g); Cholesterol 124 mg; Sodium 1,967 mg; Carbohydrate 4 g (Dietary Fiber 0.5 g); Protein 33 g.

This recipe has been vetted by the team at Whole9 (http://whole9life.com) and is considered acceptable for a cleansing 30-day Paleo launch.

Thai Green Curry Chicken

Prep time: 5 min • **Cook time:** 15 min • **Yield:** 4 servings

Ingredients	Directions
3-inch piece of lemongrass	**1** Thinly slice the pale yellow portion of the lemongrass and process it in a blender or small food processor.
2 tablespoons coconut oil	
½ white onion, thinly sliced	**2** Heat the coconut oil over medium heat in a sauté pan. Sauté the onions until translucent. Add the garlic, lemongrass puree, and ginger and sauté for 1 to 2 minutes until fragrant.
2 cloves garlic, crushed	
1-inch piece of fresh ginger, grated (about 1 tablespoon)	
1 pound boneless, skinless chicken thighs, cut into 1-inch chunks	**3** Sprinkle the chicken with the salt and pepper and add it to the pan. Brown the chicken on all sides, adding more coconut oil if needed.
1 teaspoon sea salt	
½ teaspoon ground black pepper	**4** Stir in the green curry paste, coating all the chicken. Add the rest of the vegetables and the kaffir lime leaves and cook for 2 minutes.
2 tablespoons green curry paste	
1 small zucchini, sliced	
1 red bell pepper, sliced	**5** Add the coconut milk and simmer on low for 15 minutes or until the chicken is cooked through and the vegetables are cooked but still firm and colorful.
2 cups white mushrooms, sliced	
4 kaffir lime leaves, chopped	**6** Top with the basil and serve.
2 cups coconut milk	
½ cup fresh basil, chopped	

Per serving: Calories 473 (From Fat 335); Fat 37 g (Saturated 28 g); Cholesterol 95 mg; Sodium 737 mg; Carbohydrate 13 g (Dietary Fiber 2.5 g); Protein 27 g.

Note: Kaffir lime leaf, also known as lime leaf, is a key ingredient in Thai cooking as well as other Southeast-Asian cuisines. Your local grocery store may carry Thai Kitchen brand lime leaves and green curry paste, or you can look for these items at an Asian market.

Recipe courtesy Arsy Vartanian, author of Rubies & Radishes (www.rubiesandradishes.com)

This recipe has been vetted by the team at Whole9 (http://whole9life.com) and is considered acceptable for a cleansing 30-day Paleo launch.

Tandoori Chicken Thighs

Prep time: 10 min, plus marinating time • **Cook time:** 40 min • **Yield:** 6 servings

Ingredients	*Directions*
4 pounds bone-in, skin-on chicken thighs	*1* Liberally season the chicken with salt and pepper in a large bowl.
Kosher salt	
Ground black pepper	*2* Combine the coconut milk, tandoori seasoning, and the juice of 1 lime in a large zip-top bag; mix well. Add the chicken to the bag, shake it around to coat, and marinate in the fridge for 8 hours.
1 cup coconut milk	
1½ tablespoons tandoori seasoning	
4 limes	*3* When you're ready to cook the chicken, preheat the oven to 400 degrees. Place a wire rack on a foil-lined rimmed baking tray and grease the rack with coconut oil.
1 tablespoon coconut oil	
	4 Arrange the chicken skin-side down on the rack and bake for 20 minutes. Flip the pieces over and bake for another 20 minutes until it has some charred bits.
	5 Cut the remaining limes into wedges. The chicken is done when the juices run clear when you pierce the meat with a fork or knife near the bone. Serve immediately with the lime wedges.

Per serving: *Calories 774 (From Fat 525); Fat 58 g (Saturated 22 g); Cholesterol 227 mg; Sodium 301 mg; Carbohydrate 6 g (Dietary Fiber 1.5 g); Protein 57 g.*

Tip: You can throw this simple Indian dish together in 10 minutes and leave it to marinate while you're at work; the chicken will be ready to bake when you get home.

*Recipe courtesy Michelle Tam, author of Nom Nom Paleo (*http://nomnompaleo.com*)*

*This recipe has been vetted by the team at Whole9 (*http://whole9life.com*) and is considered acceptable for a cleansing 30-day Paleo launch.*

Slow-Roasted Rack of Lamb

Prep time: 10 min, plus resting time • **Cook time:** 60–90 min • **Yield:** 2 servings

Ingredients	Directions
2-pound rack of lamb (approximately 2 servings, with bones removed) **Kosher salt** **3 tablespoons dukkah** **Black pepper**	**1** Dry the lamb thoroughly with paper towels. Liberally sprinkle it all over with salt and refrigerate it for 4 hours to 2 days. **2** Remove the lamb from the fridge at least 1 hour before you cook it. Preheat the oven to 250 degrees with the oven rack set in the middle. Place a wire rack on a foil-lined baking tray. **3** Coat the lamb with the dukkah and the pepper and place it on the wire rack. **4** Insert an instant-read, in-oven thermometer probe into the thickest part of the lamb. Aim it toward the center, away from the rib bones. Place the lamb in the oven. **5** Bake for 60 to 90 minutes. Remove the lamb as soon as the thermometer registers 130 degrees for medium rare or 140 degrees for medium. **6** Remove the lamb from the oven and let rest for 15 minutes. Slice between the ribs before serving.

Per serving: *Calories 229 (From Fat 92); Fat 10 g (Saturated 4 g); Cholesterol 80 mg; Sodium 334 mg; Carbohydrate 0.5 g (Dietary Fiber 0.5 g); Protein 34 g.*

Note: *Dukkah* is an Egyptian spice blend. Book III, Chapter 3, has a recipe for homemade dukkah.

Tip: Instant-read, in-oven thermometers let you keep track of your food temperature without having to continually open and close the oven (letting out heat).

Recipe courtesy Michelle Tam, author of Nom Nom Paleo (http://nomnompaleo.com)

This recipe has been vetted by the team at Whole9 (http://whole9life.com) and is considered acceptable for a cleansing 30-day Paleo launch.

Spicy Stuffed Eggplant

Prep time: 10 min • **Cook time:** 20 min • **Yield:** 4 servings

Ingredients	Directions
2 large eggplants	*1* Preheat the oven to 400 degrees.
5 tablespoons olive oil, divided	
1 onion chopped	*2* Wash the eggplants and cut them in half lengthwise. Remove the pulp, chop it coarsely, and set it aside. Leave a scooped shell about ½ inch thick.
2 cloves garlic, minced	
One 14.5-ounce can diced tomatoes, drained	*3* In a large skillet, heat half the oil. Place the eggplant shells cut-side-down in the oil and cook for about 5 minutes. With tongs, transfer the shells cut-side-up to a shallow, ovenproof dish.
One 8-ounce can tomato sauce	
½ teaspoon dried thyme	
½ teaspoon ground cayenne pepper	*4* Add the remaining oil to the skillet and sauté the onion and garlic for 2 minutes over medium heat.
Pinch of salt	
Pinch of ground black pepper	*5* Add the eggplant pulp, tomatoes, tomato sauce, thyme, cayenne, salt, and pepper and cook over medium heat until most of the moisture evaporates and a stew-like mixture remains.
½ pound ground beef, cooked	
2 tablespoons chopped fresh parsley	
	6 Remove the skillet from the heat and mix in the beef. Stuff the eggplant shells with the meat mixture and bake for 15 minutes.
	7 Top with the parsley and serve.

Per serving: Calories 539 (From Fat 356); Fat 40 g (Saturated 7 g); Cholesterol 38 mg; Sodium 306 mg; Carbohydrate 33 g (Dietary Fiber 10 g); Protein 21 g.

Recipe courtesy Mark Sisson, author of Primal Blueprint and Mark's Daily Apple (www.marksdailyapple.com)

This recipe has been vetted by the team at Whole9 (http://whole9life.com) and is considered acceptable for a cleansing 30-day Paleo launch.

Grilled Buffalo Shrimp

Prep time: 5 min • **Cook time:** 6–8 min • **Yield:** 4 servings

Ingredients	Directions
1 clove garlic, minced	**1** Combine all the ingredients except the shrimp in a bowl and mix well. Add the shrimp and mix well, ensuring an even coating.
¼ cup hot sauce	
1 teaspoon coconut oil, melted	
1 teaspoon crushed red pepper	**2** Grease the grill with coconut oil spray or a little extra melted coconut oil. Preheat your grill to about 400 degrees. Use a grill rack if you have it so your shrimp don't fall through the grates; preheat the rack on the grill. If you don't have a rack, arrange the shrimp on skewers.
1 teaspoon Italian Seasoning (see recipe in Book III, Chapter 3)	
¼ teaspoon cayenne pepper	**3** When your grill is heated, place the shrimp on the grill and close the lid. Allow to cook for 1 to 2 minutes, and then flip and finish cooking for 1 to 2 minutes on the other side.
¼ teaspoon Celtic sea salt	
¼ teaspoon ground black pepper	
24 medium shrimp, peeled and deveined	**4** Serve and enjoy.

Per serving: Calories 43 (From Fat 15); Fat 1.5 g (Saturated 1 g); Cholesterol 53 mg; Sodium 690 mg; Carbohydrate 1 g (Dietary Fiber 0 g); Protein 6 g.

Tip: If you have time, let the shrimp marinate in the fridge for 30 minutes or so before moving to Step 2. If you use skewers, double skewer the shrimp — use two parallel skewers — to prevent the shrimp from twisting around the skewers as you flip them over. You can broil the shrimp if you don't have an outdoor grill or if the temperature outside is too cold to use one.

Recipe courtesy George Bryant, CEO and author of Civilized Caveman Cooking Creations (http://civilizedcavemancooking.com)

This recipe has been vetted by the team at Whole9 (http://whole9life.com) and is considered acceptable for a cleansing 30-day Paleo launch.

Coconut Shrimp with Sweet and Spicy Sauce

Prep time: 10 min • **Cook time:** 5 min • **Yield:** 2 servings

Ingredients	Directions
1 cup chopped fresh pineapple	**1** Preheat the oven to 450 degrees. Line a baking sheet with aluminum foil, shiny side down.
1 jalapeño, seeded (optional) and chopped	
Juice of 1 lime	**2** Blend the pineapple, jalapeño, lime juice, and onion in a blender or food processor on high until the consistency of the sauce is smooth with small bits. Set this sauce aside.
¼ medium white or red onion, chopped	
½ cup almond flour	
½ cup unsweetened shredded coconut	**3** In a gallon-size zip-top bag, combine the almond flour, coconut, garlic, cumin, salt, and pepper. Beat the egg white in a small bowl.
1 clove garlic, minced	
½ teaspoon ground cumin	**4** Coat the shrimp generously in the egg wash and then place them in the zip-top bag. Shake the bag so all the shrimp are evenly coated with the breading mixture.
¼ teaspoon salt	
¼ teaspoon ground black pepper	
1 egg white	**5** Remove the shrimp from the bag and place on the baking sheet. Bake for 2 minutes on the middle rack of your oven. Flip the shrimp over and bake for 3 minutes.
12 large shrimp, peeled, deveined, and butterflied	
	6 Remove from the oven and serve with the sauce.

Per serving: Calories 451 (From Fat 206); Fat 23 g (Saturated 7 g); Cholesterol 214 mg; Sodium 1,290 mg; Carbohydrate 32 g (Dietary Fiber 7 g); Protein 33 g.

Note: Leaving the seeds in the jalapeño will make the sauce spicier.

Tip: You can use this dipping sauce on all kinds of food. Try it on eggs or chicken for a delicious twist.

Recipe courtesy George Bryant, CEO and author of Civilized Caveman Cooking Creations (http://civilizedcavemancooking.com)

This recipe has been vetted by the team at Whole9 (http://whole9life.com) and is considered acceptable for a cleansing 30-day Paleo launch.

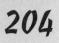

Creamy Baked Scallops

Prep time: 10 min • **Cook time:** 10 min • **Yield:** 2 servings

Ingredients	*Directions*
12 medium sea scallops	*1* Preheat the oven to 475 degrees.
1 cup chopped red onion	
1 teaspoon coconut oil	*2* Evenly space the scallops in the bottom of an 8-x-8-inch baking dish.
3 cloves garlic, minced	
½ cup tomato sauce	*3* In a large skillet, sauté the onions over medium-high heat in the coconut oil until they start to turn opaque.
¼ cup coconut milk	
¼ teaspoon dried oregano	*4* Lower the heat to medium-low. Add the garlic, tomato sauce, coconut milk, oregano, salt, and pepper, and mix well. Pour the mixture over the scallops in the baking dish. Cover with the chopped tomatoes.
¼ teaspoon salt	
¼ teaspoon ground black pepper	
1 cup diced tomatoes	*5* Bake 10 to 15 minutes until the tomatoes start to brown and the sauce is bubbling.
	6 Remove from the oven and serve in a bowl with plenty of sauce.

Per serving: Calories 367 (From Fat 107); Fat 12 g (Saturated 8 g); Cholesterol 70 mg; Sodium 1,942 mg; Carbohydrate 28 g (Dietary Fiber 3.5 g); Protein 39 g.

Tip: Any tomato sauce you have in your pantry works for this dish. Just be sure it's unsweetened.

Recipe courtesy George Bryant, CEO and author of Civilized Caveman Cooking Creations (http://civilizedcavemancooking.com)

This recipe has been vetted by the team at Whole9 (http://whole9life.com) and is considered acceptable for a cleansing 30-day Paleo launch.

Roasted Oysters

Prep time: 15 min • **Cook time:** 25 min • **Yield:** 6 servings

Ingredients	Directions
5 ounces frozen spinach	*1* Preheat the oven to 450 degrees. Prepare the spinach according to the package instructions.
12 oysters	
4 tablespoons olive oil, divided	*2* Shuck the oysters and release the meat from the cup portion of the shell; be careful to retain the liquor, or juice, in the oyster shell.
½ cup minced garlic	
½ cup minced shallots	
1 bell pepper, seeded and finely diced	*3* Press the shucked oysters securely into a bed of foil on a baking sheet so as to not spill any juice.
Kosher salt and black pepper to taste	*4* Preheat a large skillet over high heat. Add 2 tablespoons of olive oil, the garlic, and the shallots and sauté for 2 minutes. Add the bell pepper and cooked spinach; mix well, breaking up the spinach. Cook for 2 more minutes.
Chili powder to taste	
Juice of ¼ lemon	
2 slices prosciutto, each cut into six pieces	*5* Season with salt, pepper, and chili powder to taste. Stir in the lemon juice and remove the skillet from the heat.
	6 Spoon the vegetable mixture into the oyster cups. Top each oyster with a piece of prosciutto and then the place the pan on the bottom rack of the oven.
	7 Bake for 7 minutes and then transfer to the top rack of the oven. Reset the oven temperature to broil to finish cooking and crisp up the prosciutto.
	8 Remove the oysters from the oven, drizzle lightly with the remaining olive oil, and allow to rest for a few minutes before serving.

Per serving: Calories 146 (From Fat 96); Fat 11 g (Saturated 2 g); Cholesterol 20 mg; Sodium 227 mg; Carbohydrate 11 g (Dietary Fiber 1 g); Protein 5 g.

Vary It! Be creative with this recipe. You can substitute partially cooked bacon for the prosciutto; add fresh herbs to the veggie mixture; or garnish with fresh herbs, lemon zest, lobster claws, or a slice of delicately seared sea scallop. Just be sure to keep added seafood in the shellfish family.

Recipe courtesy Nick Massie, chef and author of Paleo Nick (http://paleonick.com)

This recipe has been vetted by the team at Whole9 (http://whole9life.com) and is considered acceptable for a cleansing 30-day Paleo launch.

Macadamia Nut Crusted Mahi-Mahi

Prep time: 10 min, plus marinating time • **Cook time:** 10 min • **Yield:** 2 servings

Ingredients	Directions
Two 6- to 8-ounce mahi-mahi fillets	*1* Place the fillets in a zip-top bag with the coconut milk and let sit at room temperature for 30 to 60 minutes.
1 cup coconut milk	
¼ cup roasted macadamia nuts	*2* Preheat the oven to 425 degrees.
1 tablespoon coconut flour	*3* Grind the macadamia nuts in a blender or food processor until they're coarsely ground. Add the coconut flour and almond flour and process further to mix well. Transfer the nut mixture to a bowl.
1 tablespoon almond flour	
2 tablespoons coconut oil, melted and divided	
Pinch of salt	*4* Add 1 tablespoon of melted coconut oil to the nut mixture and mix well.
Pinch of ground black pepper	
½ cup shredded unsweetened coconut	*5* Line a baking sheet with aluminum foil and brush with the remaining coconut oil so your fish doesn't stick. Place the fillets on the baking sheet and salt and pepper each side of the fish to your liking.
	6 Bake the fish for 5 minutes and then remove it from the oven. Flip the fillets over and spread the nut mixture over them, pressing it down so it sticks. Sprinkle the shredded coconut on top to your liking.
	7 Bake for an additional 8 to 10 minutes or until the coconut and macadamia nuts are nicely browned.
	8 Remove from the oven and let sit for 10 minutes before serving.

Per serving: Calories 781 (From Fat 585); Fat 65 g (Saturated 45 g); Cholesterol 146 mg; Sodium 488 mg; Carbohydrate 15 g (Dietary Fiber 8 g); Protein 42 g.

Tip: Serve this dish with fresh pineapple for an absolutely delicious meal.

Recipe courtesy George Bryant, CEO and author of Civilized Caveman Cooking Creations (http://civilizedcavemancooking.com)

This recipe has been vetted by the team at Whole9 (http://whole9life.com) and is considered acceptable for a cleansing 30-day Paleo launch.

Olive-Oil Braised Albacore

Prep time: 10 min • **Cook time:** 30 min • **Yield:** 4 servings

Ingredients	Directions
2 pounds skinless fresh albacore fillet	**1** Preheat the oven to 350 degrees.
Pinch of kosher salt **Pinch of ground black pepper**	**2** Cut the albacore crosswise into 1½-inch steaks. Season both sides with salt and pepper.
4 cloves garlic, roughly chopped **⅔ cup extra-virgin olive oil** **1 medium lemon, quartered**	**3** Place the steaks in a single layer in a casserole dish and top with the garlic. Pour the olive oil in the dish until it reaches halfway up the sides of the fish. (Use more or less oil as needed.)
	4 Cover the dish with foil and bake for 10 minutes. Carefully flip the fish and bake for another 10 minutes, covered. The albacore is finished when it's barely cooked through.
	5 Let the tuna cool to room temperature and serve with the olive-oil braising liquid and a squeeze of lemon juice.

Per serving: *Calories 610 (From Fat 372); Fat 41 g (Saturated 5 g); Cholesterol 100 mg; Sodium 771 mg; Carbohydrate 4 g (Dietary Fiber 1.5 g); Protein 65 g.*

Tip: This dish stores well in the fridge. Just keep the fish in the olive-oil braising liquid and you'll have emergency protein ready to eat.

Note: You can pair this dish with the delicious salads in Book II, Chapter 2. You can also turn to a vegetarian side, such as the Italian Broccoli or the Cocoa Cauliflower in Book II, Chapter 5.

Recipe courtesy Michelle Tam, author of Nom Nom Paleo (http://nomnompaleo.com)

This recipe has been vetted by the team at Whole9 (http://whole9life.com) and is considered acceptable for a cleansing 30-day Paleo launch.

Salmon a L'Afrique du Nord

Prep time: 5 min, plus marinating time • **Cook time:** 6–7 min • **Yield:** 8 servings

Ingredients	Directions
1 tablespoon coconut oil, melted	**1** Mix the coconut oil, orange juice, ginger, cumin, coriander, paprika, salt, and cayenne in a small bowl to form a paste the consistency of thick salad dressing.
1 tablespoon fresh orange juice	
1½ teaspoons dried ginger	**2** Place the salmon in a glass baking dish and massage the marinade over the salmon. Cover and refrigerate for 30 minutes.
1½ teaspoons ground cumin	
1½ teaspoons ground coriander	**3** Preheat a gas grill on high with the lid closed for about 10 minutes.
½ teaspoon paprika	
1½ teaspoons salt	**4** Place the salmon skin-side-down on the grill, close the lid, and cook for 3 minutes. Check the salmon; the skin should be a little blackened and starting to separate from the pink flesh.
¼ teaspoon ground cayenne pepper	
1½ pounds skin-on salmon fillets	**5** Flip the salmon, close the lid, and cook an additional 3 minutes. Serve immediately.

Per serving: Calories 169 (From Fat 97); Fat 11 g (Saturated 3 g); Cholesterol 49 mg; Sodium 485 mg; Carbohydrate 1 g (Dietary Fiber 0 g); Protein 17 g.

This recipe has been vetted by the team at Whole9 (http://whole9life.com) and is considered acceptable for a cleansing 30-day Paleo launch.

Chapter 4

Paleo Life in the Slow (Cooker) Lane

In This Chapter

▶ Making Paleo meal magic with just one pot

▶ Simplifying your life with easy, tasty slow-cooked meals

Recipes in This Chapter

▶ Beef Bone Broth

▶ Slow Cooker Pork and Sauerkraut

▶ Chicken Cacciatora

▶ Mango Coconut Chipotle Chicken

▶ Slow Cooker BBQ Pulled Pork

▶ Kalua Shredded Pork

▶ Cheater Pork Stew

▶ Pineapple Pork Ribs

▶ Pineapple and Mango Sweet Heat Chicken Wings

▶ Meatloaf

▶ Sausage-Stuffed Peppers

▶ Slow Cooker Moroccan Apricot Chicken

▶ Easy Chicken Curry with Cabbage

▶ Creamy Red Shrimp and Tomato Curry

↻ Roasted Red Pepper and Sweet Potato Soup

🌶 🍲 🥄 🧄 🌿

Back in the day, before prescriptions were abundant and medical treatments far-reaching, people used slow-cooked foods to get deep healing. Every nutrient was retained in the preparation, and the outcome was steamy, robust flavors. All the nutrition provided people's cells with the best raw material possible. It was natural healing at its finest. Getting back to using broths and slow-cooked meals to heal the body is a benefit of living and cooking Paleo.

As you prepare these easy yet decadent meals, know that you're giving your body simply the best. Bonus: Slow cooking is convenient. You can cook your meals while you're at work, at play, or even sleeping. Now that's a good deal!

Getting the Scoop on Slow Cooking

Whether you're a busy parent or just a busy person, do yourself a favor and get a slow cooker. Making meals this way is both convenient and wholesome. The slow cooker frees your oven and stove top for other uses, and it makes cooking for large gatherings or holiday meals easy! Sauces and gravies cook really well in a slow cooker too.

Even at the low setting, internal temperatures of foods are raised well above 140 degrees, the minimum temperature at which bacteria are killed. If you're concerned about food safety, bring the food up to temperature by cooking on high for the first hour. (In most slow cookers, one hour on high is equal to two hours on low.)

Here are some general tips to get you fired up on slow cooking; be sure to also consult the user manual for your particular slow cooker model:

- **Working with a new slow cooker:** When using a new slow cooker, keep an eye on it during the first few uses. These slow cookers can have a mind of their own on high and on low — they can actually boil food, burn food, or just overheat — so don't leave one unattended until you have a better idea of its idiosyncrasies. Place the cooker on a cookie sheet, a granite countertop, the stovetop, or a similar surface that won't burn; the bottom can get pretty hot on some models.

- **Cooking fish:** Fish and seafood generally aren't good candidates for the slow cooker. If you use them, put them in at the very end of cooking, as with the Creamy Red Shrimp and Tomato Curry later in this chapter.

- **Cooking dense carbohydrates:** Cut Paleo-approved dense carbohydrates, such as sweet potatoes, carrots, squash, and turnips, into small pieces (about 1 to 1½ inches). In most dishes, you should layer these root vegetables on the bottom of the crock, under the meat and other ingredients, so they begin to cook as soon as the liquids heat.

- **Browning meats:** Browning many meats helps reduce the fat content and can enhance the flavor and texture of dishes, but doing so isn't necessary. However, you should cook ground meats in a skillet before adding them to a slow cooker.

- **Using spices:** Stir in spices during the last hour of cooking. They lose their flavor if you cook them with the rest of the food or for a long period.

- **Stirring:** Try to refrain from lifting the lid to stir unnecessarily, especially if you're cooking on the low setting. Each time you lift the lid, enough heat escapes that you should extend the cooking time by 20 to 30 minutes.

Beef Bone Broth

Prep time: 10 min • **Cook time:** 10 hr • **Yield:** 12 servings

Ingredients	Directions
2 unpeeled carrots, scrubbed and roughly chopped	**1** Place all the vegetables and the garlic, bones, and bay leaves into a slow cooker. Sprinkle on the salt, drizzle with the vinegar, and add enough water to cover everything by 1 inch (about 13 cups).
2 stalks celery, including leafy part, roughly chopped	
1 medium onion, roughly chopped	**2** Cook for 8 to 10 hours on low.
7 cloves garlic, peeled and smashed	**3** Use a shallow spoon to carefully skim the film off the top of the broth. Pour the broth through a fine strainer and discard the solids. Taste the broth and add more salt as needed.
3½ pounds grass-fed beef bones (preferably joints and knuckles)	
2 dried bay leaves	
2 teaspoons kosher salt	**4** The broth will keep for 3 days in the fridge and for 3 months in your freezer.
2 tablespoons apple cider vinegar	

Per serving: Calories 285 (From Fat 126); Fat 14 g (Saturated 5 g); Cholesterol 78 mg; Sodium 477 mg; Carbohydrate 2.5 g (Dietary Fiber 0.5 g); Protein 36 g.

Vary It! Feel free to substitute chicken, fish, or pork bones or to combine them all. Also, adding dried mushrooms or using 2 tablespoons of fish sauce in place of the salt (add it in Step 1) dramatically boosts the flavor of the broth.

*Recipe courtesy Michelle Tam, author of Nom Nom Paleo (*http://nomnompaleo.com*)*

*This recipe has been vetted by the team at Whole9 (*http://whole9life.com*) and is considered acceptable for a 30-Day Reset Paleo cleanse.*

Slow Cooker Pork and Sauerkraut

Prep time: 15 min • **Cook time:** 8–10 hr • **Yield:** 8 servings

Ingredients	Directions
2 pounds boneless pork shoulder, trimmed of excess fat and blotted dry	*1* Cut the pork shoulder into 3- to 4-inch chunks and season generously with salt and pepper. Heat a large skillet over medium-high heat and add the coconut oil.
Salt and pepper	
½ tablespoon coconut oil	
2 medium onions, thinly sliced	*2* When the oil is melted, add the pork, browning on all sides. You'll probably need to cook the pork in two batches so you don't overcrowd the pan. Transfer the pork to the slow cooker.
3 cloves garlic, minced	
1 bay leaf	*3* In the same pan, cook the onion until translucent, about 5 minutes. Add the garlic and cook until fragrant, about 30 seconds. Transfer the onion and garlic to the slow cooker. Add the bay leaf.
Three 14.5-ounce cans sauerkraut	
	4 Place the sauerkraut in a colander and rinse with cold water. Squeeze out the excess moisture and pile the sauerkraut on top of the pork. Cover the slow cooker and cook on low until the pork is fork tender, about 8 to 10 hours.

Per serving: Calories 203 (From Fat 98); Fat 11 g (Saturated 4 g); Cholesterol 66 mg; Sodium 831 mg; Carbohydrate 6 g (Dietary Fiber 3 g); Protein 20 g.

Note: You can use sauerkraut from a can or bag; just check the ingredient label for non-Paleo ingredients.

Tip: Serve with unsweetened applesauce and Mashed Cauliflower (Book II, Chapter 5).

Chicken Cacciatora

Prep time: 10 min • **Cook time:** 6 hr • **Yield:** 4 servings

Ingredients	Directions
1 medium white onion, sliced	*1* Line the bottom of the slow cooker with the onions.
1 pound boneless, skinless chicken breasts, halved	*2* Add all the remaining ingredients, pouring the tomatoes over everything last.
3 tablespoons olive oil	
1 large green bell pepper, seeded and sliced	*3* Cook on low for 6 hours.
1 large red bell pepper, seeded and sliced	
1 large yellow bell pepper, seeded and sliced	
2 cups sliced mushrooms	
1 stalk celery, chopped	
3 large cloves garlic	
1 teaspoon Italian Seasoning (see recipe in Book III, Chapter 3)	
2 cups chopped or crushed tomatoes	

Per serving: Calories 375 (From Fat 135); Fat 15 g (Saturated 3 g); Cholesterol 96 mg; Sodium 391 mg; Carbohydrate 21 g (Dietary Fiber 5 g); Protein 40 g.

Recipe courtesy Jason Crouch, chef and author of PaleoPot (http://paleopot.com)

This recipe has been vetted by the team at Whole9 (http://whole9life.com) and is considered acceptable for a cleansing 30-day Paleo launch.

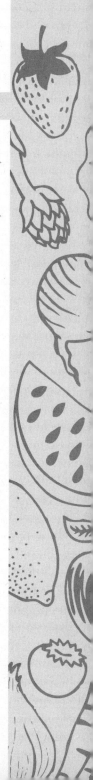

Mango Coconut Chipotle Chicken

Prep time: 10 min • **Cook time:** 4–6 hr • **Yield:** 4 servings

Ingredients	*Directions*
One 14-ounce can coconut milk	*1* Pour the coconut milk into the bottom of the slow cooker.
1 large mango	
1 pound chicken breasts	*2* Peel the mango, pit it, and cut the fruit into large and medium cubes. Add the flesh and the pit to the coconut milk (the meat on the pit adds flavor).
1 tablespoon dried chipotle flakes	
	3 Cube the chicken and add it to the slow cooker. Add the chipotle flakes and stir well.
	4 Cook on low for 4 to 6 hours.

Per serving: Calories 454 (From Fat 270); Fat 30 g (Saturated 21 g); Cholesterol 95 mg; Sodium 94 mg; Carbohydrate 11 g (Dietary Fiber 1 g); Protein 36 g.

Tip: You can also use chicken thighs. If you can't find dried chipotle flakes, you can substitute an equal amount of red pepper flakes.

Recipe courtesy Jason Crouch, chef and author of PaleoPot (http://paleopot.com)

This recipe has been vetted by the team at Whole9 (http://whole9life.com) *and is considered acceptable for a cleansing 30-day Paleo launch.*

Slow Cooker BBQ Pulled Pork

Prep time: 15 min • **Cook time:** 8–10 hr • **Yield:** 4 servings

Ingredients	Directions
2 tablespoons smoked paprika	*1* In a small bowl, mix the paprika, pepper, cumin, cocoa, and salt with a fork.
2 tablespoons ground black pepper	
2 tablespoons ground cumin	*2* Cut the pork into 2-inch chunks and place in a large bowl.
1 tablespoon unsweetened cocoa powder	
1 tablespoon salt	*3* Add the spices to the pork and toss until evenly coated.
2 pounds boneless pork shoulder, trimmed of excess fat and blotted dry	*4* Transfer the pork to the slow cooker, cover, and cook on low for 8 to 10 hours, until the pork is browned and fork tender.

Per serving: Calories 370 (From Fat 191); Fat 21 g (Saturated 7 g); Cholesterol 132 mg; Sodium 1,862 mg; Carbohydrate 6 g (Dietary Fiber 3 g); Protein 39 g.

Tip: Use two forks to shred the pork and toss with Tangy BBQ Sauce (Book III, Chapter 2). Serve with Classic Cole Slaw (Book II, Chapter 2) and Sweet Potato Shoestring Fries (Book II, Chapter 5).

Vary It! Use this spice blend on baby back ribs, beef roast, beef short ribs, or chicken. You can mix and match various meats in the same slow cooker for a BBQ feast.

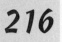

Kalua Shredded Pork

Prep time: 10 min • **Cook time:** 9–12 hr • **Yield:** 10 servings

Ingredients	*Directions*
3 slices bacon (no sugar added)	*1* Line the bottom of a slow cooker with the bacon.
1½ tablespoons coarse red Hawaiian sea salt **5-pound Boston butt pork roast**	*2* Salt the roast evenly, massaging the salt into the nooks and crannies. Place the seasoned roast skin-side-up on top of the bacon.
	3 Cook the roast on low for 9 to 12 hours.
	4 Remove the pork to a large platter and shred with two forks.
	5 Taste to check for seasoning, using the cooking liquid to season.

Per serving: Calories 608 (From Fat 360); Fat 40 g (Saturated 15 g); Cholesterol 222 mg; Sodium 1,438 mg; Carbohydrate 0 g (Dietary Fiber 0 g); Protein 59 g.

Note: Kalua is a traditional Hawaiian cooking method that uses an underground oven. This recipe lets you mimic it at home without digging up the backyard.

Tip: If you don't have red Hawaiian sea salt, any coarse salt will work. Keep leftovers of this dish handy in your fridge and freezer as an "emergency protein" for quick meals.

Recipe courtesy of Michelle Tam, author of Nom Nom Paleo (http://nomnompaleo.com)

This recipe has been vetted by the team at Whole9 (http://whole9life.com) and is considered acceptable for a cleansing 30-day Paleo launch.

Cheater Pork Stew

Prep time: 15 min • **Cook time:** 8–10 hr • **Yield:** 6 servings

Ingredients	Directions
2 small onions, thinly sliced	*1* Put the onions, carrots, and garlic in a 6-quart slow cooker. Season with ¼ teaspoon each of the salt and pepper and toss well.
½ pound baby carrots	
6 cloves garlic, peeled and smashed	
¾ teaspoon kosher salt, divided	*2* In a large bowl, combine the pork cubes, herb seasoning, fish sauce, and ¼ teaspoon each of the salt and pepper. Mix to combine.
¾ teaspoon ground black pepper, divided	
3 pounds pork shoulder, cut into 1½-inch cubes	*3* Pile the seasoned pork on top of the vegetables in the slow cooker. Arrange the cabbage wedges to cover the top of the pork, drizzle with the marinara sauce, and add the remaining salt and pepper.
1 tablespoon any herb seasoning blend	
1 tablespoon fish sauce	
1 small cabbage, cut into 8 wedges	*4* Cover and cook on low for 8 to 10 hours or until the pork is fork tender.
1 cup marinara sauce	
1 tablespoon aged balsamic vinegar	*5* When the stew is finished cooking, adjust for seasoning with the balsamic vinegar and/or salt and pepper to taste. Top with the parsley before serving (if desired).
¼ cup finely chopped Italian parsley (optional)	

Per serving: Calories 639 (From Fat 297); Fat 33 g (Saturated 11 g); Cholesterol 195 mg; Sodium 966 mg; Carbohydrate 23 g (Dietary Fiber 7 g); Protein 60 g.

Tip: Throw this stew in the slow cooker before heading to work, and a comforting, rib-sticking meal will await you when you get home.

Recipe courtesy of Michelle Tam, author of Nom Nom Paleo (http://nomnompaleo.com)

This recipe has been vetted by the team at Whole9 (http://whole9life.com) and is considered acceptable for a cleansing 30-day Paleo launch.

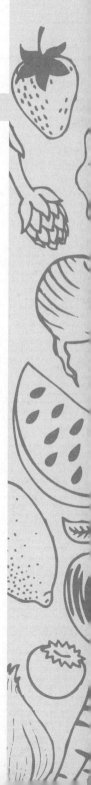

Pineapple Pork Ribs

Prep time: 10 min • **Cook time:** 6 hr • **Yield:** 4–6 servings

Ingredients	Directions
1 to 2 pounds pork ribs	**1** Cut the ribs as needed so they fit in your slow cooker and trim away any excess fat. Cut the pineapple into 1-inch cubes.
1 medium fresh pineapple	
2 tablespoons Spanish smoked paprika	**2** In a small bowl, combine the paprika, cayenne, mustard, and honey. Cover the ribs with this sauce as evenly as possible and arrange them in the bottom of the slow cooker. Top with the pineapple.
1 teaspoon cayenne pepper	
2 tablespoons sugar-free Dijon mustard	
2 tablespoons honey	**3** Cook on low for 6 hours.

Per serving: *Calories 518 (From Fat 315); Fat 35 g (Saturated 13 g); Cholesterol 137 mg; Sodium 227 mg; Carbohydrate 16 g (Dietary Fiber 1 g); Protein 33 g.*

Tip: Choose leaner cuts of ribs, and the excess fat will simply cook off.

Recipe courtesy Jason Crouch, chef and author of PaleoPot (http://paleopot.com)

Pineapple and Mango Sweet Heat Chicken Wings

Prep time: 30 min • **Cook time:** 4 hr, 15 min • **Yield:** 8 servings

Ingredients	Directions
1 tablespoon coconut oil	*1* Heat the coconut oil in a large saucepan over medium-low heat.
2 jalapeño peppers, seeded and minced	
1 habanero pepper, seeded and minced	*2* Add the peppers and garlic and let them sweat down for a few minutes. Add the mango and pineapple and cook for a few more minutes, until the fruit softens.
4 cloves garlic, chopped	
1 cup chopped mango	*3* Stir in all remaining ingredients except the chicken. Reduce the heat to low and allow the sauce to reduce for 15 minutes
2 cups crushed pineapple	
One 6-ounce can tomato paste	
1 cup beef stock	*4* Blend the sauce in a blender or food processor until it's a uniform consistency, being careful not to let the hot sauce splatter.
2 tablespoons apple cider vinegar	
2 teaspoons paprika	*5* Set the oven to broil and arrange the wings on a foil-lined baking sheet. Broil for about 5 minutes per side, until they're just browned and crisp, working in batches if you can't fit all the wings on one sheet.
2 teaspoons cayenne pepper	
3 to 4 pounds chicken wings	
	6 Transfer the wings to the slow cooker and cover them with the sauce, stirring to coat.
	7 Cook on low for 4 hours.

Per serving: Calories 691 (From Fat 387); Fat 43 g (Saturated 14 g); Cholesterol 167 mg; Sodium 392 mg; Carbohydrate 19 g (Dietary Fiber 2 g); Protein 56 g.

Recipe courtesy Jason Crouch, chef and author of PaleoPot (http://paleopot.com)

This recipe has been vetted by the team at Whole9 (http://whole9life.com) and is considered acceptable for a cleansing 30-day Paleo launch.

Meatloaf

Prep time: 10 min • **Cook time:** 4–6 hr • **Yield:** 8 servings

Ingredients	Directions
2 pounds lean grass-fed ground beef	**1** In a large bowl, combine the beef, eggs, bacon, veggies, oregano, pepper, thyme, 2 teaspoons of the paprika, and 2 teaspoons of the garlic powder.
2 eggs, beaten	
5 strips cooked bacon, chopped (no sugar added)	**2** Mix everything together by hand, forming a loaf that will fit into your slow cooker.
1 small white onion, diced	
4 scallions, chopped	**3** Place the loaf into the slow cooker and press it down so the top is flat and you have about an inch of space between the loaf and the sides of the slow cooker.
2 stalks celery, chopped	
2 teaspoons dried oregano	
1 teaspoon ground black pepper	**4** In a medium bowl, combine the tomato paste, mustard, vinegar, and remaining paprika and garlic powder; stir well. Spoon the mixture over the loaf, spreading to cover the loaf as evenly as possible.
1 teaspoon dried thyme	
4 teaspoons smoked paprika, divided	
4 teaspoons garlic powder, divided	**5** Cook on low for 4 to 6 hours.
One 8-ounce can tomato paste	
2 tablespoons sugar-free Dijon mustard	
1 teaspoon apple cider vinegar	

Per serving: Calories 293 (From Fat 153); Fat 17 g (Saturated 7 g); Cholesterol 119 mg; Sodium 454 mg; Carbohydrate 10 g (Dietary Fiber 3 g); Protein 26 g.

Tip: For a spicy kick, add 2 teaspoons cayenne pepper to the meatloaf mix in Step 1.

Vary It! Ground chicken or turkey is a great option in place of the beef.

Recipe courtesy Jason Crouch, chef and author of PaleoPot (http://paleopot.com)

This recipe has been vetted by the team at Whole9 (http://whole9life.com) *and is considered acceptable for a cleansing 30-day Paleo launch.*

Sausage-Stuffed Peppers

Prep time: 15 min • **Cook time:** 6 hr • **Yield:** 4–6 servings

Ingredients	Directions
4 to 6 bell peppers, any color	**1** Cut the tops off however many peppers will fit in your slow cooker. Scoop out and discard the seeds. Poke a hole in the bottom of each pepper to allow liquid to drain out. Save the tops.
½ head cauliflower	
6 cloves garlic, minced	
1 small white onion, diced	**2** Process the raw cauliflower in a food processor or blender until it's the size of rice. Transfer it to a large mixing bowl.
2 teaspoons dried basil	
2 teaspoons dried oregano	**3** Add the garlic, onion, basil, oregano, and thyme to the cauliflower and mix by hand.
2 teaspoons dried thyme	
1 pound ground Italian hot sausage	**4** Add the sausage and tomato paste to the seasoned cauliflower and mix with your hands. Be sure to wash your hands thoroughly afterward.
One 8-ounce can tomato paste	
	5 Spoon as much of the sausage mixture into the peppers as possible. Place them upright in the slow cooker.
	6 Cook on low for 6 hours.

Per serving: Calories 295 (From Fat 162); Fat 18 g (Saturated 7 g); Cholesterol 37 mg; Sodium 937 mg; Carbohydrate 20 g (Dietary Fiber 5 g); Protein 16 g.

Tip: To enhance the flavor of the sausage, lightly brown it in a large skillet over high heat and drain it before mixing it with the tomato and cauliflower.

Tip: Get the kids involved! Getting hands messy in Step 4 is necessary — a spoon just won't cut it — so let little ones have fun and help with dinner while you keep your hands clean.

Recipe courtesy Jason Crouch, chef and author of PaleoPot (http://paleopot.com)

This recipe has been vetted by the team at Whole9 (http://whole9life.com) *and is considered acceptable for a cleansing 30-day Paleo launch.*

Slow Cooker Moroccan Apricot Chicken

Prep time: 1 hr • **Cook time:** 5½ hr • **Yield:** 8 servings

Ingredients	Directions
4 cloves garlic, minced	*1* In a large bowl, combine garlic, ginger, coriander, cumin, pepper, and salt. Add the chicken and toss to coat.
½ tablespoon dried ginger	
2 teaspoons ground coriander	
1 teaspoon ground cumin	*2* Heat a large skillet over medium-high heat and add the coconut oil. When it's melted, add the chicken in batches and brown on all sides. Transfer the chicken to the slow cooker.
1 teaspoon ground black pepper	
¾ teaspoon salt	
2 pounds boneless, skinless chicken thighs	*3* To the slow cooker, add the chicken broth, lemon juice, and cinnamon stick. Cover and cook on low for 4 to 5 hours, until the chicken is tender.
1 tablespoon coconut oil	
¾ cup chicken broth	
¼ cup lemon juice	*4* Add the apricots and lemon zest to the slow cooker. Cover and cook on high for 30 minutes to allow the flavors to meld.
1 cinnamon stick	
16 pitted, dried apricots (about ½ cup)	*5* To serve, sprinkle with almonds and chopped cilantro (if desired).
1 tablespoon grated lemon zest (about 2 lemons)	
¼ cup sliced almonds, toasted	
Garnish: chopped fresh cilantro leaves (optional)	

Per serving: Calories 224 (From Fat 108); Fat 12 g (Saturated 4 g); Cholesterol 76 mg; Sodium 377 mg; Carbohydrate 6 g (Dietary Fiber 1 g); Protein 22 g.

Tip: Serve over Cauliflower Rice or Mashed Cauliflower (Book II, Chapter 5).

Vary It! Replace the chicken thighs with cubed, boneless lamb. You can also substitute dried prunes or dates for the apricots.

Easy Chicken Curry with Cabbage

Prep time: 10 min • **Cook time:** 4 hr • **Yield:** 6 servings

Ingredients	*Directions*
Two 14-ounce cans coconut milk	*1* Pour the coconut milk into the slow cooker and stir in the curry paste until dissolved.
3 tablespoons red curry paste	
1 to 1½ pounds boneless chicken thighs	*2* Cut the chicken thighs into 1-inch cubes and add to the slow cooker.
1 small yellow onion, chopped	*3* Stir in the onions and peppers.
1 medium green bell pepper, chopped	
½ head cabbage	*4* Cut the cabbage half into quarters, and then chop each wedge into long, thin strips. Break the strips apart with your hands.
	5 Stir in the cabbage, making sure it becomes coated with the curry mixture. (The cabbage doesn't need to be submerged in the coconut milk; it will cook down).
	6 Cover and cook on low for 4 hours.

Per serving: Calories 465 (From Fat 360); Fat 40 g (Saturated 27 g); Cholesterol 98 mg; Sodium 798 mg; Carbohydrate 12 g (Dietary Fiber 2 g); Protein 22 g.

Tip: If you have extra cabbage, simply leave it on top of the curry mixture and it will cook down.

*Recipe courtesy Jason Crouch, chef and author of PaleoPot (*http://paleopot.com*)*

*This recipe has been vetted by the team at Whole9 (*http://whole9life.com*) and is considered acceptable for a cleansing 30-day Paleo launch.*

Creamy Red Shrimp and Tomato Curry

Prep time: 10 min • **Cook time:** 6 hr • **Yield:** 6 servings

Ingredients	*Directions*
4 cups crushed tomatoes One 14-ounce can coconut milk	*1* Combine the tomatoes and coconut milk in the slow cooker.
3 tablespoons red curry paste 1 teaspoon ground cayenne or habanero pepper (optional)	*2* Stir in the curry paste and cayenne or habanero (if desired). Add the vegetables and stir well.
½ head cauliflower, cut into large chunks	*3* Cook on low for 6 hours.
1 large yellow or orange bell pepper, seeded and cut into strips 1 cup chopped scallions 1 cup chopped celery 1 pound large uncooked shrimp, peeled and deveined	*4* Add the shrimp to the slow cooker 10 minutes before serving. (Shrimp don't take long to cook, so don't forget about them.)

Per serving: Calories 281 (From Fat 153); Fat 17 g (Saturated 13 g); Cholesterol 95 mg; Sodium 1,364 mg; Carbohydrate 21 g (Dietary Fiber 5 g); Protein 16 g.

Tip: You can use precooked frozen shrimp — just thaw and add it to the pot a few minutes before serving.

Recipe courtesy Jason Crouch, chef and author of PaleoPot (http://paleopot.com)

This recipe has been vetted by the team at Whole9 (http://whole9life.com) and is considered acceptable for a cleansing 30-day Paleo launch.

Roasted Red Pepper and Sweet Potato Soup

Prep time: 10 min • **Cook time:** 4–6 hr • **Yield:** 6 servings

Ingredients	Directions
2 large sweet potatoes, peeled and cubed (about 6 cups)	*1* Add all the ingredients to the slow cooker and stir well.
One 14-ounce jar roasted red peppers in water, drained	
One 14-ounce can coconut milk	*2* Cook on low for 4 to 6 hours.
1 cup vegetable broth	*3* Transfer the soup to a blender and puree before serving. You can also transfer the soup to another container and use an immersion blender.
1 small yellow onion, chopped	
2 cloves garlic	
½ teaspoon ground black pepper	
½ teaspoon red pepper flakes	

Per serving: Calories 199 (From Fat 126); Fat 14 g (Saturated 12 g); Cholesterol 0 mg; Sodium 283 mg; Carbohydrate 16 g (Dietary Fiber 2 g); Protein 3 g.

Tip: If you're using store-bought vegetable broth, check the label for sugar, preservatives, soy, or additives of any kind. These are ingredients to avoid.

Recipe courtesy Jason Crouch, chef and author of PaleoPot (`http://paleopot.com`*)*

This recipe has been vetted by the team at Whole9 (`http://whole9life.com`*) and is considered acceptable for a cleansing 30-day Paleo launch.*

Chapter 5

Vegetable Dishes That Satisfy

Recipes in This Chapter

- ↻ Sesame Kale
- ↻ Creamy Kale
- ↻ Sweet Potato Shoestring Fries
- ↻ Spaghetti Squash Fritters
- ↻ Mashed Cauliflower
- ↻ Cauliflower Rice
- ↻ Cocoa Cauliflower
- ↻ Zucchini Pasta with Fire-Roasted Tomato Sauce
- ↻ Creamy Spiced Broccoli
- ↻ Italian Broccoli
- ↻ Sautéed Kohlrabi
- ↻ Brussels Sprouts with Cranberries and Almonds
- ↻ Kimchi
- ↻ Vegetable Latkes
- ↻ Lemon Cucumber Noodles with Cumin

🍴 🥄 🥢 🌶 🍃

In This Chapter

▶ Cooking veggies with flavor, snap — and so many nutrients
▶ Teasing your taste buds with unexpected combinations

*I*f you're one of those people who just can't seem to get on board with eating your vegetables, here's a solid reason to embrace them: Eating vegetables boosts your immunity. Everything rises and falls on your immune system. When it's strong, you avoid the pitfalls of disease, and your body expresses vitality and health.

Vegetables provide *super immunity,* which occurs when your body's greatest protector (your immune system) is working to the best of its ability to get and keep you well. Super immunity can even save your life, protecting you from the simplest of challenges, such as the common cold, to the most threatening, such as cancer.

No matter your health goals — getting well, staying well, losing weight, or fighting aging — attaining them starts with creating the healthiest cells possible. Discovering foods like the vegetable side dishes in this chapter helps your body produce these healthy cells.

Evolving Past Starches: Paleo-Friendly Hot Side Dishes

The right side dish can elevate a boring pork chop or bunless hamburger to favorite-dinner status. The hot vegetable side dishes in this chapter are ambitious and step away from the norm of steamed-and-buttered to deliver lots of flavor and interesting texture. We cover all the favorite variations of the starch family — mashed, fries, fritters, noodles, and rice — without a problematic grain in sight.

If your family is skeptical about replacing grains with vegetables, try a new spin. Instead of telling them that you're substituting their old favorites with vegetables, promote the new side dish as the latest gourmet invention. If your family ate Cauliflower Rice or Zucchini Noodles in a restaurant, they'd probably be impressed. So put on your chef's hat and talk up your new menu like a pro.

Sesame Kale

Prep time: 15 min • **Cook time:** 12 min • **Yield:** 4 servings

Ingredients	*Directions*
1 tablespoon sesame seeds	*1* Heat a large sauté pan or wok over medium-high heat. When the pan is hot, add the sesame seeds and stir constantly until they're lightly toasted, about 3 to 5 minutes. Remove from the pan and reserve for later.
1 bunch fresh kale, washed, ribs removed, coarsely chopped	
⅓ cup water	*2* Wash the kale and remove any tough and/or thick ribs, and then roughly chop or tear the leaves. Place the water in the skillet and bring to a boil over high heat.
1 tablespoon sesame oil	
½ teaspoon ginger	
Dash cayenne pepper	*3* Add half the kale to the boiling water and stir with a wooden spoon until it begins to wilt, and then add the rest of the leaves. Cover and allow the kale to steam until tender, about 5 to 6 minutes.
Salt and pepper to taste	
	4 Remove the lid and allow any remaining water to evaporate. Turn off the heat and drizzle the kale with the sesame oil, tossing to coat. Sprinkle with ginger, cayenne pepper, salt, and black pepper; toss again. Sprinkle with sesame seeds just before serving.

Per serving: Calories 76 (From Fat 44); Fat 5 g (Saturated 1 g); Cholesterol 0 mg; Sodium 174 mg; Carbohydrate 8 g (Dietary Fiber 3 g); Protein 3 g.

Vary It! This basic recipe works well with other greens, like collards, beet tops, chard, and spinach. You can also vary the flavors with different oils. For Italian flair, use olive oil in place of sesame oil, and replace the ginger with crushed garlic.

Creamy Kale

Prep time: 5 min • **Cook time:** 10 min • **Yield:** 2 servings

Ingredients	Directions
1 large bunch kale (about 12 leaves)	**1** Wash the kale and shake off any excess water. Remove the tough stems with the tip of a sharp knife. Roughly chop or tear the leaves.
1 teaspoon ground cumin	
½ teaspoon ground coriander	**2** Heat a large skillet over medium-high heat. Toss in about half the kale. Stir with a wooden spoon until the kale begins to wilt, and then add the remaining kale. Stir and cover with a lid.
2 cloves garlic, crushed	
Pinch of salt	
1 teaspoon coconut oil	**3** In a small bowl, mix the cumin, coriander, garlic, and salt. Set aside.
½ cup coconut milk	
	4 When the kale is dark green and beginning to wilt, remove the lid and let any remaining water evaporate.
	5 When the pan is mostly dry, push the kale to the side and add the coconut oil. Let the oil heat and then pour the spices directly into the pool of oil to release their fragrance, about 20 seconds.
	6 Pour the coconut milk into the pan (not directly into the oil), stirring to combine the kale, seasonings, and milk. Sauté until the sauce begins to thicken.

Per serving: Calories 131 (From Fat 90); Fat 10 g (Saturated 8 g); Cholesterol 0 mg; Sodium 58 mg; Carbohydrate 10 g (Dietary Fiber 2 g); Protein 3 g.

Tip: You can substitute another sturdy leafy green for the kale.

This recipe has been vetted by the team at Whole9 (http://whole9life.com) and is considered acceptable for a cleansing 30-day Paleo launch.

Sweet Potato Shoestring Fries

Prep time: 10 min • **Cook time:** 40 min • **Yield:** 4 servings

Ingredients	Directions
2 large sweet potatoes	*1* Preheat the oven to 450 degrees. Cover two baking sheets with parchment paper.
1 tablespoon arrowroot powder	
2 tablespoons coconut oil	*2* Cut the sweet potatoes into ⅛ - to ¼-inch strips. Place in a large bowl, add the arrowroot powder, and toss until the fries are lightly coated.
½ tablespoon ground cumin	
1 teaspoon chili powder	*3* In a small bowl, combine the coconut oil, cumin, chili powder, cinnamon, thyme, salt, and pepper. Heat in the microwave for 15 to 20 seconds until the coconut oil is melted. Stir with a fork to combine.
¼ teaspoon ground cinnamon	
¼ teaspoon dried thyme	
¼ teaspoon salt, plus more to taste	*4* Add the seasoned coconut oil to the sweet potatoes and toss with two wooden spoons to evenly coat the fries with the oil.
¼ teaspoon ground black pepper	
	5 Arrange the coated fries on the baking sheets, making sure the fries aren't touching. Bake for 15 minutes, and then flip and bake an additional 15 to 20 minutes, until desired crispness.
	6 Remove from the oven, sprinkle with additional salt, and serve immediately.

Per serving: Calories 164 (From Fat 65); Fat 7 g (Saturated 6 g); Cholesterol 0 mg; Sodium 164 mg; Carbohydrate 24 g (Dietary Fiber 3 g); Protein 2 g.

Note: If using organic sweet potatoes, keep the skin on. If using conventionally grown potatoes, peel them.

Tip: These fries are great with bunless burgers, Slow Cooker BBQ Pulled Pork (Book II, Chapter 4), or eggs for a fun and fancy brunch. Dip them in Mark's Daily Apple Ketchup, or eat them the Belgian way with seasoned Olive Oil Mayo (both recipes in Book III, Chapter 2).

Vary It! Change the seasonings! Try Garam Masala or Morning Spice (both recipes in Book III, Chapter 3), smoked paprika, or a little garlic powder for extra zing.

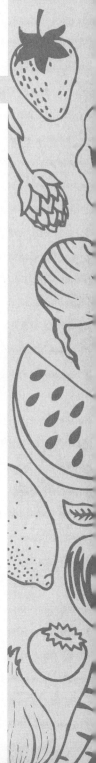

Spaghetti Squash Fritters

Prep time: 10 min • **Cook time:** 5 min • **Yield:** 4 servings

Ingredients	Directions
1 spaghetti squash	**1** Preheat the oven to 375 degrees. Cover a large baking sheet with parchment paper.
½ onion, finely minced	
½ cup almond flour	**2** Cut the squash in half lengthwise, and scoop out the seeds with a large spoon. Place the squash cut-side-down on the baking sheet.
3 large eggs	
½ teaspoon salt	**3** Place the baking sheet in the oven and roast for 35 to 40 minutes.
½ teaspoon ground black pepper	
1 to 2 tablespoons coconut oil	**4** Remove the squash from the oven and, using a hot pad to hold it, scrape the inside with a fork to shred the squash into spaghetti-like strands.
	5 In a large bowl, mix the onion, almond flour, eggs, salt, and pepper with a whisk until combined. Squeeze any excess moisture from the squash with a clean dish towel or paper towels, add to the bowl, and mix well. Allow the batter to rest 10 minutes.
	6 Place ½ tablespoon coconut oil in a nonstick skillet and heat over medium-high heat until the oil is melted and shimmers. Swivel the pan to coat the bottom.
	7 Drop ¼-cup servings of batter into the pan, making sure they don't touch. Cook until browned on the bottom and starting to set, about 4 to 5 minutes. Flip gently and cook the other side until browned, an additional 3 to 4 minutes.
	8 Cook in batches, adding more coconut oil to the pan as necessary. Serve hot.

Per serving: Calories 197 (From Fat 130); Fat 14 g (Saturated 5 g); Cholesterol 140 mg; Sodium 359 mg; Carbohydrate 8 g (Dietary Fiber 3 g); Protein 9 g.

Vary It! Substitute shredded zucchini for the spaghetti squash; just follow the instructions for Zucchini Noodles (later in this chapter) to prep the zucchini.

Mashed Cauliflower

Prep time: 5 min • **Cook time:** 5 min • **Yield:** 2–4 servings

Ingredients	Directions
2 garlic cloves **One 16-ounce bag frozen cauliflower florets** **1½ tablespoons coconut oil** **½ cup coconut milk** **2 teaspoons dried thyme leaves** **Salt and pepper to taste**	**1** Peel the garlic and cook along with the cauliflower, following the package directions, until the cauliflower is very soft but not waterlogged. **2** In a microwave-safe bowl or small saucepan, heat the coconut oil, coconut milk, thyme, salt, and pepper about 1 minute. **3** Meanwhile, puree the cauliflower in a food processor, scraping down the sides. Add the coconut milk and process about 10 seconds. Taste and adjust seasonings.

Per serving: Calories 289 (From Fat 227); Fat 25 g (Saturated 22 g); Cholesterol 0 mg; Sodium 356 mg; Carbohydrate 16 g (Dietary Fiber 7 g); Protein 6 g.

Note: You can use fresh cauliflower for this recipe, but frozen cauliflower packs the same nutritional punch and reaches a creamy texture faster and easier than fresh.

Vary It! Try substituting parsley or chives for the dried thyme. You may also use chicken broth in place of the coconut milk.

Cauliflower Rice

Prep time: 10 min • **Cook time:** 10 min • **Yield:** 4–6 servings

Ingredients	*Directions*
1 large head fresh cauliflower	**1** Break the cauliflower into florets, removing the stems. Place the florets in a food processor and pulse until the cauliflower looks like rice, about ten to fifteen 1-second pulses. You may need to do this step in two batches.
1½ tablespoons coconut oil	
½ medium onion, diced (about ½ cup)	**2** Heat a large skillet over medium heat, about 3 minutes. Add the coconut oil and allow it to melt. Add the onion and garlic, and cook gently until the onions are translucent, about 7 minutes.
1 clove garlic, minced (about 1 teaspoon)	
Salt and pepper to taste	
	3 Add the riced cauliflower to the pan and sauté until the cauliflower is tender, about 5 to 7 minutes. Taste and season with salt and pepper.

Per serving: Calories 106 (From Fat 50); Fat 6 g (Saturated 5 g); Cholesterol 0 mg; Sodium 209 mg; Carbohydrate 13 g (Dietary Fiber 6 g); Protein 5 g.

Vary It! Make curry fried rice by adding 1 teaspoon of curry powder to the cooked Cauliflower Rice, along with 2 tablespoons each of sliced almonds and raisins.

Cocoa Cauliflower

Prep time: 5 min • **Cook time:** 40 min • **Yield:** 4 servings

Ingredients	*Directions*
1 head fresh cauliflower	*1* Preheat the oven to 400 degrees. Cover a baking sheet with parchment paper or aluminum foil.
1 teaspoon paprika	
1 teaspoon unsweetened cocoa powder	*2* With a sharp knife, remove the core of the cauliflower and break the head into florets. Place the florets in a large mixing bowl.
¼ teaspoon salt	
¼ teaspoon ground black pepper	*3* In a small, microwave-safe bowl, mix the paprika, cocoa, salt, pepper, and garlic with a fork. Add the coconut oil and microwave for 15 to 20 seconds until the coconut oil is melted and the spices are fragrant.
1 clove garlic, minced	
2 tablespoons coconut oil	
	4 Drizzle the spiced oil over the cauliflower in the bowl and toss until well coated.
	5 Spread the cauliflower in a single layer on the baking sheet and roast in the oven for 25 to 30 minutes, until it's tender and beginning to brown.

Per serving: Calories 81 (From Fat 63); Fat 7 g (Saturated 6 g); Cholesterol 0 mg; Sodium 168 mg; Carbohydrate 5 g (Dietary Fiber 2 g); Protein 2 g.

Tip: If you don't care for the somewhat bitter taste of unsweetened cocoa, you can make this dish without it; the cauliflower will still be tasty!

This recipe has been vetted by the team at Whole9 (http://whole9life.com) and is considered acceptable for a cleansing 30-day Paleo launch.

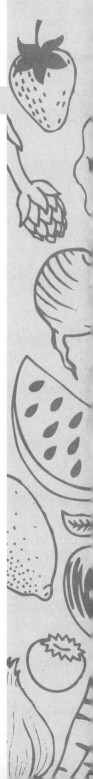

Zucchini Pasta with Fire-Roasted Tomato Sauce

Prep time: 5–20 min • **Cook time:** 5 min • **Yield:** 2 servings

Ingredients	Directions
2 whole zucchini, peeled	**Cooked Version**
Salt for draining, plus more to taste	*1* Use a spiral slicer or mandoline to make pasta out of the zucchini. If you don't have a spiral slicer, you can use a julienne peeler or vegetable peeler and make thicker noodles.
¼ cup pecans, roasted	*2* Place the zucchini noodles in a colander in the sink and heavily salt them. Let them sit for 20 minutes to drain all the water.
One 14.5-ounce can fire-roasted tomatoes	*3* Pulse the pecans in a blender or food processor until you have small chunks — not quite a flour consistency.
1 tablespoon coconut oil	*4* Add the fire-roasted tomatoes and process on high to make a smooth sauce.
Pepper to taste	*5* Preheat a saucepan on medium heat. Simmer the tomato sauce in the saucepan, covered, until hot.
	6 Preheat a sauté pan on medium heat. Add the coconut oil to the sauté pan and sauté the noodles for 1 to 2 minutes to warm them up. Transfer the noodles to a plate, dress with the sauce, and serve.

Raw Version

1 Complete Steps 1, 3, and 4 from the preceding Cooked Version recipe. Don't include Step 2 (the salting-and-draining step).

2 Plate the noodles and dress with the sauce.

3 Sprinkle with salt and pepper to taste and serve.

Per serving: *Calories 217 (From Fat 144); Fat 16 g (Saturated 7 g); Cholesterol 0 mg; Sodium 683 mg; Carbohydrate 17 g (Dietary Fiber 5 g); Protein 5 g.*

Tip: This dish is a wonderful complement to any protein for a complete meal, or you can serve it as a main course.

Recipe courtesy George Bryant, CEO and author of Civilized Caveman Cooking Creations (`http://civilizedcavemancooking.com`)

This recipe has been vetted by the team at Whole9 (`http://whole9life.com`) *and is considered acceptable for a cleansing 30-day Paleo launch.*

Creamy Spiced Broccoli

Prep time: 5 min • **Cook time:** 10 min • **Yield:** 4 servings

Ingredients	Directions
1 large bunch broccoli, broken into small florets	*1* Heat a large skillet over medium-high heat, and add the broccoli and water. Bring to a boil and cover, steaming the broccoli until it's bright green and beginning to soften, about 5 to 7 minutes.
¼ cup water	
2 teaspoons Garam Masala (see recipe in Book III, Chapter 3)	*2* In a small bowl, mix the Garam Masala, garlic, and salt with a fork. Set aside.
2 cloves fresh garlic, minced	
Pinch of salt	*3* Remove the lid from the broccoli and allow any remaining water to evaporate. When the pan is mostly dry, push the broccoli to the side and add the coconut oil. Let the oil warm up, and then pour the spices directly into the pool of oil to release their fragrance and flavor, about 20 seconds.
1 teaspoon coconut oil	
½ cup coconut milk	
	4 Pour the coconut milk into the pan, stirring to combine the broccoli, seasonings, and liquid. Sauté until the sauce begins to thicken and serve immediately.

Per serving: Calories 105 (From Fat 78); Fat 9 g (Saturated 7 g); Cholesterol 0 mg; Sodium 60 mg; Carbohydrate 7 g (Dietary Fiber 3 g); Protein 3 g.

Tip: Make this dish a complete meal by adding cooked chicken, beef, lamb, pork, or seafood during the last step.

Vary It! Substitute green beans or braising greens, such as chard, kale, or collards, for the broccoli.

Italian Broccoli

Prep time: 5 min • **Cook time:** 20 min • **Yield:** 4 servings

Ingredients	Directions
¼ cup macadamia nut oil or coconut oil	*1* Heat the oil in a large skillet over medium heat.
2 cloves garlic, crushed	*2* Add the garlic and cook for a few minutes, stirring constantly.
One 14.5-ounce can diced tomatoes	
1 tablespoon balsamic vinegar	*3* Pour in the tomatoes with their juices, the vinegar, and the basil, and simmer until the liquid has reduced by about half.
¼ teaspoon dried basil	
1 pound broccoli, trimmed and cut into spears	*4* Place the broccoli on top of the tomatoes and season with a little salt and pepper.
Salt and pepper to taste	
	5 Cover and simmer over low heat for 10 minutes or until the broccoli is tender. Don't overcook the broccoli; it should be a vibrant green.
	6 Pour the cooked broccoli into a serving dish and toss to blend with the sauce before serving.

Per serving: Calories 180 (From Fat 126); Fat 14 g (Saturated 12 g); Cholesterol 0 mg; Sodium 196 mg; Carbohydrate 14 g (Dietary Fiber 4 g); Protein 4 g.

Tip: If you use coconut oil, the dish will take on a bit of coconut flavor. If you use the macadamia nut oil, it will have a richer, buttery taste.

This recipe has been vetted by the team at Whole9 (`http://whole9life.com`*) and is considered acceptable for a cleansing 30-day Paleo launch.*

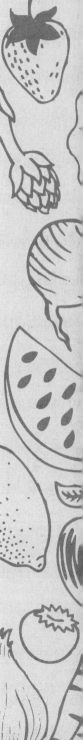

Sautéed Kohlrabi

Prep time: 10 min • **Cook time:** 10 min • **Yield:** 2 servings

Ingredients	Directions
2 kohlrabies	**1** Trim the stalks from the kohlrabies and slice off the bottoms. Peel the bulbs and cut into ¼-inch-thick slices.
1 tablespoon butter	
2 cloves garlic, crushed	
Pinch of salt	**2** Bring a pot of water to a boil. Add the kohlrabies and cook until tender but still firm, about 4 to 5 minutes. Drain the kohlrabies and run them under cold water to stop the cooking. Dry them on a paper towel.
Pinch of ground black pepper	
Chopped parsley for garnish	
	3 Heat the butter in a large skillet and add the garlic. Sauté until fragrant, stirring constantly. Add the kohlrabies to the skillet, along with the salt and pepper, and sauté until they're golden brown on both sides.
	4 Sprinkle with the parsley and serve.

Per serving: Calories 92 (From Fat 54); Fat 6 g (Saturated 4 g); Cholesterol 15 mg; Sodium 319 mg; Carbohydrate 10 g (Dietary Fiber 5 g); Protein 3 g.

Recipe courtesy Arsy Vartanian, author of *Rubies & Radishes* (www.rubiesandradishes.com)

This recipe has been vetted by the team at Whole9 (http://whole9life.com) and is considered acceptable for a cleansing 30-day Paleo launch.

Brussels Sprouts with Cranberries and Almonds

Prep time: 10 min • **Cook time:** 30 min • **Yield:** 4 servings

Ingredients	Directions
3 tablespoons coconut oil 1 medium onion, chopped	**1** Preheat a large skillet on medium-low heat for 1 to 2 minutes. Add the coconut oil.
2 cloves garlic, minced Pinch of salt, plus more to taste	**2** Add the onions and garlic and season with the salt and pepper. Cook for a few minutes until the onions are translucent.
Pinch of ground black pepper, plus more to taste 4 cups Brussels sprouts, trimmed and sliced ½ cup almonds, chopped	**3** Add the Brussels sprouts and stir to thoroughly coat with the oil. Sauté, adding more oil if the pan starts to dry out and brown. After a couple of minutes, add the almonds, cranberries, and flaxseed (if desired).
¼ cup dried cranberries (no sugar added) Pinch of flaxseed (optional)	**4** Stir thoroughly and cook until the sprouts are lightly caramelized. Salt and pepper to taste.

Per serving: *Calories 265 (From Fat 180); Fat 20 g (Saturated 10 g); Cholesterol 0 mg; Sodium 129 mg; Carbohydrate 21 g (Dietary Fiber 6 g); Protein 7 g.*

Vary It! Try adding chopped celery and napa cabbage to the sprouts for a different flavor and texture.

Tip: You can use this fabulous vegetable dish as the foundation for many different meals, so make extra! Not only is it a great side dish, but it's also an awesome meal. Add grilled chicken or steak or top with eggs.

This recipe has been vetted by the team at Whole9 (`http://whole9life.com`) and is considered acceptable for a cleansing 30-day Paleo launch.

Kimchi

Prep time: 10 min, plus marinating time • **Yield:** 6 servings

Ingredients	Directions
1 medium to large napa cabbage, shredded	**1** Toss all the ingredients together in a mixing bowl. Cover and allow the mixture to sit in a cool, dark place overnight or for at least a few hours for the flavors to mingle.
1 cup shredded carrot	
½ cup diced red bell peppers	
½ cup shredded onion	**2** After the mixture is done marinating, serve immediately. Store any leftovers in the fridge for 5 to 7 days.
1 tablespoon apple cider vinegar	
1 tablespoon minced ginger	
1 teaspoon honey	
¼ teaspoon red chili flakes	
1 tablespoon salt	

Per serving: Calories 26 (From Fat 0); Fat 0 g (Saturated 0 g); Cholesterol 0 mg; Sodium 1,180 mg; Carbohydrate 6 g (Dietary Fiber 1 g); Protein 1 g.

Note: Kimchi is an Asian pickled condiment. It really works at healing your intestines.

Tip: Kimchi is a great dish to have with your eggs in the morning! You can add even more red chili flakes if you really like it hot.

Vary It! Omit the honey if you're doing the 30-Day Paleo Reset in Book I, Chapter 1.

Recipe courtesy Alissa Cohen, chef and author of Living on Live Food (www.alissacohen.com)

Vegetable Latkes

Prep time: 15 min • **Cook time:** 4–6 min • **Yield:** 5 servings

Ingredients	Directions
3 cups grated carrot, turnip, daikon radish, or zucchini	*1* Wrap a thin dish towel around the grated vegetables, 1 cup at a time, and squeeze out as much water as possible.
2 eggs, beaten	
Pinch of Celtic sea salt	*2* In a bowl, mix the grated vegetables with the eggs, salt, and pepper. Preheat the oven to 250 degrees.
Pinch of ground black pepper	
½ cup macadamia nut oil	*3* Heat the oil in skillet over medium-high heat. Toss a pinch of the grated vegetable mixture into the pan; if it sizzles immediately, the oil is hot enough.
	4 Scoop ½ to ¾ cup of the grated vegetable mixture (slightly less than ¼ of the total mixture) into your hand and form it into a very loose patty.
	5 Set the patty into the hot pan and press it down gently with a fork. Cook at least 2 to 3 minutes on each side until nicely browned, keeping the cooked latkes warm in the heated oven. Sprinkle with a pinch of salt before serving.

Per serving: Calories 71 (From Fat 27); Fat 3 g (Saturated 2 g); Cholesterol 74 mg; Sodium 125 mg; Carbohydrate 7 g (Dietary Fiber 2 g); Protein 3 g.

Vary It! You can add cinnamon to the carrot latkes, curry powder to the turnip, or fresh herbs to the zucchini.

Tip: If the oil starts to smoke or becomes dark in color, carefully discard it, clean the pan, and start fresh with new oil before frying any more latkes. Burnt oil is definitely not healthy or Paleo-approved.

Recipe courtesy Mark Sisson, author of Primal Blueprint and Mark's Daily Apple (www.marksdailyapple.com)

This recipe has been vetted by the team at Whole9 (http://whole9life.com) *and is considered acceptable for a cleansing 30-day Paleo launch.*

Lemon Cucumber Noodles with Cumin

Prep time: 5 min • **Cook time:** 5 min • **Yield:** 2 servings

Ingredients	Directions
1 whole cucumber	**1** Use a spiral slicer or mandoline to make pasta out of the cucumber. If you don't have a spiral slicer, you can use a julienne peeler or vegetable peeler and make thicker noodles.
1 whole lemon, zested and juiced	
1 tablespoon sea salt	**2** Place the noodles in a bowl and toss with the lemon juice, salt, and cumin.
1 teaspoon ground cumin	
	3 Transfer to a bowl and garnish with lemon zest.

Per serving: Calories 39 (From Fat 5); Fat 0.5 g (Saturated 0 g); Cholesterol 0 mg; Sodium 3,514 mg; Carbohydrate 12 g (Dietary Fiber 4 g); Protein 2 g.

Tip: Double the batch for your lunch the next day.

Recipe courtesy George Bryant, CEO and author of Civilized Caveman Cooking Creations (http://civilizedcavemancooking.com)

This recipe has been vetted by the team at Whole9 (http://whole9life.com) and is considered acceptable for a cleansing 30-day Paleo launch.

Chapter 6

Paleo for Kids: Recipes Your Littles Will Love

In This Chapter

▶ Satisfying the toughest critics in the household

▶ Smoothing the Paleo transition with surefire recipes

Recipes in This Chapter

↻ Spiced Sweet Potato Fries

▶ Barbecue-Flavored Kale Chips

↻ Lunchbox Stuffed Peppers

▶ Parsnip Hash Browns

▶ Sautéed Kale with Bacon and Mushrooms

↻ Raspberry Peppermint Sorbet

↻ Raspberry Cheesecake Bites

↻ Star Fruit Magic Wands

🍴 🍽 🥄 ✻ 🥕

*P*arents face plenty of hurdles when it comes to getting kids to eat healthy. At times, the task can be downright daunting, but it's a necessary one.

In 2004, the then-surgeon general asserted that modern U.S. children will be the first generation to have a shorter life expectancy than their parents. This statement was a catalyzing moment for a lot of parents, who knew they had to take action and make a difference, starting in their very own kitchens.

Teaching children about nutrition and making them aware of healthier foods at a young age can have lasting effects. (If your kids are older, have no fear; as the saying goes, better late than never.) Have good food available and make it a part of your everyday life; kids absorb everything, and someday their understanding of the importance of nutrition may surprise you. The recipes in this chapter (plus one for Make-Your-Own Cobb Salads available online at www. dummies.com/extras/paleocookbook) get you off on the right foot.

Packing Kid-Friendly Paleo Lunches

Taking the time to pack your kids (and yourself) a nourishing lunch is one of the best ways to set them up for optimal concentration. By thoughtfully combining foods in packed lunches, your kids will feel fuller for longer and be better able to concentrate on schoolwork and other tasks without being distracted by hunger or by blood sugar crashes.

Try to anchor your lunches with a high-quality animal protein. Protein helps you to feel fuller for longer.

Paleo lunch-packing is a matter of being able to easily pull from three sources: your leftovers, your fresh foods, and your nonperishables. Here are some great ideas from Audrey Olson of www.primalkitchen.blogspot.com on how to stay stocked up on all fronts.

- **Leftovers**
  - Make double for dinner. This way, you always have at least a day's worth of leftovers to throw in everyone's lunchbox.
  - Intentionally decide which night's meal will become the next day's lunch. This smooths your menu and grocery planning.

- **Fresh to-go options**
  - Precut vegetables and fruit. Buy snack packs or cut them yourself and pack them in portion-sized containers.
  - Buy single-serve packets of guacamole.
  - Make a week's worth of Paleo quiches and egg muffins that you can easily grab and go.
  - Pre-boil eggs for a fast protein option available throughout the week. You can eat them straight up or devil them (check out Book III, Chapter 1, for a deviled eggs recipe).
  - Pack chicken, egg, or tuna salad (made with a Paleo-friendly mayo like the ones in Book III, Chapter 2) in individual containers or stuffed into peppers.
  - Make DIY plantain chips or other homemade or dehydrated veggie chips.

- **Nonperishables**
  - Put together small premade containers of homemade trail mix with nuts, coconut flakes, dried fruit, and so on.
  - Consider jerky. Grass-fed beef jerky in particular makes a great option for high-quality protein you can toss into a lunchbox when you've run out of everything, including eggs!
  - Keep individual packets of raw, unsweetened nut butters handy.
  - Pick up dried fruits such as banana chips. Watch out for added sugars and other iffy ingredients, though!

Spiced Sweet Potato Fries

Prep time: 5 min • **Cook time:** 35 min • **Yield:** 6 servings

Ingredients	Directions
3 medium sweet potatoes **2 tablespoons coconut or macadamia oil, melted** **1 teaspoon garlic powder** **½ teaspoon garam masala spice blend** **¼ teaspoon ground sea salt**	*1* Preheat the oven to 425 degrees. Line a baking sheet with parchment paper. *2* Cut the sweet potatoes lengthwise into ½-inch-wide fries. (Each potato should make 6 to 8 fries.) *3* In a gallon-sized zip-top bag, combine the sliced fries with the remaining ingredients. Shake vigorously for at least 1 minute to ensure that the oil and spices evenly combine and coat each fry. *4* Spread the fries evenly on the baking sheet. *5* Bake for 35 minutes; check the fries to be sure they're browning evenly. *6* Serve the fries while they're hot.

Per serving: *Calories 105 (From Fat 45); Fat 5 g (Saturated 4 g); Cholesterol 0 mg; Sodium 130 mg; Carbohydrate 14 g (Dietary Fiber 2 g); Protein 1 g.*

Tip: If you like your fries to be a little crisp on the ends, you can set your oven to broil and broil them for a couple of minutes after you check them for browning in Step 5.

Vary It! Garam masala blends usually contain cumin and other warm spices. You can find it in stores or make your own with the recipe in Book III, Chapter 3. Omit the garam masala if your family doesn't enjoy spicy foods.

Recipe courtesy Audrey Olson, author of Primal Kitchen: A Family Grokumentary (www.primalkitchen.blogspot.com)

This recipe has been vetted by the team at Whole9 (http://whole9life.com) and is considered acceptable for a cleansing 30-day Paleo launch.

Barbecue-Flavored Kale Chips

Prep time: 10 min • **Cook time:** 20 min • **Yield:** 2 servings

Ingredients	Directions
4 cups chopped fresh kale (stems removed)	*1* Preheat the oven to 350 degrees.
2 tablespoons cashew butter	*2* Wash the chopped kale, and then use paper towels to remove as much moisture as possible. Put the kale in a gallon-sized zip-top bag.
1 tablespoon bacon fat or coconut oil, melted	
1 tablespoon macadamia oil	*3* Blend the remaining ingredients in a blender or food processor until smooth.
2 teaspoons apple cider vinegar	
4 drops organic stevia extract (optional)	*4* Add the blended seasoning mixture to the bag with the kale. Close the bag and massage it for a couple of minutes to get the seasoning mix into as many crannies of the kale as possible.
½ teaspoon garlic powder	
2 teaspoons onion powder	
2 teaspoons paprika	*5* Spread the kale chips out on a baking sheet. Bake for 20 minutes, gently stirring the chips after 10 minutes. The kale will get a little limp before it starts to dry and crisp up during this process.
4 drops fish sauce (optional)	
Sea salt to taste	
	6 Watch the kale carefully as it approaches the 20-minute mark to make sure it doesn't burn; you're looking for crispy chips that are dark brown on the edges, not black all the way through!

7 If needed, stir the chips and continue baking. If desired, finish the chips for 1 minute under the broiler to crisp them a little more.

8 Enjoy your kale chips hot, fresh, and crispy straight out of the oven.

Per serving (2 cups): *Calories 297 (From Fat 207); Fat 23 g (Saturated 13 g); Cholesterol 0 mg; Sodium 694 mg; Carbohydrate 22 g (Dietary Fiber 4 g); Protein 8 g.*

Tip: Red Boat fish sauce is a premium fish sauce made with only anchovies and sea salt. It's a great addition to your pantry for this and many other Paleo recipes!

Tip: If you don't care for stevia but still want a little sweetness to your barbecue flavor, you can substitute a teaspoon of maple syrup or honey in your seasoning mixture.

Recipe courtesy Audrey Olson, author of Primal Kitchen: A Family Grokumentary (www.primalkitchen.blogspot.com)

This recipe has been vetted by the team at Whole9 (http://whole9life.com) *and is considered acceptable for a cleansing 30-day Paleo launch.*

Lunchbox Stuffed Peppers

Prep time: 35 min • **Yield:** 4 servings

Ingredients	Directions
¼ **cup Paleo mayonnaise (see recipe in Book III, Chapter 2)**	*1* In a medium bowl, combine the mayo, eggs, and relish. Season with salt and pepper to taste.
5 hard-boiled eggs, diced	
¼ **cup unsweetened pickle relish**	*2* Using a small spoon, scoop the egg salad into the peppers until just filled to the top.
Salt and pepper to taste	
8 mini sweet peppers, about 3 inches long, tops and seeds removed	*3* Enjoy immediately or save in the fridge for a future packed lunch.

Per serving (2 peppers): Calories 192 (From Fat 126); Fat 14 g (Saturated 3 g); Cholesterol 246 mg; Sodium 317 mg; Carbohydrate 8 g (Dietary Fiber 1 g); Protein 9 g.

Note: Bubbies relish (www.bubbies.com/kosher_dill_relish) is one option for a live, lacto-fermented relish that is free of sugar.

Vary It! Substitute canned tuna in water or leftover baked chicken (diced) for the eggs.

Recipe courtesy Audrey Olson, author of Primal Kitchen: A Family Grokumentary (www.primalkitchen.blogspot.com)

This recipe has been vetted by the team at Whole9 (http://whole9life.com) and is considered acceptable for a cleansing 30-day Paleo launch.

Parsnip Hash Browns

Prep time: 15 min • **Cook time:** 15 min • **Yield:** 3 servings

Ingredients	Directions
3 parsnips, peeled	**1** Using a box shredder, shred the parsnips until you reach the core.
4 tablespoons coconut oil	
½ teaspoon ground cloves	**2** In a large skillet over medium-high heat, melt the coconut oil and then add the spices.
½ teaspoon ground nutmeg	
½ teaspoon ground cinnamon	**3** Toss the parsnip shreds into the pan. Stir and turn frequently. The parsnips will begin to brown, crisp, and clump together. Use a spatula to shape them into three hash brown cakes about the size of your palm.
	4 Continue turning the parsnip cakes for another couple of minutes, until golden brown and slightly crispy on the outside. Serve immediately.

Per serving (1 parsnip cake): Calories 274 (From Fat 171); Fat 19 g (Saturated 16 g); Cholesterol 0 mg; Sodium 395 mg; Carbohydrate 28 g (Dietary Fiber 7 g); Protein 2 g.

Note: Because parsnips are naturally slightly sweet but not overly starchy, this recipe is a palate-pleasing yet less-carby alternative to potato hash browns.

Vary It! You can substitute butter or ghee for the coconut oil. You can also try replacing the spices with garlic powder, onion powder, and salt before pan-frying for a savory take.

Recipe courtesy Audrey Olson, author of Primal Kitchen: A Family Grokumentary (www.primalkitchen.blogspot.com)

This recipe has been vetted by the team at Whole9 (http://whole9life.com) and is considered acceptable for a cleansing 30-day Paleo launch.

Sautéed Kale with Bacon and Mushrooms

Prep time: 5 min • **Cook time:** 10–15 min • **Yield:** 6–8 servings

Ingredients	Directions
6 cups chopped fresh curly kale, stems removed	*1* Wash the chopped kale and then use paper towels to remove as much moisture as possible.
4 tablespoons macadamia oil	
8 ounces mushrooms, cleaned and sliced	*2* In a large skillet, heat the oil over medium-high heat. Sauté the mushrooms, onions, and garlic for about 5 minutes, until the onions are translucent and browning.
1 large yellow onion, sliced into 1-inch pieces	
2 cloves garlic, sliced	*3* Add the bacon and maple syrup to the pan and stir to combine, sautéing an additional 1 to 2 minutes.
6 slices cooked bacon, crumbled	
1 tablespoon maple syrup	*4* Add the kale. Add the chicken broth ¼ cup at a time and cook until the kale is fully wilted, about 4 minutes. (Adding the broth gradually keeps the other ingredients from boiling.)
1 cup chicken broth	
Splash of balsamic vinegar	
	5 Drizzle with the balsamic vinegar, stir briefly, and serve hot.

Per serving (1 cup): Calories 123 (From Fat 81); Fat 9 g (Saturated 6 g); Cholesterol 3 mg; Sodium 156 mg; Carbohydrate 10 g (Dietary Fiber 1 g); Protein 4 g.

Tip: Adding bacon to cooked greens is a magical way to mask the earthy flavor of the greens and even inspire those you're serving to ask for seconds.

Tip: Substitute butter or ghee for the macadamia oil.

Recipe courtesy Audrey Olson, author of Primal Kitchen: A Family Grokumentary (www.primalkitchen.blogspot.com)

Raspberry Peppermint Sorbet

Prep time: 15 min, plus churning time • **Yield:** 6 servings

Ingredients	*Directions*
4 to 5 cups watermelon flesh, frozen solid	*1* Process all ingredients with ½ cup water in a blender until perfectly smooth.
12 ounces frozen raspberries	
½ cup unsweetened applesauce	*2* Pour the mixture into an ice-cream maker and churn for about 30 minutes.
Pinch sea salt	
3 large fresh mint leaves, plus more for garnish	*3* Serve immediately; garnish with leftover mint leaves if desired.

Per serving (1 cup): Calories 72 (From Fat 4); Fat 0.5 g (Saturated 0 g); Cholesterol 0 mg; Sodium 50 mg; Carbohydrate 18 g (Dietary Fiber 4 g); Protein 1 g.

Note: If you don't have an ice-cream machine available, you can serve the mixture just after the blending step. It makes this recipe a delicious and kid-friendly raspberry peppermint smoothie.

Tip: Four to five cups of watermelon equals about ten ice-cream scoops full.

Tip: If you want the sorbet a little firmer, put it in the freezer in another container for an hour or so. If you don't want seeds, you can puree the raspberry and then strain it before adding it to the other ingredients.

Recipe courtesy Audrey Olson, author of Primal Kitchen: A Family Grokumentary (www.primalkitchen.blogspot.com)

Raspberry Cheesecake Bites

Prep time: 45 min, plus refrigerating time • **Yield:** 8 servings

Ingredients	Directions
8 to 10 ounces dark chocolate, divided	**1** Melt half of the chocolate in a double boiler. When the chocolate is melted, stir it with a clean, dry spoon until it's entirely smooth.
⅔ cup cashew butter	
⅓ cup palm shortening	**2** Line 8 cavities of a mini muffin pan with paper liners. Spoon the melted chocolate into the cavities.
2 teaspoons apple cider vinegar	
½ teaspoon fresh lemon juice	**3** Let sit for 5 minutes. Reheat the chocolate in the double boiler and repeat Step 2 to thicken the chocolate base in each cavity.
¼ teaspoon ground sea salt	
⅓ cup maple syrup, or to taste	**4** In a large bowl, combine the cashew butter, palm shortening, vinegar, lemon juice, and salt. Using a stand mixer or hand mixer, whip the mixture until you achieve a cream cheese consistency. Beat in the maple syrup and vanilla.
½ tablespoon vanilla extract	
8 fresh raspberries	
	5 Spoon ½ teaspoon of the cream cheese mixture onto the chocolate in each cavity.
	6 Press a fresh raspberry into the center of the cream cheese mixture in each cavity. Top each raspberry with another ½ teaspoon of the cream cheese mixture.

7 Put the pan in the freezer for at least 30 minutes.

8 Repeat Step 1 to melt the remaining (previously unmelted) chocolate. Spoon the melted chocolate over the cream cheese mixture in each cavity; the melted chocolate should be level with the top of the cavity.

9 Place the pan in the fridge until the chocolate sets fully.

10 Remove the cheesecake bites from the pan and very gently peel off the paper liner. Serve the cheesecake bites within 24 hours of creation so the raspberries are at their juicy best.

Per serving (1 cheesecake bite): Calories 422 (From Fat 270); Fat 30 g (Saturated 12 g); Cholesterol 1 mg; Sodium 80 mg; Carbohydrate 32 g (Dietary Fiber 1 g); Protein 6 g.

Tip: If you don't have a double boiler or don't want to mess with one, warm the chocolate in the microwave for 2 minutes at half power.

Vary It! Try other fresh berries (such as chopped strawberries or blueberries) or small pieces of fresh fruit in place of the raspberry. To make the bites nut-free, substitute unsweetened organic sunflower seed butter for the cashew butter. For sweetness without carbs, substitute a few drops of stevia extract for the maple syrup.

Recipe courtesy Audrey Olson, author of Primal Kitchen: A Family Grokumentary (www.primalkitchen.blogspot.com)

Star Fruit Magic Wands

Prep time: 10 min • **Yield:** 6–8 servings

Ingredients	Directions
2 large star fruits	**1** Wash the star fruits and slice them ¾ inch thick.
	2 Use a toothpick or steak knife to gently pry out any large seeds from the slices.
	3 Insert the pointy end of a bamboo skewer into the bottom of each star fruit slice, about 1 inch deep.
	4 Serve immediately or freeze for 20 minutes to create popsicle-style treats.

Per serving (1 skewer): Calories 7 (From Fat 0); Fat 0 g (Saturated 0 g); Cholesterol 0 mg; Sodium 0 mg; Carbohydrate 1.5 g (Dietary Fiber 1 g); Protein 0 g.

Recipe courtesy Audrey Olson, author of Primal Kitchen: A Family Grokumentary (www.primalkitchen.blogspot.com)

This recipe has been vetted by the team at Whole9 (http://whole9life.com) and is considered acceptable for a cleansing 30-day Paleo launch.

Book III

Paleo Extras: Snacks, Sauces, Spice Mixes, and Sweets

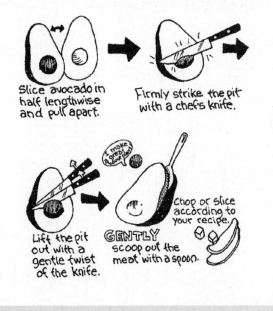

Illustration by Elizabeth Kurtzman

 Discover the supplements that boost your health without breaking from the Paleo lifestyle at www.dummies.com/extras/paleoaio.

Contents at a Glance

Chapter 1: Snacks That Fuel Your Body, Sugar Crash Not Included .... .259

Making Sure Your Snacks Are Healthy...259

Chapter 2: Spicing Up Paleo Cooking with Sauces, Dressings, and Salsas.................................... .275

Making Your Own Dressings and Condiments 275
Adding Flavor with Sugar-Free Spice Blends...276

Chapter 3: Mixing Rubs and Paleo Seasonings .... .295

Tapping the Healing Power of Spices...295

Chapter 4: Satisfying Your Sweet Tooth .... .307

Spotting Sugar in Its Sneakiest Forms...308

Chapter 1

Snacks That Fuel Your Body, Sugar Crash Not Included

In This Chapter

▶ Grab-and-go options for your Paleo lifestyle

▶ High-nutrient snacks to keep you energized and on track

Recipes in This Chapter

↻ Crispy Kale Chips

↻ Roasted Rosemary Almonds

↻ Southwest Deviled Eggs

↻ Sweet Potato Chips

↻ Fried Sage Leaves

▶ Meatball Poppers

↻ Seaweed with a Kick

↻ Avocado Cups

↻ Tropical Mango Parfait

↻ Grilled Spiced Peaches

↻ Ginger-Fried Pears

↻ Fudge Bombs

↻ Cocoa-Cinnamon Coconut Chips

↻ Nutty Fruit Stackers

🍗 🌶 🥄 🌰 🦐

The foods on the Paleo "yes" list (see Book I, Chapter 2) are among the tastiest you can eat, but every once in a while, even the most devoted cave man (or woman) wants a treat with that little something extra. The key to living Paleo is choosing treats that are based on healthful, natural ingredients that don't make you feel like you swallowed a bowling ball.

In this chapter, you discover recipes for healthy snacks that satisfy your craving for a salty crunch or a sweet treat. From toasty coconut chips and a fresh take on deviled eggs to chocolaty fudge balls, you see how deliciously easy it is to adapt tasty snacks and treats to fit into your new lifestyle.

Making Sure Your Snacks Are Healthy

When you eat foods from the Paleo "yes" list, you most likely find avoiding snacks between meals effortless, because Paleo foods are more filling and satisfying. But if a workout leaves you particularly hungry or your stomach is growling between lunch and dinner, the snack and treat recipes in this chapter will help ensure that you treat your body — and your taste buds — right.

Remember the Paleo Big Three: proteins, fats, and carbs. Snacks should be half the size of your standard meals and, ideally, should include protein, healthy fats, and a veggie or fruit to maintain steady blood sugar levels. In a pinch, combine at least two of the three, but avoid eating fruit on its own. For more on the Paleo Big Three, see Chapter 3 of Book I.

Nothing's wrong with enjoying something a little sweet from time to time. But when you decide to indulge, make sure to savor every bite and to choose treats that include nutritious ingredients.

The fruit and nut flour–based recipes in this chapter are best enjoyed with protein and fat, so eat them as part of your meal rather than as a snack between meals or before bed.

To make the most of your dessert, keep your serving sizes small and relish every single bite.

Crispy Kale Chips

Prep time: 2 min • **Cook time:** 10–12 min • **Yield:** 3 servings

Ingredients	Directions
4 cups raw kale, washed, dried, and torn into 2-inch pieces	*1* Preheat the oven to 350 degrees.
1 tablespoon coconut oil, melted	*2* Place the kale in a large bowl and pour the coconut oil over the top. Toss the leaves with two wooden spoons until completely coated with oil, about 2 minutes.
Salt to taste	*3* Spread the kale on a baking sheet in a single layer and sprinkle generously with salt.
	4 Bake for 10 to 12 minutes until crispy and lightly browned on the edges. Keep an eye on the kale chips! They can change from brown to burnt quite quickly.
	5 Remove the kale from the baking sheet and allow to cool on a cooling rack for 3 minutes. The chips are crispier after they cool.

Per serving: Calories 84 (From Fat 46); Fat 5 g (Saturated 4 g); Cholesterol 0 mg; Sodium 232 mg; Carbohydrate 9 g (Dietary Fiber 2 g); Protein 3 g.

Tip: Eat these chips fairly soon after baking — they can begin to wilt after about 30 minutes out of the oven.

Vary It! Adapting your favorite potato chip flavors to kale chips is easy! Just add additional spices along with the salt before baking. For barbecue flavor, add ½ teaspoon chili powder mixed with ½ teaspoon paprika. For onion flavor, replace the plain salt with onion salt.

Roasted Rosemary Almonds

Prep time: 5 min • **Cook time:** 8–12 min • **Yield:** 2 cups

Ingredients	Directions
1 tablespoon ghee (see recipe in Book III, Chapter 2) 2 cups whole, raw, skin-on almonds 2 tablespoons dried rosemary 2 teaspoons kosher salt ¼ teaspoon ground black pepper	**1** Melt the ghee in a large skillet over medium-low heat. **2** Add the almonds and stir until they're coated with ghee. Mix in the rosemary, salt, and pepper, and then shake the pan to arrange the almonds in a single layer. **3** Toast the almonds, stirring often, until they're slightly darkened and aromatic (about 8 to 12 minutes). **4** Transfer to a plate and cool to room temperature. Serve right away or store in an airtight container for up to one week.

Per serving (¼ cup): Calories 210 (From Fat 162); Fat 18 g (Saturated 1.5 g); Cholesterol 0 mg; Sodium 493 mg; Carbohydrate 8 g (Dietary Fiber 5 g); Protein 8 g.

Tip: You can substitute fresh rosemary for a stronger, earthier flavor; adjust the quantity according to your preference.

Recipe courtesy Michelle Tam, author of Nom Nom Paleo (http://nomnompaleo.com)

This recipe has been vetted by the team at Whole9 (http://whole9life.com) and is considered acceptable for a cleansing 30-day Paleo launch.

Southwest Deviled Eggs

Prep time: 25 min • **Yield:** 12 egg halves

Ingredients	Directions
6 large eggs	**1** Place the eggs in a saucepan and cover with water. Bring to a boil over high heat. Remove the pan from the heat, cover, and let sit for 10 minutes.
2 tablespoons Olive Oil Mayonnaise (see recipe in Book III, Chapter 2)	
½ teaspoon white wine vinegar	**2** Drain the water from the eggs and shake the pan to lightly crack the shells. Fill the pan with cold water and allow the eggs to cool for 5 minutes.
¼ teaspoon dry mustard	
¼ teaspoon chipotle pepper powder	**3** Peel the eggs and slice in half lengthwise. Using a spoon, gently remove the yolks and place in a mixing bowl. Add the mayonnaise, vinegar, mustard, chipotle pepper powder, salt, and black pepper. Mix well with a fork, mashing until the yolks form a smooth paste.
⅛ teaspoon salt	
⅛ teaspoon ground black pepper	
¼ ripe avocado, finely diced	**4** Arrange the egg whites on a serving platter and fill the wells with the seasoned yolk, making a small mound about ½ inch above the whites. Top with a little avocado, tomato, and scallion. Serve immediately.
½ ripe tomato, finely diced	
1 scallion, green only, thinly sliced	

Per serving: Calories 63 (From Fat 46); Fat 5 g (Saturated 1 g); Cholesterol 94 mg; Sodium 65 mg; Carbohydrate 1 g (Dietary Fiber 0 g); Protein 3 g.

Note: You can find chipotle pepper powder in many grocery stores and through online spice vendors. If you have trouble finding it, chili powder is a good replacement. You can also substitute 1 teaspoon finely minced canned chipotle pepper; be sure to check the label for non-Paleo ingredients.

Tip: Very fresh eggs are difficult to peel. For success with hard-boiled eggs, buy a dozen and let them rest in the refrigerator for about a week before hard boiling; just keep an eye on their expiration date.

Sweet Potato Chips

Prep time: 5 min • **Yield:** 10 servings

Ingredients	Directions
¼ cup coconut oil	**1** Preheat the oven to 400 degrees.
2 teaspoons cayenne pepper	**2** Combine the oil and cayenne pepper in a medium bowl. Add the sweet potatoes and toss to coat them with the oil mixture.
3 sweet potatoes, peeled and thinly sliced	
	3 Spread the sweet potatoes in a single layer on a parchment-lined baking sheet.
	4 Bake for approximately 20 minutes, flipping halfway through, until the sweet potatoes begin to brown. Check frequently to avoid burning smaller pieces. They will shrink in size and crisp up as they cook.
	5 Let the chips cool for about 3 minutes before serving.

Per serving: Calories 82 (From Fat 54); Fat 6 g (Saturated 5 g); Cholesterol 0 mg; Sodium 22 mg; Carbohydrate 8 g (Dietary Fiber 1 g); Protein 1 g.

This recipe has been vetted by the team at Whole9 (http://whole9life.com) and is considered acceptable for a cleansing 30-day Paleo launch.

Fried Sage Leaves

Prep time: 5 min • **Cook time:** 5 min • **Yield:** 2 servings

Ingredients	Directions
1 tablespoon ghee (see recipe in Book III, Chapter 2) **15 fresh whole sage leaves**	**1** Heat the ghee in a medium cast iron skillet. **2** Place the sage leaves flat in the skillet and cook until slightly crispy, only about a minute or two. Don't let them burn.

Per serving: Calories 24 (From Fat 14); Fat 1.5 g (Saturated 0.5 g); Cholesterol 2 mg; Sodium 1 mg; Carbohydrate 2 g (Dietary Fiber 0 g); Protein 1 g.

Tip: Fried sage adds a gourmet garnish to just about any dish!

Recipe courtesy Arsy Vartanian, author of Rubies & Radishes (www.rubiesandradishes.com)

This recipe has been vetted by the team at Whole9 (http://whole9life.com) and is considered acceptable for a cleansing 30-day Paleo launch.

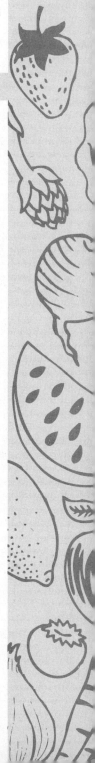

Meatball Poppers

Prep time: 20 min • **Cook time:** 25–30 min • **Yield:** 12 servings

Ingredients	Directions
2 pounds ground beef	**1** Preheat the oven to 425 degrees. Line an 11-x-17-inch rimmed baking pan with parchment paper.
2 tablespoons ground black pepper	
½ teaspoon cayenne pepper	**2** In a medium mixing bowl, combine the beef, black pepper, cayenne, and chili powder. Use your hands to mix well.
½ teaspoon chili powder	
2 teaspoons coconut oil	**3** Melt the coconut oil in a large skillet over medium heat; add the onions, celery, and carrots and cook until they're translucent, about 4 minutes. Add the walnuts and sauté for an additional 2 minutes.
¼ cup minced onion	
¼ cup minced celery	
¼ cup minced carrot	**4** Set the onion mixture aside until it's cool enough to handle. Combine the cooled mixture with the meat and form it into 24 meatballs, roughly 1 inch in size.
¼ cup chopped walnuts	
	5 Place the meatballs on the lined baking pan and bake 25 to 30 minutes.
	6 Serve warm with Moroccan Dipping Sauce (see the recipe in Book III, Chapter 2) if desired.

Per serving: Calories 214 (From Fat 126); Fat 14 g (Saturated 5 g); Cholesterol 65 mg; Sodium 68 mg; Carbohydrate 2 g (Dietary Fiber 1 g); Protein 19 g.

Tip: These meatballs are the best grab-and-go snacks! Freeze these and stock up.

This recipe has been vetted by the team at Whole9 (http://whole9life.com) and is considered acceptable for a cleansing 30-day Paleo launch.

Seaweed with a Kick

Prep time: 5 min • **Cook time:** 4 min • **Yield:** 2–4 servings

Ingredients	Directions
6 nori sheets	*1* Preheat the oven to 350 degrees.
3 tablespoons melted coconut oil	*2* Spread out the nori sheets on a flat surface and rub each with ½ tablespoon of the oil. Season with the cayenne and salt.
1 teaspoon cayenne pepper	
1 teaspoon Celtic sea salt	*3* Arrange the sheets side by side on a baking sheet and bake for 3 to 4 minutes.
	4 Break the sheets into whatever size pieces you prefer and enjoy.

Per serving: Calories 95 (From Fat 90); Fat 10 g (Saturated 9 g); Cholesterol 0 mg; Sodium 407 mg; Carbohydrate 2 g (Dietary Fiber 1 g); Protein 1 g.

Tip: Nori, or edible seaweed, is definitely a smart food (we like SeaSnax brand). It's loaded with iodine, which is a trace mineral you need for healthy thyroid function. If you're not using processed iodized table salt, then you need to make sure you're getting iodine from other sources, such as this snack. Add some protein like a hard-boiled egg for a completely balanced snack!

This recipe has been vetted by the team at Whole9 (http://whole9life.com) and is considered acceptable for a cleansing 30-day Paleo launch.

Avocado Cups

Prep time: 5 min • **Yield:** 4 servings

Ingredients	Directions
2 avocadoes	*1* Halve the avocadoes and remove the pits. Use a spoon to scoop out the flesh.
2 tomatoes, diced	
½ medium cucumber, diced	*2* In a large bowl, mash the avocado with the back of a fork and then mix in the tomatoes, cucumber, and chives. Spread this mixture into the avocado shells.
1 bunch (about 2 ounces) chives, diced	
1 tablespoon apple cider vinegar	*3* Combine the vinegar, olive oil, garlic, coconut aminos, and cayenne and pour over the avocado halves.
4 tablespoons olive oil	
1 clove garlic, minced	
½ teaspoon coconut aminos	
Dash of cayenne pepper	

Per serving: Calories 198 (From Fat 171); Fat 19 g (Saturated 2.5 g); Cholesterol 0 mg; Sodium 21 mg; Carbohydrate 8 g (Dietary Fiber 4 g); Protein 2 g.

Note: Coconut aminos are fermented coconut nectar; they're a bit like soy sauce and are a great Paleo replacement for it (because soy isn't Paleo-approved and many soy sauces also contain wheat ingredients). You can find them in some traditional grocers or online at Amazon.

Vary It! You can also mix some canned tuna into the avocado mixture for a more-balanced snack!

This recipe has been vetted by the team at Whole9 (http://whole9life.com) and is considered acceptable for a cleansing 30-day Paleo launch.

Tropical Mango Parfait

Prep time: 15 min • **Yield:** 4 servings

Ingredients	Directions
2 to 3 ripe mangoes	**1** Peel and core the mangoes and cut into ½-inch dice and place in a small bowl. You should have about 2 cups of diced mango. Add the lime zest and juice, and toss lightly to combine.
1 teaspoon lime zest	
1 teaspoon fresh lime juice	
Whipped Coconut Cream (see recipe in Book III, Chapter 4)	**2** To serve, spoon ¼ cup mango into a parfait glass or bowl. Top with 1 to 2 tablespoons Whipped Coconut Cream; repeat layers. Sprinkle with ½ tablespoon macadamia nuts.
2 tablespoons dry-roasted macadamia nuts, finely chopped	

Per serving: Calories 302 (From Fat 229); Fat 25 g (Saturated 20 g); Cholesterol 0 mg; Sodium 16 mg; Carbohydrate 21 g (Dietary Fiber 3 g); Protein 3 g.

Vary It! This dessert is also delicious with other fruits and nuts. Replace the mango with berries, omit the lime, and substitute almonds for the macadamia nuts to make another summery sweet treat.

Grilled Spiced Peaches

Prep time: 10 min • **Cook time:** 15 min • **Yield:** 4 servings

Ingredients	Directions
1 tablespoon coconut oil, melted	*1* Preheat a grill on high heat.
2 teaspoons raw organic honey, melted	*2* While the grill is preheating, thoroughly mix all the ingredients except the peaches in a medium bowl.
½ teaspoon ground cinnamon	
⅛ teaspoon ground nutmeg	*3* Add the peaches to the honey sauce and toss to ensure they're evenly coated.
Pinch of chili powder	
4 white peaches, pitted and halved	*4* When the grill is warm, carefully place the peaches on the grill grates, ensuring they don't fall through. Grill for 5 minutes on each side or until they're nicely browned.
	5 Allow to cool before serving.

Per serving: *Calories 100 (From Fat 36); Fat 4 g (Saturated 3 g); Cholesterol 0 mg; Sodium 0 mg; Carbohydrate 17 g (Dietary Fiber 2 g); Protein 1 g.*

Tip: You can turn these peaches into a sweet treat by topping them off with any of the Paleo ice creams in Book III, Chapter 4.

Recipe courtesy George Bryant, CEO and author of Civilized Caveman Cooking Creations (http://civilizedcavemancooking.com)

Ginger-Fried Pears

Prep time: 10 min • **Cook time:** 5 min • **Yield:** 4 servings

Ingredients	Directions
2 tablespoons blanched, sliced almonds	**1** Heat a nonstick skillet over medium-high heat. Add the sliced almonds and stir with a wooden spoon until toasted, about 3 to 4 minutes. Remove from pan.
1 tablespoon coconut oil	
2 large, ripe pears, cored and sliced (about 2 cups)	**2** In the same skillet, heat the coconut oil over medium-high heat. Add the pear slices and sauté until the pears begin to soften, about 3 to 4 minutes.
¼ teaspoon powdered ginger	
½ teaspoon lemon zest	**3** In a small bowl, mix the ginger, lemon zest, and salt with a fork, and then add to the pears. Continue cooking until the pears are golden and fragrant, about 5 minutes.
Generous pinch of salt	
	4 To serve, spoon the pears into dessert dishes and sprinkle with the sliced almonds.

Per serving: *Calories 109 (From Fat 48); Fat 5 g (Saturated 3 g); Cholesterol 0 mg; Sodium 72 mg; Carbohydrate 17 g (Dietary Fiber 3 g); Protein 1 g.*

Tip: To make this dish even more decadent and to increase the healthy fats, drizzle each serving with 1 or 2 tablespoons of warm coconut milk.

Vary It! Substitute apples for the pears and replace the ginger with cinnamon.

Fudge Bombs

Prep time: 15 min, plus chilling time • **Yield:** 32 servings

Ingredients	*Directions*
1 cup whole pecans	**1** Place pecans, dates, vanilla, and cocoa in a food processor. Process on high until the mixture forms a paste, about 5 to 7 minutes.
18 pitted dates	
1 teaspoon pure vanilla extract	
4 tablespoons unsweetened cocoa powder	**2** Wet your hands with water and shake off the excess, and then roll the dough into 1-inch balls. Set on a baking sheet.
Garnishes: coarse sea salt, unsweetened shredded coconut, very finely chopped pecans (optional)	**3** Top the balls with a few grains of sea salt or roll them in either coconut flakes or additional nuts (if desired).
	4 Place the Fudge Bombs in the refrigerator until firm, about 30 to 60 minutes. Allow the Fudge Bombs to come to room temperature before eating, but store them covered in the refrigerator.

Per serving: Calories 39 (From Fat 23); Fat 3 g (Saturated 0 g); Cholesterol 0 mg; Sodium 0 mg; Carbohydrate 4 g (Dietary Fiber 1 g); Protein 1 g.

Note: These Fudge Bombs are essentially Paleo candy and should be reserved for special occasions — and they're definitely meant to be shared with friends. This recipe also works well when cut in half (if you have a problem resisting the temptation of a whole batch).

Vary It! Give these bombs a spicy bite by adding ¼ teaspoon cayenne pepper to the dough.

Cocoa-Cinnamon Coconut Chips

Prep time: 1 min • **Cook time:** 3 min • **Yield:** 1 cup

Ingredients	*Directions*
¼ teaspoon salt	*1* In a small bowl, mix the salt, cocoa, and cinnamon with a fork; set aside.
¼ teaspoon unsweetened cocoa powder	
¼ teaspoon ground cinnamon	*2* Heat a nonstick skillet over medium-high heat, about 2 minutes. Add the coconut flakes and distribute evenly so they form a single layer in the bottom of the pan. Stir frequently. When the flakes start to golden, remove the pan from the heat.
1 cup unsweetened coconut flakes	
	3 Sprinkle the spices on the hot coconut flakes and toss until evenly seasoned. Transfer to a plate, arrange in a single layer, and allow them to cool and crisp. Store in an air-tight container.

Per serving (1 teaspoon): Calories 40 (From Fat 33); Fat 4g (Saturated 3g); Cholesterol 0mg; Sodium 38mg; Carbohydrate 1g (Dietary Fiber 1g); Protein 0g.

Tip: These chips are great on their own for a snack, or you can sprinkle them over fresh fruit for a dessert treat.

Vary It! Tickle your taste buds by seasoning these chips with other flavors. Just replace the cocoa and cinnamon with ¼ teaspoon of another spice. Other tempting options include garlic powder, chili powder, or Morning Spice or Garam Masala (recipes in Book III, Chapter 3). Toss these savory chips in a salad for a healthy alternative to croutons.

Nutty Fruit Stackers

Prep time: 2 min • **Yield:** 2 servings

Ingredients	Directions
1 raw apple	**1** With a sharp knife, cut the apple into six equal slices.
2 tablespoons almond butter	
¼ teaspoon pure vanilla extract	**2** In a small bowl, mix the almond butter, vanilla, cinnamon, and salt with a fork until combined.
¼ teaspoon ground cinnamon	**3** Spread each slice of apple with 1 teaspoon of almond butter. Pile slices to form stacks of three slices each. Sprinkle the top of each stack with ½ tablespoon raisins.
Dash of salt	
1 tablespoon raisins	
	4 Chill in the refrigerator for 5 minutes before eating.

Per serving: Calories 159 (From Fat 88); Fat 10 g (Saturated 1 g); Cholesterol 0 mg; Sodium 73 mg; Carbohydrate 18 g (Dietary Fiber 3 g); Protein 3 g.

Tip: This snack is also a sweet treat, so be sure to serve it with some protein to balance the sugars. A piece of grilled chicken breast or a hard-boiled egg is a good accompaniment.

Vary It! This recipe also works great with pears! Or change the flavor by swapping out the almond butter with another Paleo-friendly option, such as sunflower seed butter with a few sunflower seeds sprinkled on with the raisins. You may also like cashew or pecan butter. Or try coconut butter and add a sprinkle of shredded, unsweetened coconut to the top.

Chapter 2

Spicing Up Paleo Cooking with Sauces, Dressings, and Salsas

Recipes in This Chapter

⟳ Ghee
⟳ Cashew Butter Satay Sauce
⟳ Moroccan Dipping Sauce
⟳ Sri Lankan Curry Sauce
⟳ Classic Stir-Fry Sauce
⟳ Tangy Carrot and Ginger Salad Dressing
⟳ Smooth and Creamy Avocado Dressing
⟳ Paleo Ranch Dressing
⟳ Sweet and Spicy Vinaigrette
⟳ Cilantro Vinaigrette
⟳ Olive Oil Mayo
⟳ Cooked Olive Oil Mayo
⟳ Mark's Daily Apple Ketchup
⟳ Tangy BBQ Sauce
⟳ Orange Coconut Marinade
⟳ Basil and Walnut Pesto
⟳ Cucumber Avocado Salsa

🎣 🍶 🍳 🌶 🥢 🌿

In This Chapter

▶ Finding ways to add zip and zing to whatever you cook
▶ Bringing flavor without added sugar or other Paleo no-nos

*T*he right sauces and seasonings can mean the difference between a delectable meal and a dull one. Simple ingredients like chicken, beef, and vitamin-rich vegetables become exciting when they're dipped into something creamy or dusted with something spicy — and the right seasonings can take your taste buds on a world tour.

Think living Paleo means giving up creamy ranch dressing or luscious Asian dipping sauce? Think again. In this chapter, you find recipes for salad dressings, condiments, and spice blends that add personality and flavor to every dish on your table.

Making Your Own Dressings and Condiments

Most commercial condiments include added ingredients that make them poor choices for living Paleo. Sweet-tasting favorites like ketchup and BBQ sauce often contain high-fructose corn syrup and other sweeteners, while classics like mayonnaise and bottled salad dressing are usually based on poor quality industrial oils.

But homemade condiments can be a good source of healthy, Paleo-approved fats and naturally occurring sugars that don't wreak havoc on your blood sugar levels — and the homemade versions taste even better than the factory-produced varieties found in the grocery store.

Adding Flavor with Sugar-Free Spice Blends

The fastest way to liven up a meal is to add the right amount of spice. A sprinkle of Garam Masala or Italian Seasoning can make a standard weeknight meal feel like a weekend feast. But many spice blends include sneaky forms of sugar, soy, or wheat, along with preservatives that make them decidedly unfriendly to Paleo cooks.

Homemade spice blends take less than five minutes to throw together, and they last almost indefinitely in your pantry. Doubling or tripling batches of your favorites is easy and in your favor because then you always have some on hand. And a jar of a homemade spice blend, along with a recipe for how to use it, makes a great gift for a friend or family member who's considering the Paleo lifestyle.

Buy spices in bulk to save money and to ensure that you never run out of your favorites!

Ghee

Prep time: 5 min • **Cook time:** 15 min • **Yield:** ¾ cup

Ingredients	Directions
1 cup unsalted butter, preferably from grass-fed cows	*1* Place a fine mesh strainer on top of a heat-safe bowl or measuring cup and tuck a triple layer of cheesecloth in the strainer.
	2 Melt the butter in a medium pan over low heat. When the surface of the butter resembles foam and the milk solids have turned a deep golden brown (about 8 to 10 minutes), remove the pan from the heat.
	3 Carefully strain the ghee through the cheesecloth.
	4 Discard the milk solids left in the cheesecloth and store the ghee in a sealed glass jar.

Per serving (1 tablespoon): Calories 136 (From Fat 135); Fat 15 g (Saturated 10 g); Cholesterol 41 mg; Sodium 2 mg; Carbohydrate 0 g (Dietary Fiber 0 g); Protein 0 g.

Note: Ghee is a versatile lactose- and casein-free, high-heat cooking fat that's deliciously nutty and shelf-stable for months.

Recipe courtesy Michelle Tam, author of Nom Nom Paleo (`http://nomnompaleo.com`*)*

This recipe has been vetted by the team at Whole9 (`http://whole9life.com`*) and is considered acceptable for a cleansing 30-day Paleo launch.*

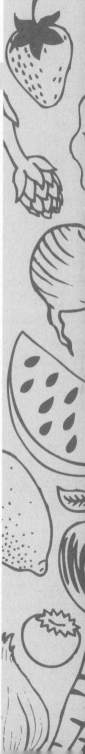

Cashew Butter Satay Sauce

Prep time: 5 min • **Yield:** 1 cup

Ingredients	Directions
½ cup cashew butter (no sugar added)	*1* Place all the ingredients except the coconut milk in a food processor or blender and process until smooth.
3 tablespoons coconut aminos	
2 tablespoons lime juice	*2* Scrape down the sides of the bowl with a rubber scraper, and then add the coconut milk. Process until blended.
1 clove garlic, minced (about 1 teaspoon)	
1 teaspoon crushed red pepper flakes	*3* Allow flavors to meld for 10 minutes before serving. Store covered in the refrigerator for up to five days.
½ teaspoon powdered ginger	
Dash of ground cayenne pepper (optional)	
½ cup coconut milk	

Per serving (1 tablespoon): Calories 97 (From Fat 52); Fat 6 g (Saturated 2 g); Cholesterol 0 mg; Sodium 66 mg; Carbohydrate 9 g (Dietary Fiber 0 g); Protein 2.

Tip: Serve Cashew Butter Satay Sauce along with grilled meats, like chicken, pork, and beef, or with seafood, like shrimp, scallops, and white fish. This sauce is especially nice with kabobs. Cashew Butter Satay Sauce is also a tasty addition to a raw vegetable and fruit platter.

Vary It! Try substituting sunflower butter or almond butter in place of cashew butter for a slightly different but still deliciously creamy flavor.

Moroccan Dipping Sauce

Prep time: 5 min • **Yield:** ½ cup

Ingredients	*Directions*
Juice of 2 lemons	**1** In a small bowl, whisk together the lemon juice, garlic, cumin, paprika, cayenne, salt, and pepper.
1 clove garlic, minced	
½ teaspoon ground cumin	
¼ teaspoon sweet, hot, or smoked paprika	**2** Continue whisking as you stream in the oil, then stir in the cilantro and parsley.
Pinch of ground cayenne pepper	**3** Serve at room temperature or refrigerate it if you're not going to eat the sauce within the hour. It keeps for two or three days in the fridge without diminishing its flavor.
½ teaspoon salt	
¼ teaspoon ground black pepper	
⅓ cup extra-virgin olive oil	
½ cup fresh cilantro leaves, minced	
½ cup fresh parsley leaves, minced	

*Per serving (**1 tablespoon**): Calories 84 (From Fat 81); Fat 9 g (Saturated 1 g); Cholesterol 0 mg; Sodium 148 mg; Carbohydrate 1 g (Dietary Fiber 0.5 g); Protein 0 g.*

This recipe has been vetted by the team at Whole9 (`http://whole9life.com`*) and is considered acceptable for a cleansing 30-day Paleo launch.*

Sri Lankan Curry Sauce

Prep time: 5 min • **Cook time:** 20 min • **Yield:** 2½ cups

Ingredients	*Directions*
2 medium jalapeño peppers, seeds and ribs removed	**1** In a blender or small food processor, blend the jalapeños, coconut, coriander, cinnamon, cumin, ginger, salt, garlic, and ¼ cup water until you have a smooth paste. Remove to a medium bowl and stir in ½ cup of the coconut milk.
¼ cup unsweetened shredded coconut	
2 teaspoons ground coriander	
1 teaspoon ground cinnamon	**2** Heat a large nonstick skillet over medium-high heat for about 3 minutes. Melt the coconut oil in the skillet and add the carrots. Sauté, stirring with a wooden spoon, until they're tender, about 3 minutes.
1½ teaspoons ground cumin	
½ teaspoon ground ginger	
¾ teaspoon salt	**3** Add the tomatoes and their juice to the carrots. Bring to a boil and then reduce the heat to simmer, stirring occasionally and crushing the tomato chunks with the back of the spoon.
2 cloves garlic, roughly chopped	
¾ cup coconut milk, divided	
1 tablespoon coconut oil	**4** Cook 7 to 10 minutes until the sauce thickens and the vegetables are soft.
3 medium carrots, grated (about 2 cups)	
Two 14.5-ounce cans diced tomatoes	**5** Stir the spice paste into the tomato mixture and add the remaining coconut milk. Stir to combine, and then remove from the heat. Use immediately or store in a covered container in the refrigerator for up to one week.

Per serving (1 tablespoon): Calories 92 (From Fat 58); Fat 7 g (Saturated 6 g); Cholesterol 0 mg; Sodium 424 mg; Carbohydrate 8 g (Dietary Fiber 2 g); Protein 1.5 g.

Tip: Try this sauce with steamed vegetables and your meat of choice.

This recipe has been vetted by the team at Whole9 (http://whole9life.com) and is considered acceptable for a cleansing 30-day Paleo launch.

Classic Stir-Fry Sauce

Prep time: 5 min • **Cook time:** 10 min • **Yield:** ⅔ cup

Ingredients	Directions
1 clove garlic, minced (about 1 teaspoon) 1 teaspoon crushed red pepper flakes 1 tablespoon Chinese five-spice powder ¼ teaspoon ground ginger 1 teaspoon rice vinegar ¼ cup unsweetened applesauce ¼ cup coconut aminos ½ tablespoon arrowroot powder ½ tablespoon water	*1* In a small saucepan, mix the garlic, red pepper flakes, five-spice powder, ginger, and rice vinegar with a fork to form a smooth paste. Stirring continuously with the fork, add the applesauce and coconut aminos. *2* In a small bowl, whisk the arrowroot powder and water together until smooth; set aside. *3* Place the saucepan over medium-high heat and bring to a boil. Add the arrowroot paste to the saucepan, stirring to combine. Return to a boil, and then reduce heat and simmer gently, uncovered, until slightly thickened, about 5 minutes. *4* Use immediately in a stir-fry or store covered in the refrigerator for up to five days.

Per serving (1 tablespoon): *Calories 69 (From Fat 2); Fat 0 g (Saturated 0 g); Cholesterol 0 mg; Sodium 127 mg; Carbohydrate 14 g (Dietary Fiber 0 g); Protein 0 g.*

Note: This stir-fry sauce works well with just about any combination of meat and vegetables. One batch is enough for about 4 servings.

Tip: Keep your freezer stocked with grab-and-go Classic Stir-Fry Sauce. Just double or triple the recipe, and then freeze the sauce in flexible plastic ice cube trays. Pop the sauce cubes into a freezer-safe bag so you'll always have fast access to individual portions of Classic Stir-Fry Sauce whenever you need them.

Vary it! If you can't find Chinese five-spice powder, you can substitute a combination of cinnamon, cloves, ginger, and nutmeg.

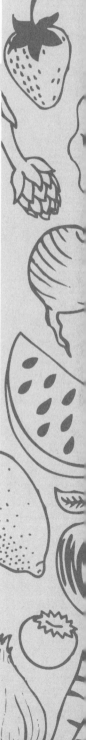

Tangy Carrot and Ginger Salad Dressing

Prep time: 5 min • **Cook time:** 5 min • **Yield:** ¾ cup

Ingredients	Directions
½ cup apple cider vinegar	*1* Combine the vinegar, carrots, ginger, scallions, and mustard in a blender on high speed until liquefied. There may still be bits of carrot in the dressing, which is fine.
2 large carrots, diced	
1-inch knob of fresh ginger, peeled and sliced	
2 scallions, white parts only	*2* Add the mayonnaise and blend on low until emulsified. Add salt and pepper to taste.
1 teaspoon kosher Dijon mustard	
⅓ cup Olive Oil Mayo (see recipe later in this chapter)	
Kosher salt to taste	
Ground black pepper to taste	

Per serving (1 tablespoon): *Calories 48 (From Fat 40); Fat 4.5 g (Saturated 0.5 g); Cholesterol 7 mg; Sodium 90 mg; Carbohydrate 2.5 g (Dietary Fiber 0.5 g); Protein 0.5 g.*

Tip: If you prefer your dressing a bit sweeter, add a touch of honey in Step 1.

*Recipe courtesy Michelle Tam, author of Nom Nom Paleo (*http://nomnompaleo.com*)*

*This recipe has been vetted by the team at Whole9 (*http://whole9life.com*) and is considered acceptable for a cleansing 30-day Paleo launch.*

Smooth and Creamy Avocado Dressing

Prep time: 10 min • **Yield:** ¾ cup

Ingredients	Directions
1 avocado, peeled, pitted, and cubed	*1* Blend all ingredients in a blender or food processor. Adjust the salt, cayenne (if desired), and vinegar to taste. Serve immediately.
½ cucumber, roughly chopped	
½ cup olive oil	
¼ cup honey	
3 teaspoons apple cider vinegar	
1 teaspoon Celtic sea salt	
Pinch of cayenne pepper (optional)	

Per serving (1 tablespoon): Calories 120 (From Fat 93); Fat 11 g (Saturated 1.5 g); Cholesterol 0 mg; Sodium 107 mg; Carbohydrate 7 g (Dietary Fiber 1 g); Protein 0.5 g.

Tip: If you want the dressing to be a little more pourable, consider adding more vinegar. You can also use this dressing as-is as a veggie dip!

Tip: For the highest-quality olive oil, look for the terms *organic* and *first-pressed*.

Recipe courtesy Alissa Cohen, chef and author of Living on Live Food (www.alissacohen.com)

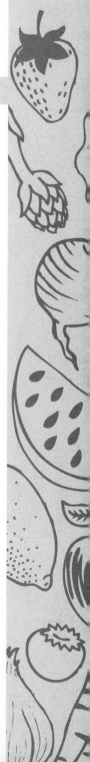

Paleo Ranch Dressing

Prep time: 15 min • **Yield:** 1½ cups

Ingredients	Directions
1 egg, room temperature	**1** Crack the egg into the bowl of a blender or food processor. Run it on medium speed, enough to whip the egg into a uniform mixture.
1 cup macadamia or avocado oil, room temperature	
2 teaspoons dried dill	**2** Turn the appliance onto high speed and very slowly and steadily drizzle in the oil (this process should take a few minutes).
1 teaspoon garlic powder	
1 teaspoon onion powder	
½ teaspoon sea salt	**3** After you've achieved a nice, thick mayo base, lower the speed to medium and add the remaining ingredients. If you want to be conservative, add a little of each at a time to suit your tastes.
¼ teaspoon chili powder	
¼ teaspoon ground black or white pepper	
2 tablespoons vinegar of choice	**4** Store the dressing in an airtight glass jar in the fridge and consume within a few days.
1½ teaspoons hot sauce	
1 teaspoon honey	
1 teaspoon yellow mustard	

Per serving (1 tablespoon): *Calories 178 (From Fat 171); Fat 19g (Saturated 2g); Cholesterol 16mg; Sodium 104mg; Carbohydrate 2g (Dietary Fiber 0g); Protein 1g.*

Vary It! Omit the vinegar for thicker dressing that makes a good dip, or omit the chili powder and hot sauce if you don't want the spicy heat. If you prefer a thinner dressing, you can adjust by adding some extra vinegar. You can also vary the flavor by substituting curry paste (for tasty heat), fish sauce (for savory), or tamari and/or coconut aminos (for even more savory).

Tip: The flavor of the dressing intensifies with time in the fridge, so keep that in mind as you add your seasonings. A batch that tastes just a little underseasoned while you're making it may be just right by the next morning.

Recipe courtesy Audrey Olson, author of Primal Kitchen: A Family Grokumentary (`www.primalkitchen.blogspot.com`*)*

Sweet and Spicy Vinaigrette

Prep time: 15 min • **Yield:** ⅔ cup

Ingredients	Directions
¼ teaspoon lemon zest	**1** Whisk together all the ingredients and serve.
⅓ cup fresh lemon juice (2–3 lemons)	
⅓ cup olive oil	
1 clove garlic, crushed	
1 teaspoon honey	
½ teaspoon Dijon mustard	
½ teaspoon minced jalapeño (optional)	
⅛ teaspoon ground black pepper	
Salt to taste	

Per serving (1 tablespoon): Calories 62 (From Fat 58); Fat 7 g (Saturated 1 g); Cholesterol 0 mg; Sodium 6 mg; Carbohydrate 1 g (Dietary Fiber 0 g); Protein 0 g.

Tip: Zest the lemon before juicing it.

Recipe courtesy Arsy Vartanian, author of Rubies & Radishes (www.rubiesandradishes.com)

Cilantro Vinaigrette

Prep time: 10 min • **Yield:** 1¾ cup

Ingredients	*Directions*
2 cups fresh cilantro leaves and stems	*1* Mix all the ingredients in a blender or food processor. Serve immediately.
1 cup apple cider vinegar	
½ cup olive oil	
1 large clove garlic	
1½ tablespoons honey	
½ teaspoon Celtic sea salt	
½ teaspoon ground black pepper	

Per serving (1 tablespoon): Calories 41 (From Fat 36); Fat 4 g (Saturated 0.5 g); Cholesterol 0 mg; Sodium 25 mg; Carbohydrate 1.5 g (Dietary Fiber 0 g); Protein 0 g.

Recipe courtesy Alissa Cohen, chef and author of Living on Live Food (www.alissacohen.com)

Olive Oil Mayo

Prep time: 5 min, plus standing time • **Yield:** 1¼ cup

Ingredients	*Directions*
1 large egg	*1* Crack the egg into the container of a blender or food processor with the lemon juice and allow the liquids 30 minutes to come to room temperature.
2 tablespoons fresh lemon juice	
½ teaspoon dry mustard	*2* Add the dry mustard, salt, and ¼ cup of the olive oil to the container and blend on medium speed until the ingredients are combined.
½ teaspoon salt	
1¼ cup light-tasting olive oil (not extra-virgin), divided	*3* With the blender running, add the remaining olive oil in a slow, steady stream until the substance resembles traditional mayonnaise, about 2 to 3 minutes.
	4 When all the oil is incorporated, transfer the mayo to a container with a lid. Mark the container with your egg expiration date — that's when the mayo expires, too.

Per serving (1 tablespoon): Calories 124 (From Fat 123); Fat 14 g (Saturated 2 g); Cholesterol 9 mg; Sodium 62 mg; Carbohydrate 0 g (Dietary Fiber 0 g); Protein 0 g.

Note: If you're using a blender, you'll hear the pitch change as the liquid begins to form the emulsion.

This recipe has been vetted by the team at Whole9 (http://whole9life.com) and is considered acceptable for a cleansing 30-day Paleo launch.

Cooked Olive Oil Mayo

Prep time: 10 min • **Yield:** 2 cups

Ingredients	Directions
2 large egg yolks 2 tablespoons water 2 tablespoons fresh lemon juice 1 teaspoon dry mustard 1 teaspoon Celtic sea salt 1 cup olive oil	**1** Heat the egg yolk, water, and lemon juice in a small saucepan over very low heat, stirring constantly. **2** At the first sign of thickness, remove the saucepan from the heat and set it in a large pan of cold water, being careful not to get water in the eggs. Continue stirring to avoid creating citrusy scrambled eggs. **3** Transfer the egg mixture to a blender or food processor and blend for a few seconds; let it sit uncovered for at least 5 minutes to cool. **4** Add the dry mustard and salt and blend on low speed. **5** With the blender running, drizzle the oil slowly into the mixture until all the ingredients are combined. Scoop into a large glass container and chill immediately. The mayonnaise should keep for one week if stored correctly.

Per serving (1 tablespoon): Calories 64 (From Fat 63); Fat 7 g (Saturated 1 g); Cholesterol 13 mg; Sodium 40 mg; Carbohydrate 0 g (Dietary Fiber 0 g); Protein 0 g.

Note: This recipe is great if you're wary of using raw eggs in your mayonnaise.

Recipe courtesy Mark Sisson, author of Primal Blueprint and Mark's Daily Apple (www.marksdailyapple.com)

This recipe has been vetted by the team at Whole9 (http://whole9life.com) and is considered acceptable for a cleansing 30-day Paleo launch.

Mark's Daily Apple Ketchup

Prep time: 5 min • **Yield:** 1⅓ cup

Ingredients	Directions
6 ounces tomato paste	**1** Combine all the ingredients in a food processor and blend until the onion disappears.
⅔ cup apple cider vinegar	
⅓ cup water	
2 tablespoons minced onion	**2** Spoon the mixture into an airtight container and store in the refrigerator.
2 cloves garlic	
1 teaspoon salt	
⅛ teaspoon ground allspice	
⅛ teaspoon ground cloves	
⅛ teaspoon ground black pepper	

Per serving (1 tablespoon): Calories 7 (From Fat 0); Fat 0g (Saturated 0g); Cholesterol 0mg; Sodium 167mg; Carbohydrate 1.5g (Dietary Fiber 0.5g); Protein 0g.

Recipe courtesy Mark Sisson, author of Primal Blueprint and Mark's Daily Apple (www.marksdailyapple.com)

This recipe has been vetted by the team at Whole9 (http://whole9life.com) and is considered acceptable for a cleansing 30-day Paleo launch.

Tangy BBQ Sauce

Prep time: 5 min • **Cook time:** 25 min • **Yield:** 1½ cups

Ingredients	Directions
1 cup Mark's Daily Apple Ketchup (see recipe earlier in this chapter)	*1* In a large bowl, whisk the Mark's Daily Apple Ketchup, water, applesauce, vinegar, coconut aminos, honey (if desired), mustard, hot pepper sauce, and black pepper until smooth.
½ cup water	
⅓ cup unsweetened applesauce	
2 tablespoons cider vinegar	*2* Heat the coconut oil in a saucepan over medium heat until shimmering. Add the garlic, chili powder, and cayenne pepper, and cook until fragrant, about 30 seconds.
2 tablespoons coconut aminos	
1 tablespoon honey (optional)	*3* Add the ketchup mixture to the saucepan, and whisk to combine. Bring to a boil, and then reduce the heat to medium-low and simmer gently, uncovered, until the sauce thickens, about 20 minutes.
1 teaspoon dry mustard	
1 teaspoon hot pepper sauce	
¼ teaspoon ground black pepper	*4* Enjoy warm or at room temperature. Store in the refrigerator for up to a week.
1 tablespoon coconut oil	
1 medium clove garlic, crushed	
1 teaspoon chili powder	
¼ teaspoon cayenne pepper	

Per serving (1 tablespoon): Calories 30 (From Fat 6); Fat 1 g (Saturated 1 g); Cholesterol 0 mg; Sodium 39 mg; Carbohydrate 5 g (Dietary Fiber 0 g); Protein 1 g.

Tip: Use this BBQ sauce to spice up grilled chicken, to toss with Slow Cooker BBQ Pulled Pork (Book II, Chapter 4), or to dollop on top of a freshly cooked beef burger.

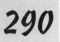

Orange Coconut Marinade

Prep time: 15 min • **Yield:** ½ cup

Ingredients	Directions
1 teaspoon orange zest	*1* Mix all the ingredients in a medium bowl. Combine with meat and marinate 2 to 6 hours for best flavor.
½ teaspoon lemon zest	
Juice of 1 orange	
2 tablespoons coconut aminos	
1 teaspoon honey	
1 teaspoon grated fresh ginger	
2 cloves garlic, crushed	
¼ cup diced white onion	
½ jalapeño, minced	
⅛ teaspoon salt	
⅛ teaspoon ground black pepper	

Per serving (1 tablespoon): *Calories 15 (From Fat 0); Fat 0 g (Saturated 0 g); Cholesterol 0 mg; Sodium 122 mg; Carbohydrate 3.5 g (Dietary Fiber 0.5 g); Protein 0 g.*

Tip: This marinade is great on chicken.

Recipe courtesy Arsy Vartanian, author of Rubies & Radishes (www.rubiesandradishes.com)

Basil and Walnut Pesto

Prep time: 5 min, plus standing time • **Yield:** 1 cup

Ingredients	*Directions*
2 cups fresh basil leaves, packed	*1* Combine all ingredients in a blender or food processor to desired consistency.
½ cup fresh parsley leaves, packed	
½ cup extra-virgin olive oil	*2* Allow the flavors to meld for about 30 minutes before eating. Store in an airtight container in the refrigerator.
⅓ cup walnuts	
3 cloves garlic, roughly chopped	
½ teaspoon salt	
⅛ teaspoon ground black pepper	

Per serving (1 tablespoon): Calories 80 (From Fat 76); Fat 8 g (Saturated 1 g); Cholesterol 0 mg; Sodium 74 mg; Carbohydrate 1 g (Dietary Fiber 0.5 g); Protein 0 g.

This recipe has been vetted by the team at Whole9 (http://whole9life.com) and is considered acceptable for a cleansing 30-day Paleo launch.

Cucumber Avocado Salsa

Prep time: 20 min • **Yield:** 5 cups

Ingredients	Directions
2 large cucumbers, peeled, seeded, and diced	*1* Combine all ingredients except the salt and pepper in a large mixing bowl and mix well.
10 Roma tomatoes, seeded and diced	
4 limes, juiced	*2* Season with salt and pepper to taste.
2 jalapeños, minced	
½ cup chopped fresh cilantro	
2 avocadoes, peeled, pitted, and diced	
Kosher salt to taste	
Ground black pepper to taste	

Per serving (1 tablespoon): *Calories 79 (From Fat 38); Fat 4.5 g (Saturated 0.5 g); Cholesterol 0 mg; Sodium 242 mg; Carbohydrate 9 g (Dietary Fiber 3.5 g); Protein 2 g.*

Tip: For milder salsa, remove the seeds from the jalapeño before mincing it.

*Recipe courtesy Nick Massie, chef and author of Paleo Nick (*http://paleonick.com*)*

*This recipe has been vetted by the team at Whole9 (*http://whole9life.com*) and is considered acceptable for a cleansing 30-day Paleo launch.*

Chapter 3

Mixing Rubs and Paleo Seasonings

....

In This Chapter

▶ Using herbs for better health and zippier flavor

▶ Leaving out non-Paleo additives but keeping the *pow!*

....

Recipes in This Chapter

↻ Grilling Spice Rub

↻ Succulent Steak Seasoning

↻ Everything Seafood Seasoning

↻ Italian Seasoning

↻ Dukkah

↻ Garam Masala

↻ Morning Spice

↻ Flame Out Blend

↻ Gremolata

Think about all the little things that make a big impact in your life — a simple walk on the beach or maybe a smile from someone you love. Well, spices are kind of like that: small things that make a big difference.

Spices crank up the flavor in any dish. Bursting with sweetness or warming with heat, spices turn the ordinary into the extraordinary. Adding spices lets you create really great dishes with few ingredients; the spices take away the need to add a lot of extras like rich sauces and condiments.

Cayenne pepper, chili pepper, chipotle powder, chili powder, and paprika are considered *nightshades*. This label means that if you have an autoimmune or inflammatory condition, these spices may aggravate your symptoms, and you should avoid them.

Tapping the Healing Power of Spices

Many cultures have used spices to heal for thousands of years. The following are top picks for healing spices:

✔ **Black pepper:** Pepper is a great spice to maximize your digestion. It helps move food along the colon at a good pace, and the quicker and smoother the ride, the healthier your colon.

If you have digestive complaints, black pepper can be irritating to the intestinal lining.

- ✔ **Cayenne:** Cayenne lowers blood pressure and has even been known to stop a heart attack! Cayenne thins phlegm and eases its passage through the lungs, and it improves digestion and relieves nausea and gas.

- ✔ **Cinnamon:** Cinnamon is serious about balancing blood sugar. Its active ingredient, *cinnamaldehyde,* decreases blood sugar, total cholesterol, and triglycerides and increases good cholesterol. This wonderful spice may also help treat cancer because it may slow the development of new blood supplies to tumors.

- ✔ **Curry:** If you've ever tasted Indian food, you've probably tried curry. It controls diabetes and can prevent or treat heart disease, infection, age-related memory loss, and inflammation. Curry has powerful antioxidants called *carbazole alkaloids* that are abundant only in the curry leaf and are responsible for preventing cell damage, which causes disease and premature aging.

- ✔ **Ginger:** Ginger rules all natural digestive aids: It relieves nausea and vomiting, settles the stomach, and eases the discomfort from gas and bloating. Research shows that ginger is one of the most effective remedies available for motion sickness, even more so than over-the-counter medications. It's also an antioxidant, antibacterial, antiviral, and anti-inflammatory that helps treat migraine headaches, arthritis, and asthma.

- ✔ **Oregano:** Oregano is your natural protection against infection. The active compounds in oregano have strong antiviral, antibacterial, and antifungal properties. Oregano helps get rid of intestinal parasites and kills the bacteria that causes food poisoning; it heals ulcers, calms intestinal irritation, and aids in digestion. Plus, oregano contains minerals, antioxidants, fiber, and omega-3 fatty acids.

- ✔ **Parsley:** Parsley contains an antioxidant called *apigenin* that helps other antioxidants work better. Parsley is used as a diuretic; can reduce high blood pressure; and is a natural agent to fight cancer, heart disease, and Type 2 diabetes.

- ✔ **Thyme:** The healing oil in thyme is a natural antiseptic. When applied to skin or the mucous membranes of the mouth, it kills germs. Thyme is great for calming coughs and helping prevent tooth decay and general infection.

- ✔ **Turmeric:** The active ingredient in turmeric is *curcumin,* which has been shown to protect and heal virtually every organ in the human body. Turmeric protects against cancer, Alzheimer's disease, Parkinson's disease, heart disease, stroke, diabetes, eye diseases, depression, and skin problems. Research at Tufts University showed that turmeric may prevent weight gain.

Grilling Spice Rub

Prep time: 5 min • **Yield:** ⅓ cup

Ingredients	Directions
2 tablespoons cumin	**1** Place all the spices in a medium bowl and mix with a fork until combined.
2 tablespoons chili powder	
1 tablespoon salt	**2** Transfer the spice blend to an airtight container.
½ tablespoon dry mustard	
½ tablespoon ground black pepper	
1 teaspoon cayenne pepper	

Per serving (1 teaspoon): Calories 9 (From Fat 4); Fat 1 g (Saturated 0 g); Cholesterol 0 mg; Sodium 448 mg; Carbohydrate 1 g (Dietary Fiber 1 g); Protein 0 g.

Tip: Use this spice blend liberally as a rub on steaks, chops, or chicken parts. You can also mix 1 tablespoon per pound into ground beef, pork, lamb, or turkey for burgers or meatballs.

Succulent Steak Seasoning

Prep time: 5 min • **Yield:** ½ cup

Ingredients	Directions
2 tablespoons ground black pepper	**1** Combine all ingredients in a container or jar (preferably glass) with a tight-fitting lid. Store in a cool, dark place, shaking the jar well to distribute the spices between uses.
2 tablespoons salt	
1 tablespoon powered garlic	
½ teaspoon curry powder	**2** Rub the seasoning well into meat before baking, grilling, or slow cooking.
½ teaspoon apple cider vinegar	
4 tablespoons dry mustard	
1 teaspoon Celtic sea salt	

Per serving: Calories 23 (From Fat 11); Fat 1 g (Saturated 0 g); Cholesterol 0 mg; Sodium 1,904 mg; Carbohydrate 2.5 g (Dietary Fiber 1 g); Protein 1 g.

Note: This spice blend really pops with grass-fed meats because they're incredibly lean.

This recipe has been vetted by the team at Whole9 (http://whole9life.com) and is considered acceptable for a cleansing 30-day Paleo launch.

Everything Seafood Seasoning

Prep time: 5 min • **Yield:** 1½ tablespoons

Ingredients	Directions
2 teaspoons celery salt	**1** Combine all ingredients in a container or jar (preferably glass) with a tight-fitting lid. Store in a cool, dark place, shaking the jar well to distribute the spices between uses.
½ teaspoon paprika	
¼ teaspoon ground black pepper	
¼ teaspoon cayenne pepper	**2** Rub the seasoning well into fish or seafood before baking, grilling, or slow cooking.
¼ teaspoon dry mustard	
¼ teaspoon ground nutmeg	
¼ teaspoon ground cinnamon	
¼ teaspoon ground cardamom	
¼ teaspoon ground allspice	
¼ teaspoon ground ginger	

Per serving: Calories 3 (From Fat 0); Fat 0 g (Saturated 0 g); Cholesterol 0 mg; Sodium 0.5 mg; Carbohydrate 0.5 g (Dietary Fiber 0.5 g); Protein 0 g.

Note: This spice blend is a home run on seafood, but it works on many other dishes as well, so feel free to experiment.

*This recipe has been vetted by the team at Whole9 (*http://whole9life.com*) and is considered acceptable for a cleansing 30-day Paleo launch.*

Italian Seasoning

Prep time: 5 min • **Yield:** ⅓ cup

Ingredients	Directions
1 tablespoon dried oregano leaves	**1** Mix all the spices with a fork until combined.
1 tablespoon dried basil leaves	**2** Transfer the spice blend to an airtight container.
1 tablespoon dried parsley leaves	
1 tablespoon dried rosemary	
2 teaspoons coarse (granulated) garlic powder	
1 teaspoon salt	

Per serving (1 teaspoon): Calories 4 (From Fat 1); Fat 0 g (Saturated 0 g); Cholesterol 0 mg; Sodium 146 mg; Carbohydrate 1 g (Dietary Fiber 0 g); Protein 0 g.

Note: When making the spice blend, toss the dried herbs gently to avoid crushing them. When using the spice blend to cook, crush the spice blend between your fingers to release the leaves' flavor.

Tip: Use the Italian Seasoning to make a quick salad dressing with extra-virgin olive oil and red wine vinegar, or sprinkle onto steamed vegetables tossed with coconut or olive oil and a freshly crushed garlic clove.

Dukkah

Prep time: 5 min • **Cook time:** 10 min • **Yield:** 1 cup

Ingredients	Directions
⅓ cup raw hazelnuts	**1** Preheat the oven to 375 degrees.
¼ cup roasted shelled pistachios	**2** Spread the hazelnuts on a foil-lined baking sheet and roast them for 5 to 7 minutes or until they turn golden brown and fragrant.
⅓ cup raw sesame seeds	
¼ cup coriander seeds	
2 tablespoons cumin seeds	**3** Transfer the roasted hazelnuts to a clean towel and allow them to cool. Use the towel to rub off the papery hazelnut skins and discard them. Transfer the skinned hazelnuts to a medium bowl and add the pistachios.
	4 Toast the sesame seeds in a dry skillet over medium-low heat for 1 minute or until they turn light brown, shaking constantly to prevent scorching. Reserve 1 tablespoon of the toasted seeds; place the rest in the bowl with the nuts.
	5 Toast the coriander seeds in the skillet until they're fragrant and place them in the bowl. Repeat with the cumin seeds.
	6 When the mixture of nuts and seeds has cooled, coarsely grind it in small batches in a spice grinder until lightly crushed. Mix in the reserved toasted sesame seeds. Store the spice blend in an airtight container in the fridge for up to 3 months.

Per serving: Calories 72 (From Fat 57); Fat 6 g (Saturated 0.5 g); Cholesterol 0 mg; Sodium 3 mg; Carbohydrate 3.5 g (Dietary Fiber 2 g); Protein 2 g.

Note: Dukkah is an Egyptian spice blend that adds a smoky, nutty flavor to roasts in particular.

*Recipe courtesy Michelle Tam, author of Nom Nom Paleo (*http://nomnompaleo.com*)*

*This recipe has been vetted by the team at Whole9 (*http://whole9life.com*) and is considered acceptable for a cleansing 30-day Paleo launch.*

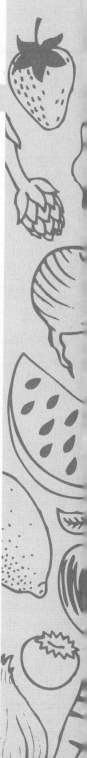

Garam Masala

Prep time: 5 min   •   **Yield:** ⅓ cup

Ingredients	Directions
1 tablespoon ground cumin	**1** Place all the spices in a medium bowl and mix with a fork until combined.
1 tablespoon ground coriander	
1 tablespoon ground cardamom	**2** Transfer the spice blend to an airtight container.
1 tablespoon ground black pepper	
1 tablespoon ground cinnamon	
1 teaspoon ground cloves	
1 teaspoon ground nutmeg	
½ teaspoon chili powder	

Per serving (1 teaspoon): Calories 8 (From Fat 3); Fat 0 g (Saturated 0 g); Cholesterol 0 mg; Sodium 2 mg; Carbohydrate 1 g (Dietary Fiber 1 g); Protein 0 g.

Tip: Mix 1 tablespoon per pound into ground beef, pork, lamb, or turkey for burgers or meatballs. It's also delicious mashed with baked sweet potatoes or roasted butternut squash.

Morning Spice

Prep time: 5 min • **Yield:** ¼ cup

Ingredients	Directions
1 tablespoon ground cinnamon	*1* Measure all the spices into a medium bowl and mix with a fork until combined.
2 teaspoons ground marjoram	
1 teaspoon ground nutmeg	*2* Transfer the spice blend to an airtight container.
1 teaspoon coarse (granulated) garlic powder	
1 teaspoon salt	
½ teaspoon ground black pepper	

Per serving (1 teaspoon): Calories 4 (From Fat 1); Fat 0 g (Saturated 0 g); Cholesterol 0 mg; Sodium 194 mg; Carbohydrate 1 g (Dietary Fiber 0 g); Protein 0 g.

Note: This spice blend is cozy and spicy-sweet. Based on traditional Russian sausage seasonings, it adds warmth to burgers, meatballs, soups, stews, and hearty vegetables.

Tip: Mix 1 tablespoon per pound into ground beef, pork, lamb, or turkey for instant "sausage." Just shape into patties or brown loose in a skillet. It also livens up baked sweet potatoes, cooked carrots, fried plantains, and roasted butternut or acorn squash.

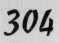

Flame Out Blend

Prep time: 5 min • **Yield:** ⅓ cup

Ingredients	Directions
2 tablespoons ground cinnamon	**1** Combine all ingredients in a container or jar (preferably glass) with a tight-fitting lid.
2 tablespoons ground ginger	
1 tablespoon orange zest	**2** Store in the refrigerator for up to 3 months.
1 tablespoon lemon zest	

Per serving: Calories 10 (From Fat 0); Fat 0 g (Saturated 0 g); Cholesterol 0 mg; Sodium 0.5 mg; Carbohydrate 2.5 g (Dietary Fiber 1.5 g); Protein 0 g.

Note: This spice blend is fantastic if you suffer from any kind of inflammatory or autoimmune conditions. The ginger helps your body cool down. You can use this spice anywhere you want a cooling blend, but it's particularly good in baking!

This recipe has been vetted by the team at Whole9 (`http://whole9life.com`*) and is considered acceptable for a cleansing 30-day Paleo launch.*

Gremolata

Prep time: 15 min • **Yield:** ⅔ cup

Ingredients	Directions
1 bunch Italian parsley, stems removed Zest of 3 lemons 4 cloves garlic, minced (about 2 teaspoons) ½ cup olive oil Kosher salt to taste Pepper to taste 1 tablespoon lemon juice	**1** Combine the parsley, lemon zest, and garlic in a blender. With the blender running, slowly drizzle in the olive oil. Blend until the consistency is slightly thicker than pickle relish, adding more parsley or using less olive oil as necessary. **2** Season with the salt, pepper, and lemon juice and enjoy!

Per serving: Calories 82 (From Fat 81); Fat 9g (Saturated 1.5g); Cholesterol 0mg; Sodium 42mg; Carbohydrate 0.5g (Dietary Fiber 0g); Protein 0g.

Note: Gremolata is a basic spice blend that's a great complement to many entrees and is particularly lovely with seafood dishes.

Tip: Instead of a blender, you can also crush the ingredients with a mortar and pestle, drizzling in the olive oil as you do.

Recipe courtesy Nick Massie, chef and author of Paleo Nick (http://paleonick.com)

This recipe has been vetted by the team at Whole9 (http://whole9life.com) and is considered acceptable for a cleansing 30-day Paleo launch.

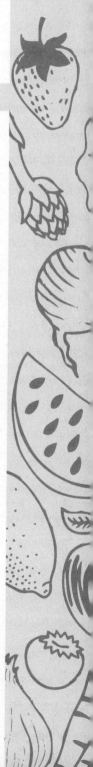

Chapter 4

Satisfying Your Sweet Tooth

Recipes in This Chapter

- Cranberry Ginger Cookies
- Almond Cookies with Cinnamon Glaze
- OMG Chocolate Chip Cookies
- Coconut Chocolate Chip Cookies
- Chocolate Chip Cookie Dough Granola Bars
- Classic Apple Crisp
- Chocolate-Strawberry Crumble Bars
- Pumpkin Cranberry Scones
- Pumpkin Pie Muffins
- Pumpkin Poppers
- Cinnamon Chocolate Chip Muffins with Honey Frosting
- Banana Cacao Muffins
- Chocolate Bacon Brownie Muffins
- Lemon Brownies with Coconut Lemon Glaze
- Blueberry Espresso Brownies
- Chocolate Zucchini Bread
- Avocado Chocolate Bread
- Maple Bacon Ice Cream
- Chocolate Ice Cream
- Coco-Mango Ice Cream
- Berries and Whipped Coconut Cream

In This Chapter

▶ Indulging in desserts without straying from your Paleo lifestyle

▶ Making tasty, healthier treats for special occasions

*W*ho wants to go through the rest of their lives feeling guilty for indulging in sweet treats or even avoiding them altogether? Boring.

The truth is that you're hard-wired to want the sweet stuff; it's part of your natural design. What you aren't hard-wired for are the grain- and sugar-laden foods most people know as desserts. Most cakes, pastries, cookies, and other treats are refined-food overkill and become a burden for your body to deal with.

Luckily, every once in a while you can have your (Paleo-approved) cake and eat it, too. You just have to redefine what sweets should be by using ingredients such as coconut flour, almond flour, fresh and dried fruits, nuts, vanilla, cinnamon, cocoa, honey, nut butters, maple syrup, and coconut milk.

Whether you go for the Blueberry Espresso Brownies, the Banana Cacao Muffins, or the Chocolate Ice Cream, you can relax. No guilt. The recipes in this chapter are super pure and super good! (The same can be said for the bonus recipe for Macadamia Nut Chocolate Chip Cookies you can find online at www.dummies.com/extras/paleocookbook.) *Note:* For all the recipes in this chapter, the serving size is one item unless otherwise noted.

Spotting Sugar in Its Sneakiest Forms

Wiping out sugar entirely is nearly impossible because all carbohydrates, even the healthy ones, are essentially sugar. However, you can control the *added sugar* and sweeteners in your food that provide no nutritional value.

Turn up your nose at these sugars and sweeteners:

- Agave
- All artificial sugars in boxes or packets
- Aspartame
- Brown sugar
- Corn syrup
- High fructose corn syrup
- Maltodextrin
- Molasses
- Raw sugar
- Rice syrup
- Sucralose
- Sugar cane
- White sugar

The absolute best way to reprogram your body to not reach for sugar or sugary carbohydrates is to go completely without sugar for 30 days. No cheating, no wavering — just 30 days of cleaning your body by getting rid of weak, unhealthy cells and building healthier cells for a stronger, more youthful body. The process is scary and difficult, yes, but it's one of those game-changers in life that's worth doing. Find out how in Book I, Chapter 1.

Cranberry Ginger Cookies

Prep time: 10 min • **Cook time:** 15 min • **Yield:** 20 cookies

Ingredients	Directions
2½ cups almond flour	**1** Preheat the oven to 350 degrees. Line a baking sheet with parchment paper.
½ cup almond butter	
½ cup unsweetened shredded coconut	**2** Combine all the ingredients except the cranberries and mix well with a hand mixer or stand mixer.
½ cup honey, melted	
¼ cup coconut oil, melted	**3** Fold in the dried cranberries by hand, ensuring they're evenly distributed.
1 egg	
1 tablespoon ground ginger	**4** Using a cookie scoop (smaller than an ice cream scoop) or two teaspoons, place scoops of dough on the baking sheet, leaving room between the cookies because they will expand slightly.
½ teaspoon sea salt	
½ teaspoon baking soda	
½ cup dried cranberries	
	5 Using your hand or the back of the scoop or spoon, slightly flatten the cookies.
	6 Bake for 10 to 15 minutes or until done.
	7 Remove from the oven and let the cookies remain on the pan for 1 minute before transferring them to wire racks to cool.

Per serving: Calories 133 (From Fat 81); Fat 9 g (Saturated 4 g); Cholesterol 9 mg; Sodium 76 mg; Carbohydrate 12 g (Dietary Fiber 1 g); Protein 2 g.

Tip: These cookies will largely retain whatever shape you put them in before baking, so shape them as desired.

Recipe courtesy George Bryant, CEO and author of Civilized Caveman Cooking Creations (http://civilizedcavemancooking.com)

Almond Cookies with Cinnamon Glaze

Prep time: 10 min • **Cook time:** 20 min • **Yield:** 12 cookies

Ingredients	Directions
2½ cups almond flour	**1** Preheat the oven to 350 degrees. Line a baking sheet with parchment paper.
¼ cup coconut flour	
2 teaspoons baking powder	**2** Combine the almond flour, coconut flour, baking powder, and 1 tablespoon of the cinnamon in a mixing bowl and stir well.
2 tablespoons ground cinnamon, divided	
¼ cup macadamia nut oil or coconut oil, melted	**3** To the dry ingredients, add the oil, 1 tablespoon of the honey, the almond extract, and the eggs and mix into a soft dough.
3 tablespoons honey, melted and divided	
1 teaspoon almond extract	**4** Dust your work surface with more almond flour and lay the dough out, pressing to just shy of ½ inch thick all around.
2 eggs	
1 tablespoon ghee or butter, melted	**5** Use a biscuit cutter or the lid of a jar to cut the dough into circles; lay them on the baking sheet.
⅓ cup unsweetened shredded coconut (optional)	
	6 Bake for 9 minutes.
	7 While the cookies bake, prepare the glaze by mixing the remaining honey, the ghee or butter, and the remaining cinnamon in a small bowl.

8 Remove the cookies from the oven and brush them with the glaze. Bake for 9 to 11 more minutes or until done.

9 Remove from the oven, sprinkle with some shredded coconut (if desired), and drizzle the remaining glaze over your cookies.

10 Serve immediately or store in an airtight container for 3 to 4 days.

Per serving: Calories 121 (From Fat 81); Fat 9 g (Saturated 6 g); Cholesterol 31 mg; Sodium 73 mg; Carbohydrate 3 g (Dietary Fiber 2 g); Protein 9 g.

Vary It! For a lighter almond flavor, substitute vanilla extract for the almond extract.

Recipe courtesy George Bryant, CEO and author of Civilized Caveman Cooking Creations (http://civilizedcavemancooking.com)

OMG Chocolate Chip Cookies

Prep time: 10 min, plus refrigerating time • **Cook time:** 10 min • **Yield:** 12 cookies

Ingredients	*Directions*
1½ cups almond flour	**1** In a large bowl, combine the almond flour, baking soda, and salt.
¼ teaspoon baking soda	
¼ teaspoon sea salt	**2** In a separate bowl, beat the coconut oil, vanilla, honey, and egg. Add the wet ingredients to the dry ingredients and mix well to combine.
2 tablespoons coconut oil, melted	
½ teaspoon vanilla extract	**3** Mix in the chocolate chips. Cover and refrigerate the cookie dough for 30 minutes.
¼ cup honey	
1 egg (room temperature)	**4** Preheat the oven to 350 degrees. Line a baking sheet with parchment paper.
¾ cup Paleo-approved chocolate chips	
	5 Roll the dough into 12 balls and arrange them on the baking sheet.
	6 Bake for 5 minutes. Remove the pan from the oven and flatten the cookies slightly with the back of a spoon. Put them back in the oven for about 5 more minutes, or until they look done. If you like soft and chewy cookies, take them out as soon as they start to turn golden brown.
	7 Remove the cookies from the oven and let the cookies remain on the pan for 1 minute before transferring them to wire racks to cool.

Per serving: Calories 134 (From Fat 72); Fat 8 g (Saturated 4 g); Cholesterol 16 mg; Sodium 66 mg; Carbohydrate 15 g (Dietary Fiber 2 g); Protein 2 g.

Note: These cookies are so good that Dr. Kellyann gave them away for holiday gifts one year to rave reviews! They're a great way to introduce your friends and family to Paleo.

Note: If you aren't sure where to find Paleo-approved chocolate chips, try the Enjoy Life brand (available online at www.enjoylifefoods.com/chocolate-for-baking). They're dairy-, soy-, and nut-free.

Coconut Chocolate Chip Cookies

Prep time: 10 min • **Cook time:** 12 min • **Yield:** 12 cookies

Ingredients	Directions
½ cup coconut oil	**1** Preheat the oven to 375 degrees. Line a baking sheet with parchment paper.
½ cup honey	
4 eggs	**2** Microwave the honey and coconut oil in a microwave-safe bowl for 30 to 60 seconds to melt them together. Add them to a large bowl with the eggs, vanilla, and salt and mix well with a hand mixer or stand mixer.
½ teaspoon vanilla extract	
⅛ teaspoon sea salt	
1 cup coconut flour	**3** Add the coconut flour. Stir in the shredded coconut and chocolate chips.
½ cup shredded unsweetened coconut	
¾ cup Paleo-approved chocolate chips	**4** Drop heaping tablespoons of cookie dough onto the baking sheet.
	5 Bake for 12 minutes or until golden brown.
	6 Remove from the oven and let the cookies remain on the pan for 1 minute before transferring them to a wire rack to cool.

Per serving: Calories 255 (From Fat 153); Fat 17 g (Saturated 13 g); Cholesterol 62 mg; Sodium 43 mg; Carbohydrate 26 g (Dietary Fiber 5 g); Protein 4 g.

Note: If you aren't sure where to find Paleo-approved chocolate chips, try the Enjoy Life brand (available online at www.enjoylifefoods.com/chocolate-for-baking). They're dairy-, soy-, and nut-free.

Tip: These cookies will largely retain whatever shape you put them in before baking, so shape them as desired.

Recipe courtesy George Bryant, CEO and author of Civilized Caveman Cooking Creations (http://civilizedcavemancooking.com)

Chocolate Chip Cookie Dough Granola Bars

Prep time: 10 min, plus chilling time • **Yield:** 5 servings

Ingredients	Directions
½ cup raw cashews ½ cup raw almonds	*1* Chop the cashews and almonds separately in a food processor and place them in a large bowl.
10 large Medjool dates ½ cup unsweetened coconut flakes	*2* Remove the pit from the dates and process the flesh in the food processor until a creamy paste forms.
1 teaspoon vanilla extract 3 tablespoons flaxseed meal	*3* Mix the date paste with the chopped nuts and the remaining ingredients by hand until fully combined.
⅓ cup Paleo-approved chocolate chips Pinch of salt	*4* Line the bottom and sides of an 8½-x-4½-inch medium loaf with parchment paper and press the mixture evenly across the bottom of the pan.
	5 Refrigerate for an hour and then cut into approximately five 2-x-4-inch bars.

Per serving: Calories 433 (From Fat 224); Fat 25 g (Saturated 10 g); Cholesterol 0 mg; Sodium 45 mg; Carbohydrate 50 g (Dietary Fiber 8 g); Protein 9 g.

Note: If you aren't sure where to find Paleo-approved chocolate chips, try the Enjoy Life brand (available online at www.enjoylifefoods.com/chocolate-for-baking). They're dairy-, soy-, and nut-free.

Classic Apple Crisp

Prep time: 15 min • **Cook time:** 40 min • **Yield:** 4–6 servings

Ingredients	Directions
1 pound apples, cut into half-moon slices (about 4 cups)	**1** Preheat the oven to 350 degrees.
½ teaspoon lemon zest	**2** In a medium bowl, mix the apples, lemon zest, and lemon juice with a wooden spoon. Allow to rest at room temperature while you prepare the topping.
½ tablespoon lemon juice	
⅓ cup almond flour	**3** Place almond flour, dates, cinnamon, nutmeg, and salt in food processor. Pulse until combined.
4 dried dates, pitted	
¼ teaspoon ground cinnamon	**4** Sprinkle the chilled coconut oil chunks over the flour mixture. Pulse about 10 times, and then process on high for 5 to 10 seconds until there are no more lumps. Pour the topping into a bowl and use a fork to mix in the chopped nuts.
⅛ teaspoon nutmeg	
⅛ teaspoon salt	
1 tablespoon coconut oil, chilled until solid, then diced	
¼ cup chopped walnuts or pecans	**5** Pour the fruit into an 8-inch square pan, pressing it gently into place with the back of a wooden spoon. Sprinkle the nut topping over the fruit and lightly press it into the fruit with the back of the spoon.
	6 Cover the crisp lightly with foil and bake for 30 minutes. Remove the foil and bake 5 to 10 more minutes, until browned.

Per serving: Calories 220 (From Fat 120); Fat 13 g (Saturated 4 g); Cholesterol 0 mg; Sodium 77 mg; Carbohydrate 24 g (Dietary Fiber 5 g); Protein 4 g.

Note: You can also bake this dish in individual ramekins. Place four ramekins on a baking sheet covered with parchment paper. Spoon generous ½-cup servings into each ramekin, press about 2 tablespoons of topping onto each, and then follow the baking instructions above.

Vary It! Substitute pears for the apples and sliced almonds for the walnuts or pecans. For extra zing, add ½ teaspoon dried ginger along with the lemon juice to the pears.

Chocolate-Strawberry Crumble Bars

Prep time: 20 min • **Cook time:** 28 min • **Yield:** 10–12 servings

Ingredients	Directions
2¼ cups blanched almond flour	*1* Preheat the oven to 350 degrees. In a large bowl, mix the almond flour, flaxseed meal, arrowroot powder, coconut sugar, baking soda, and salt.
6 tablespoons flaxseed meal	
⅔ cup arrowroot powder	*2* In a separate bowl, whisk the coconut oil, coconut milk, and vanilla.
½ cup organic coconut palm sugar	
½ teaspoon baking soda	*3* Using your hands, mix the wet and dry ingredients gently to form the dough. (You may want to wear gloves for this process.) Don't overmix.
¼ teaspoon salt	
6 tablespoons coconut oil, melted	*4* Reserve ½ cup of dough and press the remaining dough evenly across the bottom of an 8-x-8-inch baking pan lined with parchment paper.
3 tablespoons full-fat coconut milk	
2 teaspoons vanilla extract	*5* Sprinkle the chocolate chips on top of the crust. Cover the chocolate chips with the sliced strawberries and then drizzle with the lemon juice.
½ cup Paleo-approved dark chocolate chips	
1 cup fresh strawberries, sliced	*6* To make the crumble topping, mix the sliced almonds with the reserved dough by hand. Scatter the crumbs evenly over the strawberries.
1 tablespoon fresh lemon juice	
Handful of sliced almonds	*7* Bake for 18 minutes and then lower the heat to 325 degrees and bake for another 10 minutes until lightly golden.
	8 Set the pan over a wire rack to cool and then cut the bars into squares.

Per serving: Calories 415 (From Fat 268); Fat 30 g (Saturated 12 g); Cholesterol 0 mg; Sodium 136 mg; Carbohydrate 37 g (Dietary Fiber 7 g); Protein 8 g.

Note: If you aren't sure where to find Paleo-approved chocolate chips, try the Enjoy Life brand (available online at www.enjoylifefoods.com/chocolate-for-baking). They're dairy-, soy-, and nut-free.

Pumpkin Cranberry Scones

Prep time: 10 min • **Cook time:** 18 min • **Yield:** 12 scones

Ingredients	Directions
2 cups almond flour, plus more for dusting	*1* Preheat the oven to 400 degrees. Line a large baking sheet with parchment paper.
½ cup pumpkin puree	
½ cup dried cranberries	*2* Combine all the ingredients in a large mixing bowl and knead together with your hands.
¼ cup shredded unsweetened coconut	
¼ cup crushed pecans	*3* Divide the dough in half. Dust your work surface with more almond flour and press half the dough out into a circle, about ¼-inch thick.
1 egg	
3 tablespoons honey, melted	*4* Use a pizza cutter to slice the circle into equal wedges, making the pieces your desired size.
1 teaspoon sea salt	
1 teaspoon baking powder	*5* Repeat Steps 3 and 4 with the other half of the dough and put the scones on the baking sheet. Sprinkle with a little more pumpkin pie spice or cinnamon if desired.
1 teaspoon ground cinnamon	
1 teaspoon pumpkin pie spice	
½ teaspoon ground ginger	
	6 Bake for 15 to 18 minutes or until a toothpick inserted in the center of a scone comes out clean.
	7 Remove from the oven and transfer the scones to wire racks to cool.

Per serving: Calories 177 (From Fat 117); Fat 13 g (Saturated 2 g); Cholesterol 16 mg; Sodium 178 mg; Carbohydrate 15 g (Dietary Fiber 3 g); Protein 5 g.

Recipe courtesy George Bryant, CEO and author of Civilized Caveman Cooking Creations (http://civilizedcavemancooking.com)

Pumpkin Pie Muffins

Prep time: 10 min • **Cook time:** 20 min • **Yield:** 12 muffins

Ingredients	Directions
½ cup coconut flour	*1* Preheat the oven to 400 degrees. Line a muffin pan with paper liners.
2 teaspoons pumpkin pie spice	
½ teaspoon baking powder	*2* Sift the coconut flour and pie spice together. Add the baking powder.
¾ cup pumpkin puree	
½ cup coconut oil, melted	*3* In a separate bowl, mix all the remaining ingredients except the walnuts until well blended.
6 eggs	
2 teaspoons vanilla extract	*4* Add the dry ingredients to the wet ingredients. Mix well and divide the batter between the muffin cups. Sprinkle with the walnuts.
¼ cup honey, melted	
⅓ cup chopped walnuts	*5* Bake for 18 to 20 minutes or until a toothpick inserted in the center of a muffin comes out clean.

Per serving: Calories 179 (From Fat 126); Fat 14 g (Saturated 9 g); Cholesterol 93 mg; Sodium 57 mg; Carbohydrate 11 g (Dietary Fiber 3 g); Protein 4 g.

Recipe courtesy George Bryant, CEO and author of Civilized Caveman Cooking Creations
(http://civilizedcavemancooking.com)

Pumpkin Poppers

Prep time: 15 min • **Cook time:** 15 min • **Yield:** 20 poppers

Ingredients	Directions
Melted coconut oil for greasing	**1** Preheat the oven to 350 degrees. Use a little melted coconut oil to coat a 24-cup mini-muffin tin.
½ cup butter, melted	
5 eggs, beaten	**2** In a large bowl, combine the butter, eggs, vanilla, pumpkin, and honey. Add the coconut flour, salt, and spices (using ½ teaspoon of the cinnamon). Whisk to combine.
1 teaspoon vanilla extract	
½ cup pumpkin puree	
⅓ cup honey	**3** Let the batter sit for 5 minutes to allow the coconut flour to absorb the wet ingredients.
½ cup coconut flour	
¼ teaspoon sea salt	**4** Stir in the baking soda and then fill the mini-muffin tins with the batter until they're almost full.
1 tablespoon plus ½ teaspoon ground cinnamon, divided	
½ teaspoon ground nutmeg	**5** Bake for 15 minutes or until a toothpick inserted in the center of a muffin comes out clean. Tip the muffins out of the pan to cool on wire racks.
¼ teaspoon ground allspice	
⅛ teaspoon ground cloves	
½ teaspoon baking soda	**6** In a small bowl, mix the coconut sugar and remaining cinnamon.
2 tablespoons coconut sugar	
½ cup coconut butter, melted	**7** Dip the cooled muffins in the coconut butter and then roll them in the cinnamon sugar until fully coated.

Per serving: *Calories 107 (From Fat 72); Fat 8 g (Saturated 5 g); Cholesterol 59 mg; Sodium 70 mg; Carbohydrate 9 g (Dietary Fiber 2 g); Protein 2 g.*

Note: Be sure you're using pumpkin puree and not pumpkin pie filling.

Recipe courtesy Arsy Vartanian, author of Rubies & Radishes (www.rubiesandradishes.com)

Cinnamon Chocolate Chip Muffins with Honey Frosting

Prep time: 15 min • **Cook time:** 18 min • **Yield:** 18 muffins

Ingredients	Directions
Honey Frosting (see the following recipe)	**1** Preheat the oven to 375 degrees with the rack in the middle position. Line a muffin pan with paper liners.
6 eggs	**2** Whisk or beat the eggs, honey, vanilla, butter, and applesauce in a large mixing bowl or a stand mixer.
¼ cup honey, melted	
1 teaspoon vanilla extract	
8 tablespoons unsalted butter, melted	**3** Sift the coconut flour, cinnamon, baking powder, baking soda, and salt into a medium bowl.
½ cup unsweetened applesauce	**4** Add the dry ingredients to the wet ingredients and whisk until well blended.
¾ cup coconut flour	
1 tablespoon ground cinnamon	**5** Fold in the chocolate chips, ensuring they're evenly distributed. Spoon the batter into the muffin cups.
2 teaspoons baking powder	
1 teaspoon baking soda	**6** Bake for 16 to 18 minutes or until a toothpick inserted in the center of a muffin comes out clean.
Small pinch of sea salt	
½ cup Paleo-approved chocolate chips	**7** Remove the muffins from the oven and let cool. Top the cooled muffins with Honey Frosting.

Honey Frosting

1 cup palm shortening

¾ cup full-fat coconut milk, chilled

¼ cup honey, melted

1 teaspoon ground cinnamon

Orange zest for garnish (optional)

Crushed pecans (optional)

1 Combine the shortening, coconut milk, and honey in a stand mixer or mixing bowl and beat on low for 20 seconds.

2 Scrape down the sides of your bowl and then beat on high for approximately 60 seconds until the frosting thickens.

3 Fold in the cinnamon and the optional ingredients (if desired) by hand, ensuring they're evenly distributed.

Per serving: Calories 265 (From Fat 198); Fat 22 g (Saturated 9 g); Cholesterol 76 mg; Sodium 176 mg; Carbohydrate 16 g (Dietary Fiber 3 g); Protein 3 g.

Note: If you aren't sure where to find Paleo-approved chocolate chips, try the Enjoy Life brand (available online at www.enjoylifefoods.com/chocolate-for-baking). They're dairy-, soy-, and nut-free.

Recipe courtesy George Bryant, CEO and author of Civilized Caveman Cooking Creations (http://civilizedcavemancooking.com)

Banana Cacao Muffins

Prep time: 15 min • **Cook time:** 25 min • **Yield:** 9 muffins

Ingredients	Directions
2 ripe bananas	**1** Preheat the oven to 350 degrees.
3 eggs	
¼ cup honey	**2** In a mixing bowl, mash the bananas until smooth. Add the eggs, honey, coconut oil, vanilla, and almond butter and mix thoroughly.
⅓ cup coconut oil, melted	
1 teaspoon vanilla extract	
¼ cup almond butter	**3** Add the coconut flour and cinnamon and mix well. Let the batter sit for 5 to 10 minutes to allow the coconut flour to absorb the wet ingredients.
½ cup coconut flour	
1 teaspoon ground cinnamon	**4** Add the baking soda and chocolate chips. Mix until the baking soda is mixed through.
½ teaspoon baking soda	
2 tablespoons Paleo-approved chocolate chips	**5** Divide the batter among the muffin cups. These muffins will slide out of the pan without paper liners.
	6 Bake for 25 minutes or until a toothpick inserted in the center of a muffin comes out clean.
	7 Remove the muffins from the muffin pan and let cool.

Per serving: Calories 217 (From Fat 126); Fat 14 g (Saturated 8 g); Cholesterol 62 mg; Sodium 95 mg; Carbohydrate 21 g (Dietary Fiber 4 g); Protein 5 g.

Note: Don't skip the resting time in Step 3. The batter will be too thin to scoop.

Note: If you aren't sure where to find Paleo-approved chocolate chips, try the Enjoy Life brand (available online at www.enjoylifefoods.com/chocolate-for-baking). They're dairy-, soy-, and nut-free.

Recipe courtesy Arsy Vartanian, author of Rubies & Radishes (www.rubiesandradishes.com)

Chocolate Bacon Brownie Muffins

Prep time: 20 min • **Cook time:** 30 min • **Yield:** 24 muffins

Ingredients	Directions
2 cups almond butter	*1* Preheat the oven to 325 degrees. Line a muffin tin with paper liners.
2 eggs	
½ cup honey	*2* Using a hand mixer, blend the almond butter in a large bowl to make it a smoother consistency. Beat in the eggs and then the honey and vanilla.
1 tablespoon vanilla extract	
½ teaspoon sea salt	
1 teaspoon baking soda	*3* Add the salt and baking soda; slowly add in the cacao powder as you continue beating. Beat in the coconut milk.
¼ cup cacao powder	
2 tablespoons coconut milk	
8 slices crispy cooked bacon, chopped	*4* Fold in the bacon and mix well by hand to ensure it's evenly distributed.
	5 Divide the batter among the muffin cups and bake for 20 to 30 minutes or until a toothpick inserted in the center of a muffin comes out clean.

Per serving: Calories 178 (From Fat 126); Fat 14 g (Saturated 1.5 g); Cholesterol 18 mg; Sodium 142 mg; Carbohydrate 11 g (Dietary Fiber 2 g); Protein 6 g.

Note: *Cacao powder* isn't the same as cocoa powder. Cacao is raw and unsweetened (much like a spice); it contains lots of magnesium and antioxidants. Cocoa powder is processed and contains cocoa butter to enhance flavor. We like Navitas brand (http://navitasnaturals.com/product/441/Cacao-Powder.html).

Tip: Cooking your bacon in the oven on a cookie sheet yields perfect bacon. Place the bacon in a cold oven and then set the temperature to 400 degrees. Wait 15 to 18 minutes, flip the bacon, and then cook for an additional 3 to 4 minutes.

Recipe courtesy George Bryant, CEO and author of Civilized Caveman Cooking Creations (http://civilizedcavemancooking.com)

Lemon Brownies with Coconut Lemon Glaze

Prep time: 15 min • **Cook time:** 20–25 min • **Yield:** 12 servings

Ingredients	Directions
Coconut Lemon Glaze (see the following recipe)	**1** Preheat the oven to 350 degrees. In a large bowl, mix the almond flour, arrowroot powder, baking soda, and salt.
2 cups blanched almond flour	
1 tablespoon arrowroot powder	**2** In a separate bowl, whisk the eggs, lemon juice, lemon zest, honey, coconut oil, coconut milk, coconut butter, and vanilla.
½ teaspoon baking soda	
¼ teaspoon salt	
2 room temperature eggs	**3** Add the dry ingredients into the wet and gently mix with a spoon or spatula to form a batter. Don't overmix.
2½ tablespoons lemon juice	
1 tablespoon lemon zest	
4 tablespoons raw honey	**4** Spread the batter across the bottom of an 8-x-8-inch baking pan lined with parchment paper. Make sure the paper covers all four sides of the pan.
¼ cup coconut oil, melted	
⅓ cup full-fat coconut milk	**5** Bake until a toothpick inserted into the center comes out clean, about 20 to 25 minutes.
2 tablespoons coconut butter	
1 teaspoon vanilla extract	**6** Set the pan on a wire rack to cool and then top with the Coconut Lemon Glaze.

Coconut Lemon Glaze

2 tablespoons full-fat
coconut milk

2½ teaspoons coconut butter

½ tablespoon lemon juice

2 teaspoons lemon zest

2 teaspoons arrowroot
powder

1 teaspoon raw honey

1 In a bowl, whisk together all the ingredients.

Per serving: Calories 271 (From Fat 199); Fat 22 g (Saturated 10 g); Cholesterol 37 mg; Sodium 147 mg;
Carbohydrate 15 g (Dietary Fiber 3 g); Protein 7 g.

Blueberry Espresso Brownies

Prep time: 10 min • **Cook time:** 30 min • **Yield:** 18 brownies

Ingredients	Directions
2 teaspoons coconut oil	**1** Preheat the oven to 325 degrees. Grease a 9-x-13-inch baking dish with the coconut oil.
1 cup coconut cream concentrate	
3 eggs	**2** Beat all the remaining ingredients except the blueberries in a large mixing bowl to mix well.
½ cup honey	
1 cup pecans, crushed	**3** Fold in the blueberries by hand so you don't crush them. Pour the batter into the greased baking dish.
¼ cup cocoa powder	
1 tablespoon ground cinnamon	**4** Bake for approximately 30 minutes. After about 25 minutes, insert a toothpick in the center and judge how much more baking time you need based on how clean it is.
1 tablespoon ground coffee or espresso	
2 teaspoons vanilla extract	**5** Remove from the oven and let cool.
½ teaspoon baking soda	
¼ teaspoon sea salt	**6** If desired, drizzle some additional melted coconut cream concentrate over the cooled brownies.
1 cup fresh blueberries	

Per serving: Calories 155 (From Fat 81); Fat 9 g (Saturated 4 g); Cholesterol 31 mg; Sodium 75 mg; Carbohydrate 19 g (Dietary Fiber 1 g); Protein 2 g.

Recipe courtesy George Bryant, CEO and author of Civilized Caveman Cooking Creations (http://civilizedcavemancooking.com)

Chocolate Zucchini Bread

Prep time: 20 min • **Cook time:** 35 min • **Yield:** 10 servings

Ingredients	Directions
1½ cups blanched almond flour	*1* Preheat the oven to 350 degrees. In a bowl, mix the almond flour, baking soda, cacao powder, cinnamon, and salt.
1½ teaspoons baking soda	
¼ cup raw cacao powder	
2 teaspoons ground cinnamon	*2* In a separate bowl, beat the egg and then add the yogurt, coconut oil, vanilla, honey, and vinegar. Mix until well combined.
¼ teaspoon salt	
1 room temperature egg	
¼ cup plain Greek yogurt	*3* Stir the zucchini, pecans, and chocolate chips into the wet ingredients.
¼ cup coconut oil, melted	
1 teaspoon vanilla extract	*4* Using a rubber spatula, gently mix the wet and dry ingredients together. Don't overmix.
3 tablespoons raw honey	
1 teaspoon apple cider vinegar	*5* Spoon the batter into an 8½-x-4½-inch medium loaf pan lined with parchment paper. Bake until a toothpick inserted into the center comes out clean, about 35 minutes.
1 cup zucchini, finely grated	
½ cup pecans, chopped	
½ cup Paleo-approved chocolate chips	*6* Cool on a wire rack. Store in an airtight container in the refrigerator.

Per serving: Calories 290 (From Fat 203); Fat 23 g (Saturated 9 g); Cholesterol 19 mg; Sodium 265 mg; Carbohydrate 19 g (Dietary Fiber 4 g); Protein 7 g.

Note: If you aren't sure where to find Paleo-approved chocolate chips, try the Enjoy Life brand (available online at www.enjoylifefoods.com/chocolate-for-baking). They're dairy-, soy-, and nut-free.

Avocado Chocolate Bread

Prep time: 20 min • **Cook time:** 45 min • **Yield:** 10 servings

Ingredients	Directions
1½ cups avocado, mashed	*1* Preheat the oven to 350 degrees. Pulse the avocado in a food processor until creamy.
3 tablespoons coconut oil, melted	
1 teaspoon vanilla extract	*2* Add the coconut oil, vanilla, coconut cream, honey, and eggs and pulse to combine.
2½ tablespoons coconut cream	
3 tablespoons raw honey	*3* In a large bowl, mix the pecans, almond flour, baking soda, cacao powder, salt, and chocolate chips.
2 eggs	
½ cup pecans, chopped	*4* Combine the wet and dry ingredients and mix gently with a rubber spatula. Don't overmix.
2 cups blanched almond flour	
1 teaspoon baking soda	*5* Spoon the batter into an 8½-x-4½-inch medium loaf pan lined with parchment paper, spreading it across the pan with a spatula. Sprinkle the top with chocolate chips.
¼ cup raw cacao powder	
½ teaspoon salt	
⅓ cup Paleo-approved chocolate chips, plus more for garnish	*6* Bake until a toothpick inserted into the center of the bread comes out clean, about 45 minutes.
	7 Let it cool on a wire rack. To preserve freshness, place inside an airtight container and store in the refrigerator.

Per serving: Calories 342 (From Fat 243); Fat 27 g (Saturated 8 g); Cholesterol 0 mg; Sodium 269 mg; Carbohydrate 21 g (Dietary Fiber 6 g); Protein 8 g.

Note: If you aren't sure where to find Paleo-approved chocolate chips, try the Enjoy Life brand (available online at www.enjoylifefoods.com/chocolate-for-baking). They're dairy-, soy-, and nut-free.

Maple Bacon Ice Cream

Prep time: 20 min, plus freezing time • **Yield:** 4 servings

Ingredients	Directions
One 15.5-ounce can full-fat coconut milk, chilled	**1** Combine the coconut milk, maple syrup, and vanilla in a blender until mixed well.
⅓ cup pure maple syrup	
1 teaspoon vanilla extract	**2** Set up your ice-cream maker according to its operating instructions. Turn it on and pour in the coconut milk mixture.
3 slices crispy bacon, chopped	
	3 When your ice cream starts to solidify (about 10 to 15 minutes), add the bacon.
	4 Transfer the ice cream to another bowl and put it in the freezer for 30 minutes to 1 hour.

Per serving: Calories 310 (From Fat 238); Fat 27 g (Saturated 22 g); Cholesterol 6 mg; Sodium 126 mg; Carbohydrate 19 g (Dietary Fiber 0 g); Protein 4 g.

Recipe courtesy George Bryant, CEO and author of Civilized Caveman Cooking Creations (http://civilizedcavemancooking.com)

Chocolate Ice Cream

Prep time: 20 min, plus chilling and freezing time • **Yield:** 2 servings

Ingredients	Directions
¼ cup honey	*1* Warm the honey and stir in the cocoa powder. Combine this mixture with the coconut milk and vanilla in a blender until the honey is fully dissolved. Chill the coconut milk mixture for 30 to 60 minutes.
2 tablespoons cocoa powder	
1 cup full-fat coconut milk, chilled	
1 teaspoon vanilla extract	*2* Set up your ice-cream maker according to its operating instructions. Turn it on and pour in the coconut milk mixture.
	3 Let the ice-cream maker work for 10 to 20 minutes, until the ice cream is partially set.
	4 Transfer the ice cream to another bowl and place in the freezer for 30 minutes to 1 hour.

Per serving: Calories 368 (From Fat 225); Fat 25 g (Saturated 22 g); Cholesterol 18 mg; Sodium 18 mg; Carbohydrate 41 g (Dietary Fiber 2 g); Protein 3 g.

Recipe courtesy George Bryant, CEO and author of Civilized Caveman Cooking Creations (http://civilizedcavemancooking.com)

Coco-Mango Ice Cream

Prep time: 10 min, plus freezing time • **Yield:** Five 1-cup servings

Ingredients	Directions
4 ripe bananas, peeled and roughly chopped	**1** Blend the bananas, mangos, and coconut milk in a food processor until smooth.
4 ripe mangos, peeled and roughly chopped	**2** Chop the chocolate into chunks your desired size and stir it into the banana mixture.
½ cup full-fat coconut milk, chilled	
1.75 ounces at least 70 percent dark chocolate	**3** Divide into 1-cup portions and freeze.
	4 Remove the portions from the freezer 15 minutes before serving to allow them time to soften. (The low fat content compared to regular ice cream makes this ice cream freeze hard, like ice.)

Per serving: Calories 287 (From Fat 90); Fat 10 g (Saturated 7 g); Cholesterol 0 mg; Sodium 8 mg; Carbohydrate 52 g (Dietary Fiber 6 g); Protein 4 g.

Note: Make sure your chocolate bar has no added soy or soy lecithin. Enjoy Life brand has a soy-free chocolate bar (www.enjoylifefoods.com/chocolate-bars/).

Recipe courtesy Nick Massie, chef and author of Paleo Nick (http://paleonick.com)

Berries and Whipped Coconut Cream

Prep time: 20 min, plus refrigerating and freezing time • **Yield:** 6–8 servings

Ingredients	Directions
2 tablespoons Caramelized Coconut Chips (see the following recipe)	*1* Refrigerate the can of coconut milk for at least 3 hours (overnight is best).
One 15.5-ounce can coconut milk	*2* When you're ready to make the dessert, place the can, a metal mixing bowl, and the beaters from a mixer in the freezer for 15 minutes.
2 cups fresh berries	
2 tablespoons sliced almonds	*3* Gently wash the berries and pat dry with paper towels.
1 teaspoon almond or vanilla extract	*4* Heat a skillet over medium-high heat, add the almonds, and stir continuously with a wooden spoon for 3 to 5 minutes, until the almonds turn golden brown. Transfer the toasted almonds to a bowl.
	5 Pour the coconut milk into the chilled mixing bowl and add the almond or vanilla extract. Whip on the mixer's highest setting until the milk is fluffy and resembles the texture of whipped cream, about 5 to 7 minutes.
	6 Divide the berries among four bowls and top each one with whipped cream, a sprinkle of toasted almonds, and Caramelized Coconut Chips.

Caramelized Coconut Chips

¼ teaspoon salt

¼ teaspoon ground cinnamon

1 cup unsweetened coconut flakes

1 Mix the salt and cinnamon with a fork in a small dish; set aside.

2 Heat a skillet over medium-high heat for about 2 minutes. Add the coconut flakes and distribute evenly in a single layer. Stir frequently, continuing to spread them in a single layer, until toasted, about 3 minutes.

3 Sprinkle the hot coconut flakes with the cinnamon mixture and toss until evenly seasoned. Transfer to a plate and allow them to cool in a single layer.

Per serving: Calories 589 (From Fat 477); Fat 53 g (Saturated 48 g); Cholesterol 0 mg; Sodium 609 mg; Carbohydrate 21 g (Dietary Fiber 12 g); Protein 5 g.

Tip: You can easily multiply this recipe to accommodate a large crowd.

*This recipe has been vetted by the team at Whole9 (*http://whole9life.com*) and is considered acceptable for a cleansing 30-day Paleo launch.*

Book IV
Primal Power Moves for a Healthier Body

Knowing the Common Categories of Paleo Exercises

- **Hinges:** These exercises require you to bend at your hips.

- **Squats:** You bend at the hips and the knees when you do squats.

- **Pushes:** This category includes the familiar push-up and works out your upper body.

- **Pulls:** These exercises require you to pull to strengthen your back and shoulders.

- **Carries:** You work out your arms, back, and shoulders when you perform carries.

- **Core exercises:** These exercises strengthen and tone your abs.

web extras

View videos of some of the exercises in the upcoming chapters at www.dummies.com/extras/paleoaio.

Contents at a Glance

Chapter 1: Hinging and Squatting Your Butt and Legs to Primal Perfection . . .337

The Lowdown on Hinges 337
Beginner Hinging Exercises 339
Intermediate Hinging Exercises 343
Advanced Hinging Exercises 346
The Lowdown on Squats 350
Beginner Squatting Exercises 352
Intermediate Squatting Exercises 356
Advanced Squatting Exercises 359

Chapter 2: Pushes and Pulls for a Strong, Solid Torso 363

All about the Primal Pushes 363
Beginner Pushes 365
Intermediate Pushes 368
Advanced Pushes 373
All about the Primal Pulls 375
Beginner Pulls 377
Intermediate Pulls 379
Advanced Pulls 382

Chapter 3: Carrying Heavy Things and Ab Exercises That Don't Suck 387

Mastering the Art of the Loaded Carry 388
Beginner Carries 389
Intermediate Carries 392
Advanced Carries: The Bottoms-Up Carry 394
Getting the Abs of Your Dreams 396
Beginner Ab Exercises 397
Intermediate Ab Exercises 400
Advanced Ab Exercises 403
An All-Around Paleo Exercise: The Turkish Get-Up 406

Chapter 4: Primal Power Moves for Explosive Athleticism 411

Understanding Primal Power 412
Beginner Power Moves 413
Intermediate Power Moves 416
Advanced Power Moves 420

Chapter 5: Beyond Strength Training and Cardio to Metabolic Conditioning. .425

Introducing Primal Strength Training 426
Gaining Strength Without Gaining Weight 429
Moving Past Chronic Cardio Syndrome 432
Developing the Recipe for a Good Exercise Program 435
Introducing Metabolic Conditioning 437
Turbocharging Fat Loss with Complexes 440

Chapter 6: Programs for Getting Started — and for Pushing Forward 447

Beginning at the Beginning: The 21-Day Primal Quick Start 448
Gearing Up for the 21-Day Program 448
Your 21-Day Primal Quick Start 455
From Average to Elite: The 90-Day Primal Body Transformation 459
Building a Balanced 90-Day Program 460
Your 90-Day Primal Body Transformation 465

Chapter 1

Hinging and Squatting Your Butt and Legs to Primal Perfection

In This Chapter

▶ Developing hinge movements

▶ Discovering how to squat deeply (without wrecking your knees)

*I*n terms of neuromuscular activation, squats and hinges soar high above most other exercises; they recruit more muscle fibers, demand more metabolically, and subsequently chop more fat and build more muscle.

To keep it simple, you can think of hinging as maximum hip bend with some knee bend, and you can think of squatting as maximum hip bend *and* knee bend. In a hinge, the butt reaches back. In a squat, the butt reaches down. Knowing the difference is important because hinges are heavily driven by the posterior chain (hamstrings, butt, lower back), whereas squats require a bit more from the anterior chain (front side) — specifically, the quads.

This chapter is dedicated to showing you the primal hinging and squatting movements you need to form, firm, and strengthen the legs, butt, and midsection. Here, you discover how to perform the choicest lower body exercises for a cast-iron posterior and legs that won't quit — all without wrecking your knees or wrenching your back.

The Lowdown on Hinges

The purpose of the hinge is to move and produce force from the hips. This is a necessary life skill. Being able to move properly from the hips allows you to lift weight safely up off the ground without wrecking your back and maximizes your athletic abilities.

The most basic, or primal, hinging pattern is the dead lift: a bending of the hips to reach down and pick something up. Conventional wisdom tells you that you shouldn't lift with your back, but in fact you *should* lift from your back — as well as from the rest of your posterior chain.

For example, when you watch a baby pick something up off the ground, the baby almost invariably reverts to the dead lift to do so. Very rarely will any baby pick something up from a squat because the dead lift (which is interchangeable with *hinge* in this book) is the natural human crane position. When the back is kept flat, the hips reach back, and the knees bend slightly, you're in position to heave a considerable load from the floor.

Perhaps the most potentially injurious way to lift any weight off the ground, especially if you're new to weight training, is to do so with a rounded (hunched) back. When hinging, push your chest up (think "proud chest") to maintain the natural curvature of your spine.

The following sections give you a few more details and benefits about the hinge.

Using your hips in the hinge

An athlete's power comes from the hips. Hinging shows you how to fully use the strength and power of your hips. Whether you aim to pick something up without wrecking your back or to jump across a creek without ruining your pants, using your hips will help you do just that.

In a properly hinged position, the hips take the load, not the back. (And often, the hinge is referred to as a *hip hinge*.) A proper hinge ensures optimum spinal alignment and transmission of force; that is, when you hinge properly, the hips do the heavy lifting and the back is kept safe. Here's how:

1. **Keep your back flat (never rounded or overarched).**

2. **Push your hips back as far as possible.**

3. **Allow your knees to bend slightly (but not so much that they come forward).**

   The bottom of a hinge should have your legs and torso looking like the less than sign (<).

Everyone's hinge will look slightly different. As long as your shins are vertical, your back is flat, and your hips are above the knees (but below the shoulders), you're good to go!

Counting the benefits of a strong hinge

Developing the hinge movement pattern is extremely important. A strong, patterned hinge makes all the heavy lifting of life easier. Literally.

But there's more to it than that. A strong hinge offers the following benefits as well:

- ✔ Less risk of back injury
- ✔ Less risk of knee injury
- ✔ More power and athletic ability
- ✔ A stronger, firmer butt
- ✔ A resilient, sturdy back
- ✔ Functional, durable hamstrings

Practice your hinge as often as possible. Whether you're picking up a pencil or 500 pounds, get those hips back and keep the back flat!

Beginner Hinging Exercises

You can express the hinge in many ways. But like most all other movements, you should start out slow with the basics. The basic dead lift is a perfect introduction to the hinge. The dead lift, which is picking something up (and putting it back down), is as fundamental as it gets.

Don't let the unpretentious nature of this movement fool you. The dead lift will be a staple in all the primal fitness programs because it's a monstrous strength-building exercise; it allows you to load the system with more weight than just about any other movement.

The following sections outline the pattern for the dead lift and the single-leg dead lift.

The dead lift

The dead lift is simply the hinge put to work. To get started practicing the dead lift, you need something to pick up. Start with a kettlebell or a dumbbell (and eventually you'll move on to a set of kettlebells, dumbbells, or a

Book IV

Primal Power Moves for a Healthier Body

barbell). Most men can start out with a weight between 35 and 40 pounds and most women between 18 and 25 pounds.

1. **Stand on top of the weight so it's positioned between your heels, assume a shoulder-width stance, and point your toes out slightly (between 10 and 20 degrees). (See Figure 1-1a.)**

2. **Push your hips back toward the wall behind you.**

   Imagine you're reaching your butt back for a bench that's just out of reach.

3. **Keep your back flat, but let your knees bend as you continue to reach your butt back as far as you possibly can without toppling backward.**

4. **When you hit maximum hip bend, grab hold of the weight and take a deep breath into your belly. (See Figure 1-1b.)**

   Be sure to keep the head and neck in line with the rest of your back as well. Focus your eyes on the ground slightly in front of you or onto the horizon where the wall meets the floor.

5. **Push your heels hard into the ground and stand up as quickly as possible. (See Figure 1-1c.)**

6. **Reverse the movement to set the weight back onto the floor. Don't round your back to set the weight down.**

   Be sure to start and finish the dead lift with good posture.

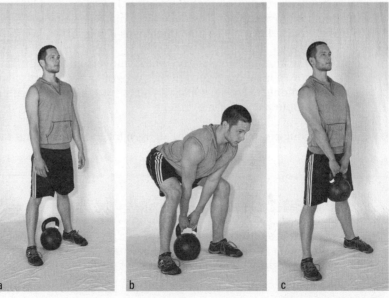

Figure 1-1: The deadlift is the fundamental hinge movement.

Photos courtesy of Rebekah Ulmer

Whether you're lifting 35 pounds or 350, respect the weight all the same. Don't get into the habit of setting the weight down lazily or with poor form. What you practice is what you'll revert to when under stress. Get in the habit of doing it right.

Sometimes mobility may be a limiting factor in the dead lift. If you feel like you have to compromise your form to reach down to the weight, bring the weight up to you! There's no point in performing an exercise unsuccessfully or with poor form when you can make small adjustments to help you train around mobility restrictions. Simply find a small box or any other implement to elevate the weight, as shown in Figure 1-2, to make the weight easier to reach until your mobility improves.

The single-leg dead lift

The single-leg dead lift is pretty much what it sounds like — the dead lift using only one leg — with a few minor tweaks, of course. Most natural and athletic movements happen from a split stance, not an even one, so it's equally important to train the one-limbed (unilateral) movements as it is the

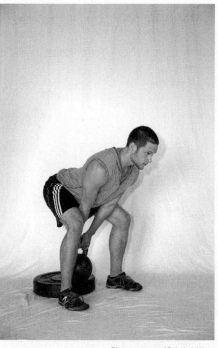

Figure 1-2: Elevating the weight makes it easier to reach.

Photo courtesy of Rebekah Ulmer

Book IV

Primal Power Moves for a Healthier Body

two-limbed (bilateral) movements. The big benefits of the single-leg dead lift that don't necessarily come with the conventional dead lift are the additional balance, coordination, and motor control components.

Start by using a kettlebell or dumbbell for this exercise, but if you want to develop extra balance and coordination, practice this movement as often as possible without weight. Here are the steps for the single-leg dead lift with a weight:

1. **Stand on top of the weight so it's positioned between your heels (refer to the setup for the dead lift in the previous section and see Figure 1-3a).**

2. **Push your heel back and up toward the ceiling.**

   Be sure to minimize any twisting and rotation throughout the movement. Both of your shoulders should fall and rise at the same rate; you want to keep them as square as possible throughout the movement.

3. **As your back heel starts to rise, naturally let yourself hinge at the hips.**

4. **Allow your knee to bend as you hinge.**

   To keep your balance, your knee may even come slightly forward in the single-leg dead lift.

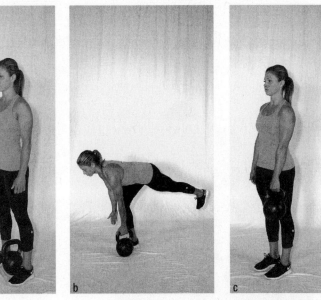

Figure 1-3:
The single-leg dead lift is all about control.

a   b   c

Photos courtesy of Rebekah Ulmer

This is a single-leg dead lift. Not a "stiff leg" single-leg dead lift. So let the knee bend! If you don't, you run the risk of overloading the hamstring.

5. **When you're able to, reach down and grab the weight with the arm opposite the planted leg.**

    For example, if your right leg is on the ground, grab the weight with your left arm (see Figure 1-3b).

6. **Finish the movement the same way you came into it, standing tall at the top, as shown in Figure 1-3c.**

7. **Be sure to place the weight back down exactly how you picked it up.**

Intermediate Hinging Exercises

The next step in hinging progressions is to add some power to the pattern. In this section, you discover the swing and the one-arm swing, two explosive hinging exercises.

Don't proceed with intermediate hinging exercises prematurely. The swing is built off the back of the dead lift, so if you don't have that pattern close to perfect yet, your swing and everything else hereafter will suffer. If you need more practice with the dead lift, refer to the "Beginner Hinging Exercises" section.

Paleo fitness is about progressing at your own pace. There's no prize for being the first person to master all the exercises. The more time you spend practicing the basics, the easier the more advanced movements will be later.

When you've mastered the dead lift, the swing comes easy, because the swing is really just a fast and continuous string of dead lifts.

The swing

Swings are as handy as hot sauce. They go well with anything and spice up even the blandest dishes. This is to say that you can pretty much add swings to any workout (foolishly assuming that you don't already do so) to instantly make it better.

The swing shows you how to generate power/explosiveness from your hips and is a marvelous all-around fat-chopping device. It blends strength and cardiovascular efforts, a trait shared by few exercises.

Book IV

Primal Power Moves for a Healthier Body

The swing also strengthens the muscles of the lower back, and strong evidence supports that swings may ward off back problems later in life. Swings also commonly lead to what has been affectionately dubbed the "kettlebutt" — a firm, strong, and aesthetically privileged backside.

The swing is best performed with a kettlebell (and it's often called a "kettlebell swing"), but you may use a dumbbell as well. A barbell is far too unwieldy for this exercise.

Here's how to do the swing:

1. **Assume a shoulder-width stance approximately one foot behind the weight you're using, and point your toes slightly outward.**

2. **Hinge at the hips like you would in a dead lift (refer to the earlier section on the dead lift), reach out, and grab hold of the weight (see Figure 1-4a).**

   Be sure to get the hips back and keep the back flat.

3. **Start the swing with a forceful hike back of the weight, like a center hiking a football (see Figure 1-4b).**

   Keep the handle of the weight above your knees at all times; otherwise, your back may round. Also, don't be shy about the hike! You have to forcefully throw the weight back to properly load the hips for the swing.

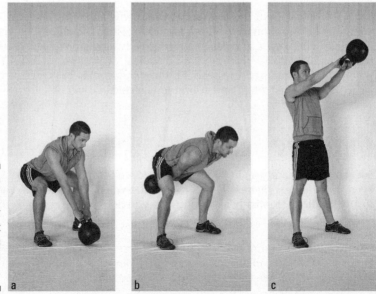

Figure 1-4:
The swing is a power movement that blends strength and cardio.

a   b   c

Photos courtesy of Rebekah Ulmer

4. **When the weight reaches the top of the backswing, immediately reverse the movement by driving your hips forward and standing up as quickly as you can.**

   Your hips and knees should extend simultaneously. Think "jump," but keep your heels planted on the ground. The hips should visibly snap forward when executing the swing. The aim is to be as explosive as possible, regardless of the weight you're using.

5. **Allow the weight to float no higher than eye level before reversing and repeating the movement. Don't lean back at the top of the swing; just stand tall. See Figure 1-4c.**

   If you have issues with your back, allow the weight to float no higher than shoulder level. When done right, the weight should float outward and upward. The movement is powered entirely by the hips. Your arms are simply loose chains connecting the weight to your body.

 While performing the swing, keep the arms relaxed but the armpits tight so your shoulders don't get pulled forward by the force of the weight. Imagine that you're squeezing a wad of cash or wringing a sponge in your armpit. This will help to keep the shoulders in a safely packed position.

The one-arm swing

The closest relative to the (two-arm/kettlebell) swing, the one-arm swing adds an additional grip challenge and rotary stability component (the ability to prevent rotation). Just like the two-arm swing, your best bet is to use a kettlebell or dumbbell for this exercise.

Because you now bear the weight by only one side of the body, a good one-arm swing can be measured directly by the amount of rotation that doesn't occur. So work to keep your shoulders square through the movement. Here are the steps to the one-arm swing:

1. **Set up like you would for a two-arm swing (see previous section), reach out, and grab the weight with one arm (see Figure 1-5a).**

   Grab the handle of the weight as close to dead center as possible.

2. **Hike the weight back as you would a two-arm swing while minimizing any twist in your torso (see Figure 1-5b).**

   With the one-arm swing, you may rotate your thumb slightly in (downward) on the backswing to ensure that the weight doesn't crash into the knees.

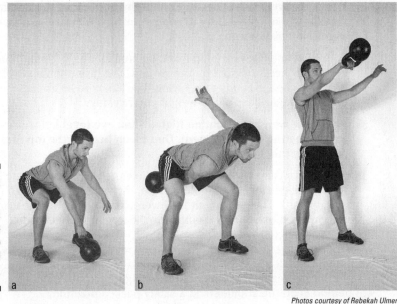

Figure 1-5:
The one-arm swing challenges your grip strength and stability.

a   b   c

Photos courtesy of Rebekah Ulmer

3. **When the weight reaches the top of the backswing, snap the hips forward and stand up as quickly as possible to complete the movement.**

4. **Allow the weight to float no higher than eye level (see Figure 1-5c) before reversing and repeating the movement.**

   If you have issues with your back, allow the weight to float no higher than shoulder level.

Remember to keep your armpit tight throughout the exercise. Don't let the weight pull your shoulder forward.

Advanced Hinging Exercises

The exercises in this section tread less stable ground, both literally and metaphorically. These movements aren't more advanced in the sense that you perform them with more weight (although that may sometimes be the case) but because of the higher levels of control, concentration, and coordination required for proper execution.

For example, you wouldn't attempt the snatch before the two-arm swing any more than you'd try to juggle before first learning to catch.

The beginner and intermediate hinging movements earlier in this chapter show you how to produce and reduce force from the hips — a necessary skill to maximize athletic potential and lessen injury risk. But there's one more skill you need to know, and that's the ability to redirect force — both toward you and away from you. To be able to both subtly and aggressively redirect force is a true exhibition of athleticism. You see this in all domains of sport; for example, the judo player who, through proper timing and subtle movement, redirects his opponent's oncoming force into a powerful hip toss.

But this is merely a hidden benefit. Cleans and snatches are markedly more infamous for building the backside, bolstering lung capacity, and butchering body fat.

The clean

The *clean,* another powerful hip-dominant movement, develops your ability to produce, reduce, and redirect force — a necessary athletic skill, even for non-athletes. The clean can also be a tremendous cardiovascular conditioner and power builder by itself. What's more is that heavy cleans, especially heavy double-kettlebell cleans, show you how to take a hit!

Cleans performed with a kettlebell or dumbbell differ slightly from cleans performed with barbells, sandbags, or other such devices that you can't easily swing between your legs. This section covers kettlebell or dumbbell cleans because they're slightly more forgiving than barbell cleans (especially for those with restricted shoulder mobility), and the learning curve is less intimidating.

The purpose of the clean is to bring the weight explosively up into the rack position, where you place the weight in front of the chest so you can easily press, squat, jerk, and so on. In the rack, or the finished position of the clean, your forearms should be vertical and pressed against your rib cage. Here are the steps to the clean:

1. **Set up exactly how you would for a one-arm swing (see the earlier section), reach out, and grab the weight with one arm.**

2. **Start the clean with a forceful hike back of the weight (see Figure 1-6a).**

   Up until this point, the movement should be identical to the one-arm swing.

3. **When the weight reaches the top of the backswing, snap your hips forward (just like you would a swing).**

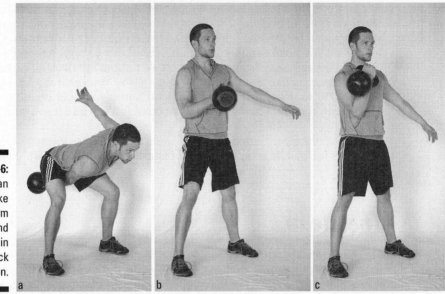

Figure 1-6:
The clean starts like the one-arm swing and finishes in the rack position.

a   b   c

Photos courtesy of Rebekah Ulmer

4. **As your hips drive forward, keep your elbow in close to your body and draw the weight up your center line (see Figure 1-6b).**

   Do your best to keep the weight as close to your body as possible. The more the weight casts outward, the less efficient the movement becomes. If it helps, imagine you're trying to zip up a big coat.

5. **Catch the weight in the rack position, with your forearm(s) against your rib cage, as shown in Figure 1-6c.**

   If you're using a kettlebell, allow it to gently roll onto the forearm before landing in the rack. A common mistake with the clean is to use the arms to curl the weight up. The hips must power the movement. Think about it like this: The hips are the engine, and the arm is the steering wheel.

Sometimes the best fix for poor clean technique is to pick up a heavier weight, which forces you to use more hips and less arms and to seek the most efficient trajectory. Most of the time, however, the best way to fix your clean is to go back and fix your swing and one-arm swing. The same goes for the snatch, which you find out about in the next section. Often, people venture into cleaning and snatching way too soon. Be sure to master the swing and one-arm swing before attempting the clean and the snatch; doing so will make the clean and the snatch that much easier.

The snatch

To perform the snatch, you swing the weight back between your legs and bring it up over your head in one smooth, uninterrupted motion. This movement brings you to the pinnacle of your primal hinging progressions.

The snatch builds on all the preceding exercises. If you haven't spent adequate time perfecting your swings, one-arm swings, and cleans, you're not ready for the snatch.

The snatch manufactures the raw power and "never say die" conditioning of an Olympian. And when applied liberally, it blasts body fat like a blowtorch. When you get into high-rep snatching, you'll see what we mean.

This section focuses primarily on kettlebell and dumbbell snatches because they're more forgiving, easier to learn, and don't require an Olympic lifting platform. Here's how to do the snatch:

1. **Set up behind the weight (kettlebell or dumbbell) like you would for a one-arm swing or clean (see earlier sections) and hike the weight forcefully back between your legs (see Figure 1-7a).**

2. **Drive your hips forward and explode out of the hinge. Imagine you're trying to jump through your heels.**

   To do the snatch right, you have to fully commit yourself to the movement; otherwise, the bell won't go where it needs to. Be sure to snap those hips!

3. **As the weight accelerates upward, keep your elbow in close to the body, guiding the weight up your center line (not letting it arch out wildly; see Figure 1-7b).**

   This portion of the snatch is sometimes referred to as the *high pull*. Notice in Figure 1-7b how the elbow is slightly bent and stays relatively in line with the body. This form ensures an efficient trajectory. The farther the weight gets away from you on the way up, the less efficient the movement, so keep it tight.

4. **If using a kettlebell, practice "punching" through the bell around eye level to ensure a smooth transfer of the weight onto the forearm (see Figure 1-7c).**

   When you go to punch through the bell, be sure to loosen your grip to avoid tearing any callouses. It may even help if you "spear" through the bell and open your hand entirely.

5. **Finish the snatch overhead in a full lockout position; that is, lock your elbow and line your bicep with or slightly behind your ear (see Figure 1-7d).**

Book IV

Primal Power Moves for a Healthier Body

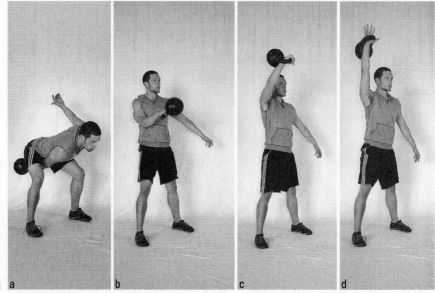

Figure 1-7:
The snatch
is the
pinnacle
of primal
hinging
progressions.

a   b   c   d

Photos courtesy of Rebekah Ulmer

It will take some time to find your groove, but in the end, the snatch should be one smooth and graceful movement.

To avoid unnecessary callous tears when using kettlebells, maintain a relatively loose grip. Hold on just tight enough to keep the bell in your possession but loose enough so the handle may rotate without grinding up your hands.

The Lowdown on Squats

It's often joked that the squat is an essential movement for eating dinner in Thailand and taking care of business in the woods. But there are other uses for the squat. The squat is the most potent of all exercises; pound for pound, it burns more calories and triggers more muscular activation than any other movement. The squat is also the king of all strength-building movements, and nothing can dethrone it.

Heavy squats are marvelous. They place a tremendous amount of stress on the body and flood the system with natural growth hormones (including natural human growth hormone).

Another benefit of the squat less talked about but equally valuable is to help you sit down, perhaps the most common application. But it should be noted that the original intention of this movement pattern was not to sit down but to stand up. People first enter the squat as babies, from the ground (oftentimes out of a crawl) and use it to stand. So like the Turkish get-up (see Book IV, Chapter 3), the squat is just as useful of a device to pick yourself up off the ground as it is to sit down onto it.

The following sections squelch some common myths about squatting and explore the many benefits of this technique.

Getting to the truth about squatting

People often think squatting is bad for your knees. But forget about that. *How* you squat may be bad for your knees, but the squat itself isn't bad for the knees. In fact, there are no bad movements, only a lack of preparation for movement. You need to strengthen the knees just like all other joints and muscles. And the only way to strengthen the knees is through movement.

If you have prior knee issues, or any issues for that matter, always get clearance from your doctor before beginning any type of fitness program.

Another common, somewhat silly myth is that your knees shouldn't cross over your toes during a squat. It's okay if your knees cross over your toes as long as they stay in line with your toes. The knee is meant to bend. In fact, it's just about the only thing it can do, so let it do just that.

Exploring the benefits of a deep squat

The deep squat is an essential pattern. Ideally, you should be able to squat butt to ankles with your heels on the ground and your knees in line with your toes, all the while keeping your back relatively flat. Go ahead and give it a try! If you have the mobility, the bottom of a squat should feel like a rest position — like you could really hang out there for a while.

The cave man probably spent a lot of time hanging out in the bottom of a bodyweight squat, and you might want to do the same. The more time you can accumulate in the bottom of the squat throughout the day, the better. This position loosens your hips, toughens your joints, and gets you up off the couch!

Book IV

Primal
Power
Moves for
a Healthier
Body

As your deep squat improves, so will your lower body strength, lower body mobility, and general usefulness in society. An uninhibited squat is a strong indicator of functional movement. It requires ample mobility of the ankles, knees, and hips and stability of the pelvis. What does that mean? Well, a lot has to be working right for someone to squat deeply. It means your working equipment is somewhat in order, so you're less likely to fall apart.

Here are a few ways to work the squat into your daily routine:

- ✔ Answer at least ten e-mails a day from a squat.

- ✔ Talk on the phone from a squat.

- ✔ Watch TV from a squat (or, at the very least, watch the commercials from a squat).

- ✔ Eat one time during the day from a squat.

- ✔ When waiting in line, get down into a squat (let 'em stare!).

Beginner Squatting Exercises

The beginner squatting exercises in this section are easy to understand and easy to use. They include the goblet squat, the bodyweight squat, and the goblet lunge. These squats are the most user-friendly variations; all intend to produce a big calorie burn while improving your squatting pattern.

Be patient with the squat, and don't get discouraged if you can't squat very low at first. The depth will come — especially when you practice the movements in Book IV, Chapter 3. And don't ever push into a range of motion where you feel uncomfortable or are unable to maintain proper form.

The goblet squat

"Well, the funny thing about the goblet squat ... is that it answers the question: What do the hips do? And if ... the kettlebell 'reverse engineers' the action of the hips, ... then in the goblet squat, the movement greases that key human motion: the squat." And there you have it in plain speech, by Dan John himself, master strength coach and originator of the goblet squat.

The goblet squat is the speediest way to get someone squatting properly and quickly. Really, it's nearly impossible to do wrong. The following steps walk you through it:

1. **Grab a kettlebell or dumbbell and hold it directly in front of the chest, like a goblet (hence, the name *goblet squat;* see Figure 1-8a).**

   Keep the weight held as snuggly to the chest as possible.

2. **Assume a little wider than hip-width stance, and point your toes slightly out. This is your squatting stance.**

3. **Start the movement by sitting down, as if you're reaching your butt down for a curb. (It may help to think that you're pulling yourself down between your legs.)**

   Keep in mind that in a squat, you sit down; in a swing, you sit back.

4. **Continue to descend for as long as you're able to keep your heels on the ground, your knees in line with your toes, and your back flat (see Figure 1-8b).**

5. **When you stand up, be sure that your hips and shoulders ascend simultaneously.**

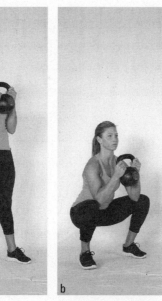

Figure 1-8: The goblet squat helps develop proper squatting form.

a

b

Photos courtesy of Rebekah Ulmer

The bodyweight squat

It may strike you as odd to find the bodyweight squat after the goblet squat in terms of progressions, but there are good reasons for that. For one thing, the bodyweight squat is horribly overworked, and people generally lack the authentic mobility and stability to properly do one.

So don't be surprised when you discover that the goblet squat comes easier than a bodyweight squat. The natural counterbalance of the weight helps compensate for mobility issues, allowing for a greater range of motion with better form.

With that being said, the bodyweight squat is still great, and it should be everyone's goal to perform one beautifully. Here's how:

1. **Assume a hip-width stance and point your toes slightly out.**

2. **Reach your arms out in front of you for balance (see Figure 1-9a) and begin to sit down, pulling yourself between your legs.**

   Your knees *will* come forward in a squat; just be sure they stay in line with your toes.

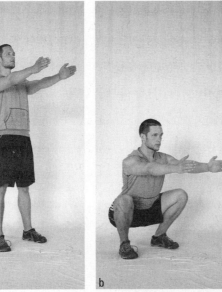

Figure 1-9:
The challenge with the bodyweight squat is maintaining balance.

a   b

Photos courtesy of Rebekah Ulmer

3. **Go as low as you can, keeping your heels on the ground, your knees in line with your toes, and your back flat (see Figure 1-9b).**

   Do your best to keep your weight evenly distributed throughout your feet.

4. **When you stand up, be sure your hips and shoulders ascend simultaneously.**

The goblet lunge

The lunge isn't a squat *per se,* but it's still a knee, or quad, dominant movement, and it's still an extremely valuable one at that. The lunge is effectively a squat taken from a split stance, or more simply, a sort of single-leg squat. Because most of your movement occurs either from a split stance or as the result of pushing off just one leg, you want to train the unilateral (one-limb) movements, such as the lunge, just as extensively as you train the bilateral (two-limb) movements, such as the squat.

You can perform the lunge with either a weight held in the goblet position (like you would a goblet squat) or with no weight at all. You may find that holding a weight in front of your chest assists with balance and posture. Follow these steps to do the goblet lunge:

1. **Assume a hip-width stance and hold the weight in front of your chest as you would a goblet squat (see the previous section).**

2. **Begin by stepping back deeply with one leg (see Figure 1-10a), maintaining the hip-width stance. Imagine you're lunging on railroad tracks.**

   Maintain a fairly square and upright torso throughout the lunge. That means don't lean forward, twist, or rotate. Also don't go too narrow with your stance, unless you want to topple over.

3. **Continue to lunge back until the knee of your back leg reaches the ground (see Figure 1-10b). You may rest your knee there, but don't bang it.**

   Notice that in the lunge, both feet are pointing forward.

4. **To come out of the lunge, push equally off your front leg and back leg and return to the starting position.**

   Be sure to keep your back toes tucked, not pointed, so you can push off the ball of your back foot when lunging.

Book IV

Primal Power Moves for a Healthier Body

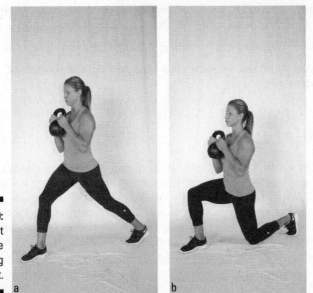

Photos courtesy of Rebekah Ulmer

Figure 1-10:
The goblet
lunge is like
a single-leg
squat.

Intermediate Squatting Exercises

After your squatting mechanics are sound, you can start to load the movement considerably. With squats, and with most movements relating to the squat, you can move a lot of weight, and sometimes that's precisely what you should do.

When you load a movement — meaning you add weight to it — you cement the pattern. Don't push the weight until your form is near faultless.

The two exercises in this section are favorite variations for adding more weight to squats and lunges in the quickest and safest manner possible.

The racked squat

With a racked squat, you perform a squat with weight held in the rack position (in front of your chest). This squat is best done with two kettlebells, two dumbbells, or a sandbag. Racked squats stress the core in a unique way and light up your abs.

When starting out with "racked" exercises, start with just one weight (either a kettlebell or dumbbell) in the rack to get accustomed to the position before moving onto two weights.

Follow these steps to do a racked squat:

1. **Clean the weight up into the rack position (see the earlier section on the clean).**

   Keep your forearms vertical and tight against your rib cage (see Figure 1-11a). Take a small step if needed to assume your squatting stance (feet shoulder-width apart; toes out).

2. **Take a deep breath into your belly and start your squat.**

   Imagine you're pulling yourself down between your legs. Keep your back flat, heels on the ground, and knees in line with the toes (see Figure 1-11b).

   Be sure to keep air in your belly throughout the movement to help keep your spine safe.

3. **When you've hit your maximum depth, push your heels into the ground, drive your hips forward, and stand up.**

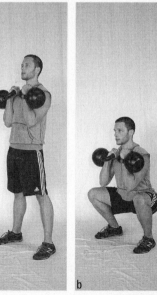

Figure 1-11: A racked squat with two weights really calls on your core muscles.

a   b

Photos courtesy of Rebekah Ulmer

The racked lunge

The racked lunge not only lets you load more weight onto the movement, but it may also provide an additional challenge for your core — especially if you're using two different size weights. You'll know it when you feel it.

And, yes, you can use two different size weights for just about any exercise, and from time to time, you should do just that. Rarely in life do you pick up anything that's perfectly even in weight. So it doesn't need to be that way at the gym either.

Here are the steps for the racked lunge:

1. **Clean the weight into the rack position and assume your squatting stance (see the earlier sections for these movements and Figure 1-12a).**

   Keep your stance approximately shoulder-width throughout the lunge to keep your balance.

2. **Step back into a deep lunge (see Figure 1-12b).**

   You may plant your hind knee on the ground; just don't bang it.

3. **Push hard from both your front and hind legs to stand up out of the lunge.**

   Be sure to keep your back toes planted (not pointed) so you can push off the ball of your foot (rather than your instep) when lunging.

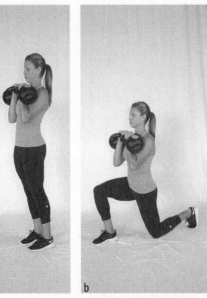

Figure 1-12:
A racked lunge with two weights requires good stability.

a   b

Photos courtesy of Rebekah Ulmer

Advanced Squatting Exercises

The front squat allows you to move a considerably larger load through the squatting pattern than the intermediate racked or goblet squats. Due to the placement of the weight, it requires more shoulder mobility, too. The second advanced exercise — the pistol squat — serves as one of the best single-leg bodyweight exercises in existence for strengthening the lower body.

The front squat

You want to perform the front squat with a barbell, solely for the reason that you can load more weight onto a barbell than you can handle with a set of kettlebells or dumbbells. But other than the amount of weight and the placement of the weight, the movement pattern is identical to the goblet squat or racked squat (discussed earlier in this chapter) — so don't move too hastily onto the front squat until you have those two movements mastered.

Note: To perform the front squat, you also need a rack to hold the barbell in between sets.

Here's how to do the front squat:

1. **Set up under the barbell so it lies across the front of your shoulders just above your clavicle and close to your throat (see Figure 1-13a).**

   Hold the barbell with a *clean grip* — where your fingers loosely grip the bar just outside of your shoulders while you drive your elbows up and in until your forearms are parallel with the ground. Support the weight with your body, not your arms; the clean grip simply acts as a placeholder for the weight across the front of your shoulders.

2. **Stand up out of the rack, and step away.**

   Get in the habit of taking as few steps as you need to find your squatting stance — there's no point in wasting time or energy messing around with your stance.

3. **Take a deep breath into your belly and start your squat (refer to the earlier section "The goblet squat" for the basic squat form, and see Figure 1-13b).**

   As always, keep your back flat, heels on the ground, and knees in line with your toes.

   It's imperative to keep air in your belly when under load. Breathe out while pushing your tongue against the roof of your mouth when coming out of your squat (to maintain intra-abdominal compression), but just don't breathe all your air out.

Book IV

Primal Power Moves for a Healthier Body

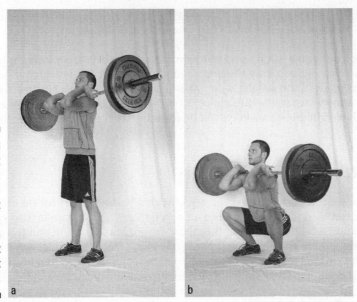

Figure 1-13
The front squat uses the standard squat pattern but with different weight placement.

Photos courtesy of Rebekah Ulmer

4. **When you've hit your maximum depth, push your heels into the ground and drive your hips forward to stand up and finish the movement.**

You're not done with the front squat until the barbell is placed safely back on the rack. Just because you've completed the rep doesn't mean you can relax. Stay tight and maintain good form the entire time you're under the bar. Keep those elbows up!

The pistol squat

The pistol squat is a full squat on one leg. It sounds simple, but, as you probably know, simple isn't always easy — and the pistol squat is an undeniable testament to that fact.

The pistol squat requires not only brute strength but also stability, mobility, balance, and coordination. It's not only a fantastic leg strengthener in itself but also a viable metric of your overall movement abilities. If you can do a pistol squat, you have gained a lot; if you can't, you have a lot to gain.

You can do the pistol squat with or without weight. Often, people find the pistol squat is more accessible when they're allowed to hold a small weight out in front as a counterbalance. Experiment and see what works best for you. Follow these steps for the pistol squat:

1. **Assume a shoulder-width stance and extend your arms out in front as a counterbalance.**

   If you choose to weight the pistol squat, hold it in the goblet or rack position (see earlier sections for these positions).

2. **Lift one leg straight up off the ground (see Figure 1-14a); the higher you can get it up, the better.**

   Try to keep your elevated leg fully extended out in front of you throughout the entire movement. It may even help to keep your toes pointed straight up. Also, be sure to start with your working leg heel on the ground.

3. **Begin to squat down as low as you can on one leg (see Figure 1-14b) while keeping your heel on the ground, your knee in line with your toes, and your back as flat as possible.**

   If you keep falling on your butt, try holding a light weight out in front of you to act as a counterbalance, as shown in Figure 1-14b.

4. **When you hit rock bottom (if you're able), push your heel hard into the ground and drive your hips forward to stand up.**

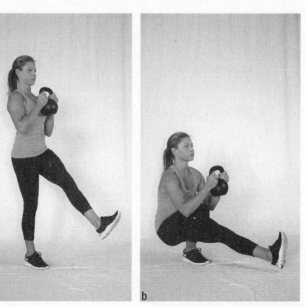

Figure 1-14:
You do the pistol squat with one leg out in front of you.

a   b

Photos courtesy of Rebekah Ulmer

Book IV

Primal Power Moves for a Healthier Body

Chapter 2

Pushes and Pulls for a Strong, Solid Torso

In This Chapter

▶ Developing a truly perfect push-up

▶ Working your way to your first pull-up — and beyond!

The chapters in this part of the book are here to help you understand movement quality. Remember not to press forward into the primal fitness programs prematurely. You need to have dominance over the fundamental primal movements before you slam it into high gear. If you don't, then it's like you're driving with the emergency brake on, and you'll progress slower than you would otherwise. Or even worse, you're driving with no brakes at all and are bound to injure yourself.

In this chapter, you find upper body movements and cover the fundamental pushing and pulling exercises found within the primal exercise programs. If you're new to exercise, this is the place to learn how to do a truly perfect push-up and how to get your first pull-up. If you're a veteran, you get the challenges of the one-arm push-up, the one-arm one-leg push-up, and the elusive one-arm chin-up.

The minor function of all these exercises, of course, is to develop raw upper body strength, inexhaustible power, and eye-catching aesthetics. The major function, and the one most overlooked, is to develop beautiful, functional movement.

All about the Primal Pushes

In the domain of pushes, there are two categories. The first is a horizontal push, such as the push-up. It's horizontal not because the push-up has you in a horizontal position but because if performed standing, the movement would be horizontal to the floor. The second is a vertical push, such as an overhead military press. Naturally, countless angles and variations exist between these two exercises.

If it's not clear by now, all the movements in this book are big, full-body movements. Paleo fitness doesn't focus on "isolation" (or bodybuilding) training because everything in the body is connected, and everything is meant to work together. Paleo fitness focuses on the big, compound movements that work multiple muscle groups simultaneously. It's better that way.

Reaping the benefits of the big pushes

Upper body strength is just one of the benefits of pushes. And with that upper body strength, you achieve robust, durable shoulders. And how about a torso that's the envy of the neighborhood? Yes, you can most assuredly expect all of this and more from the movements throughout this chapter.

But there's more: When you make your way into the more advanced pushing variations, such as the infamous one-arm one-leg push-up, you quickly discover that these pushes develop much more than upper body strength. Perhaps it'd be more appropriate to say that just about all these exercises are really full-body movements with an upper body emphasis. You see what that means when you feel how the push-ups and overhead presses sneakily attack core and lower extremities as well.

And don't let the "advanced" stuff intimidate you. Again, Paleo fitness is about progressing at your own pace. No matter what level you're at, this book gives you a starting place where you'll be challenged but successful. And that is the key.

Practicing strength

People often think that strength is the result of bigger muscles. This idea is true in part — a relatively small part, that is. Strength is more neurological than anything else, meaning it stems first from the central nervous system. A useful and common analogy is to think of your muscles as the factory, your central nervous system as the manager, and strength as the output. To increase the output, you can do one of three things: (1) Increase the size of the factory (build bigger muscles); (2) increase the efficiency of the manager (train the nervous system); or (3) do a combination of both.

In other words, you don't have to be "big" to be strong. Many athletes, like gymnasts for example, display an almost superhuman level of strength, yet they don't sport the bulky frame of a bodybuilder. That's because these athletes have a very finely tuned nervous system. They're highly efficient machines and have become so by training their nervous system first, not by bulking their muscles.

The movements in this chapter — such as the one-arm push-up — will, at first, feel very difficult. Rest assured that with much practice, they'll feel less and less difficult over time. Efficiency comes with practice.

TIP

If you want to get better at a particular movement, practice it as often as you can throughout the day. Try setting yourself a daily, or even an hourly, quota of reps. Keep the reps low, though, to avoid too much fatigue (when practicing an exercise, you want to feel as fresh as possible). For example, do you want to get better at pull-ups? Start by doing just one pull-up every hour you're awake. You'll be amazed how much stronger you feel at pull-ups even after one week!

Beginner Pushes

You probably know exactly what exercise is introduced in this section. And you'll soon have a newfound appreciation and understanding of this classic exercise: the push-up.

In this section, you find the push-up and the military press — one horizontal push and one vertical push. Together these two movements will help make you strong at just about every angle.

The push-up

Is the push-up the perfect primal exercise? In many ways, yes, it is. It hits hard not only the primary pushing muscle group — chest, triceps, and shoulders — but also many unsuspecting parts of the body, such as the abs. It can be easily scaled to accommodate all strength levels, and it's perhaps the most shoulder-friendly pushing exercise.

Unfortunately, many people discount the push-up because they feel it's too easy; they think there isn't as much to be gained with the push compared to lifting weights. They're wrong. You gain strength from working against resistance. Whether that resistance is your own body weight or external weight is irrelevant. Your muscles don't know the difference. Neither does your brain.

Yes, the push-up by itself can take you only so far, and if you can rep out 15 or so push-ups with faultless form, then it's likely time for you to move on to a more difficult variation, such as the one-arm push-up or the one-arm one-leg push-up. On the other hand, if you've had a difficult time achieving even one push-up, don't worry: You find out how to get there in the following steps.

Book IV

Primal Power Moves for a Healthier Body

1. **Set up in the top of a push-up position so your hands are directly under your shoulders and your feet are together (see Figure 2-1a).**

   The top of the push-up is identical to the top of a plank. Follow the "rule of thumb" — your thumb should be inside your shoulders when setting up for a push-up.

2. **Brace your abs/core and squeeze your butt.**

   This step often helps fix alignment issues. You should have a straight line from the back of your head all the way down through your tailbone.

3. **As you descend into the push-up, keep your elbows pointed back and tucked in to your sides (see Figure 2-1b).**

   A vertical forearm is a marker of a proper push-up form.

4. **When you hit rock bottom (elbows bent to at least 90 degrees), push hard into the ground and drive back up into a full lockout position (elbows fully extended).**

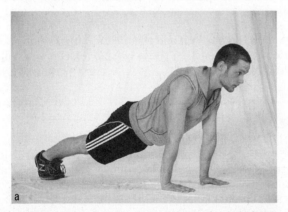

Figure 2-1:
The push-up
works a lot
of muscles
beyond the
obvious
chest,
arms, and
shoulders.

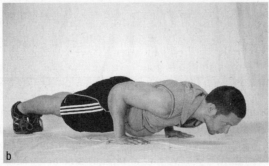

Photos courtesy of Rebekah Ulmer

If you have trouble performing a strict push-up, continue to work the push-up from your feet but do so on a slight incline. (Push-ups from the knees encourage poor mechanics and rarely help build the strength required for a full push-up.) The easiest variation is to perform push-ups on a set of stairs so your hands are elevated. As you get stronger, lessen the incline, and continue to work your way down to the floor.

Strength comes from practice. If you want to get good at push-ups, then you have to practice push-ups! The best way to practice is to perform a few push-ups intermittently throughout the day. You can even try setting yourself a daily, or hourly, push-up quota.

The military press

The military press is an old-timey strength builder, one that fell slightly out of fashion with the advent of the bench press but is slowly starting to come back. The military press is one of the most effective upper body grinding exercises found anywhere. It builds "real-world" overhead strength — some would call that "dad strength."

The military press toughens the shoulders and brutalizes the abs in a way the bench press can't. This movement is best performed with either one or two kettlebells or dumbbells or a barbell. Start out practicing this movement with a single kettlebell or dumbbell, and then work your way into double kettlebell/dumbbell and barbell pressing. All the same rules apply.

Here are the steps for the military press:

1. **Clean a kettlebell or dumbbell up into the rack position. (See Book IV, Chapter 1, for steps to the clean and check out Figure 2-2a.)**

2. **Brace the abs/core, squeeze your butt, and take in a deep breath of air.**

3. **Begin to press the weight up overhead; try to keep your forearm vertical throughout the entire press (see Figure 2-2b).**

   Don't lean back or arch your back during the military press. Keep the abs tight and the spine neutral!

4. **Press to a full lockout position, as shown in Figure 2-2c.**

   Your bicep should be in line with, or slightly behind, your ear at the top position.

5. **Pull the weight all the way back down to the rack position and repeat.**

Book IV

Primal Power Moves for a Healthier Body

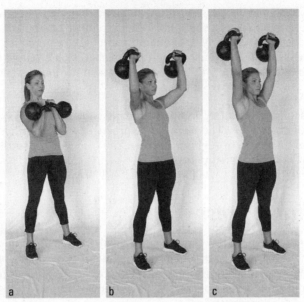

Figure 2-2:
Look straight ahead or keep your eye on the weight when doing the military press.

Photos courtesy of Rebekah Ulmer

Intermediate Pushes

The intermediate pushes are the bench press, one-arm push-up, and dip. You should have a strong handle on both the push-up and the military press to prep the shoulders and assess their tolerance before moving on to the bench press. And the one-arm push-up simply isn't possible unless you already have a strong push-up foundation.

When you're ready for these exercises, they will blast you into previously undreamt of levels of upper body strength!

The one-arm push-up

The one-arm push-up develops strength in ways few exercises can. This movement requires total body control, intense focus, and raw strength. The one-arm push-up is much more than a party trick. This exercise has tremendous carry-over into all sports and activities.

The one-arm push-up will seem near impossible at first attempt, but don't give up. Here are the steps:

1. **Set up at the top of your push-up position (refer to Figure 2-1a).**

   Be sure to set up with your hand as close to in line with your sternum (lower chest) as possible to ensure the shoulder is kept in good position throughout the push-up.

2. **Split your stance.**

   Kick your opposite leg out like a kickstand to assist with balance. The farther you kick out your opposite leg, the more assistance it will lend to the movement.

3. **Lift the non-working arm off the ground. You may want to place it on your hip for balance (see Figure 2-3a).**

4. **Begin to descend into your one-arm push-up, keeping your elbow in close to your side (see Figure 2-3b).**

   The most difficult part of the one-arm push-up is keeping everything as square as possible. Don't let your shoulders or hips rotate throughout the movement.

5. **When you hit rock bottom (see Figure 2-3c), drive back up, following the same path you took on the descent.**

Your hip may deviate outward a little bit when performing the one-arm push-up; just be sure to keep it to a little bit.

The bench press

No one can ignore the bench press or deny its effectiveness. Admittedly, this exercise isn't for everyone, but for those who have the shoulders for it, the bench press offers huge strength returns.

You may or may not have the shoulders to handle bench pressing. If you experience any pain or discomfort with this movement, stop immediately. You can also exchange push-up variations for bench pressing.

The bench press is best performed with a barbell because it allows you to load the most weight onto the movement. And really, the ability to move the most weight through the greatest range of motion is the major benefit of the bench press over the other pushing exercises. However, if you feel more comfortable bench pressing with dumbbells or kettlebells, go for it.

Book IV

Primal Power Moves for a Healthier Body

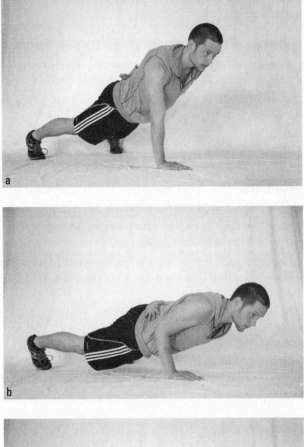

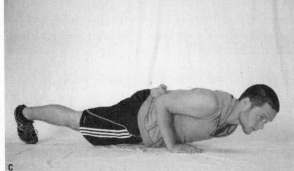

Photos courtesy of Rebekah Ulmer

Figure 2-3:
A one-arm push-up is quite a feat!

Here's how to properly execute a bench press:

1. **Lie down on the bench, planting your feet on the ground.**

   Make sure the bench touches your butt and upper back at all times, and maintain the natural curvature of your spine (neutral spine) throughout the movement.

2. **Grab the bar just outside of shoulder-width, maybe a little wider. Place the bar deep into the heel of your palm to take some stress off the wrist (see Figure 2-4a).**

   If you need to, use a spotter to help you lift the barbell up into the starting position. In fact, it's best to have a spotter at all times during the bench press.

   Don't go too wide with your grip, or you may irritate your shoulders.

3. **Keep your elbows within a 45-degree angle as you lower the bar down toward your sternum (see Figure 2-4b).**

   The forearms should be vertical or very close to vertical at the bottom of the bench press, as shown in Figure 2-4c. To help keep your shoulders in a good position and your elbows in the right spot, imagine that you're trying to bend that bar like a horseshoe throughout the bench.

4. **Drive the bar back up and over your face. The bar shouldn't travel straight up and down but rather in a C pattern.**

   Don't forget to breathe! Take a deep breath into the belly as you lower the bar, and let out a compressed breath as you press it back up. Also, be sure to press back up to a full lockout with each rep.

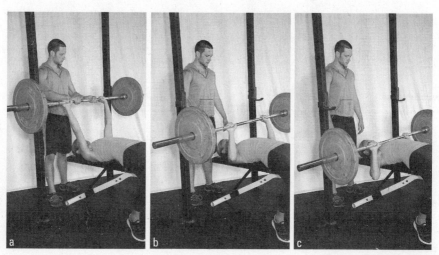

Figure 2-4: If you need to, use a spotter when doing the bench press.

Photos courtesy of Rebekah Ulmer

Book IV

Primal Power Moves for a Healthier Body

The dip

You can perform the dip on a set of parallel bars, gymnastic rings, or straps. It's a good idea to develop the dip first on the most stable surface: the parallel bars. After that, progress to gymnastic rings because they make for the greatest challenge and allow for more freedom of movement.

The dip is most commonly seen in gymnastics training. It strengthens the shoulder and the elbow joints (just be careful not to push it too far or too much at first), while building the deltoids, chest, and triceps.

Here are the steps to the dip:

1. **Stabilize yourself on top of a set of parallel bars (or rings or straps). Lock your elbows and keep your body as close to vertical as possible (see Figure 2-5a).**

   Don't let your shoulders shrug up. Press yourself away from the bars/rings.

2. **Slowly start to bend your elbows and come down into the dip.**

   To lessen the stress on your shoulders, you may begin to lean slightly forward, tilting your body into a more horizontal position. Continue until your elbows reach a 90-degree bend (see Figure 2-5b).

3. **Press back up into a full lockout position.**

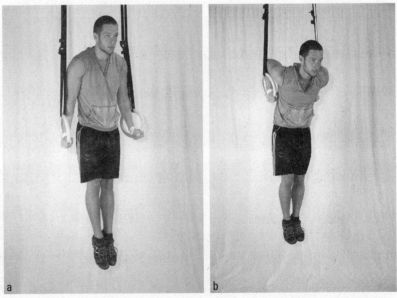

Figure 2-5: Ease your way into the dip so your shoulders get accustomed to the movement.

a   b

Photos courtesy of Rebekah Ulmer

Advanced Pushes

The two exercises in this section use only body weight, but don't underestimate their difficulty. If you aim to conquer the one-arm one-leg push-up and the handstand push-up, you need to be patient with them.

When you master these two movements, you'll pretty much have all you'll ever need as far as upper body strength goes. Sure, there are greater feats to master, but just being able to do these two movements will by default place you in the top 1 percentile. And that's not too shabby.

The one-arm one-leg push-up

The one-arm one-leg push-up calls for more core control and grinding strength than the standard one-arm push-up (see the earlier section). Not surprisingly, it develops more, too. Here's how to do it:

1. **Set up at the top of your push-up position and lift one arm and the opposite leg off the ground (see Figure 2-6a).**

   For example, if you lift your left arm, lift your right leg off the ground; if you lift your right arm, lift your left leg. Take time to stabilize yourself before moving on to the next step. You should also remain on the ball of your foot throughout the movement. Grip the ground forcefully with your fingers and toes (if you're barefoot) to help stabilize yourself.

2. **Begin to descend into the push-up position, keeping your shoulders and hips square (see Figure 2-6b).**

3. **When you hit the deck (Figure 2-6c), drive back up to the starting position.**

   Core control is vital. Keep a flat back and minimize all rotation throughout the movement. Not twisting or rotating is hard, but the less you do, the more effective the movement will be.

The handstand push-up

This section shows you how to perform a handstand push-up against a wall. But eventually, you should work up to performing the push-up from a free balancing handstand, which is by no accounts an easy feat!

Because you're inverted, this movement naturally falls into the vertical pushing category. It's more difficult than the standard push-up because you're moving a higher percentage of your body weight and you're doing so from a less advantaged position.

Book IV

Primal Power Moves for a Healthier Body

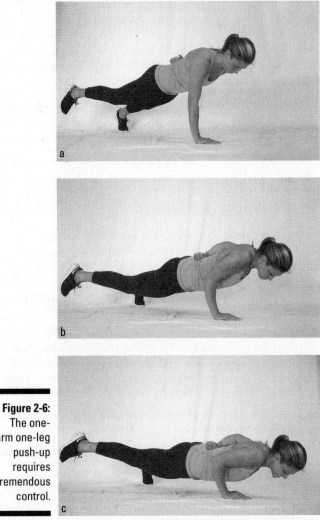

Photos courtesy of Rebekah Ulmer

Figure 2-6:
The one-arm one-leg push-up requires tremendous control.

Here are the steps to the handstand push-up:

1. **Find a spot in front of the wall, and with your back toward the wall, place your hands on the floor shoulder-width apart fairly close to the wall. Keeping your elbows locked, kick your feet up so you're inverted and balanced against the wall.**

2. **Organize yourself in this inverted position. Shrug your shoulders up so they cover your ears, keep your belly tight (try to flatten out the arch in your back), put your legs together, and point your toes (see Figure 2-7a).**

   Spend as much time as you need to get used to this position before attempting a push-up.

3. **Start to bend your elbows and lower yourself into the handstand push-up, moving your head closer to the ground, as shown in Figure 2-7b.**

   You want to get your head as close to the ground as possible, but don't bang it. Keep everything super tight and maintain the stiffness throughout your entire body. Don't force it. If something doesn't feel right, come out of the handstand.

4. **When your head reaches the floor, press back up into a full lockout to finish the movement.**

Figure 2-7:
Use a wall
or a spotter
to help you
with the
handstand
push-up.

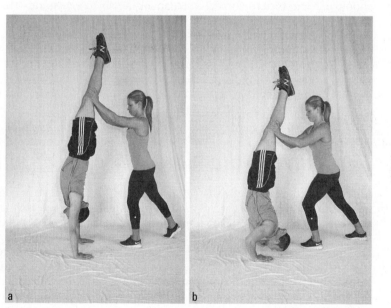

a   b

Photos courtesy of Rebekah Ulmer

Book IV

Primal
Power
Moves for
a Healthier
Body

All about the Primal Pulls

A push without a pull is as wrong as eggs without bacon. But because most people are after the "mirror muscles" — the pecs, the biceps, and the shoulders — they do way too much pushing and almost forget about pulling.

In fact, most people are so unbalanced, they would benefit from performing twice, or even three times, as many pulls as they do pushes!

In this section, you find some favorite primal pulling movements to develop a strong, sinewy back and to balance out all that pushing!

Balancing out with pulls

Overemphasizing pushing and neglecting pulling eventually lead to some unwelcome imbalances, not to mention a weak back and poor posture. After you dive into the primal fitness programs, you'll see that almost every push is balanced out with some sort of pull — either immediately or not too long after.

Sure, it'd be impossible to ever get the body perfectly balanced. But you should use exercise to correct imbalances, never to exaggerate them.

The easiest way to pair your pushes and pulls is to match the horizontal pushes with the horizontal pulls and the vertical pushes with the vertical pulls. For example, you can pair sets of push-ups with rows and sets of military presses with pull-ups. You find more ways to balance out your routine in the workout programs in Book IV, Chapters 5 and 6, but for now, get into the habit of practicing pulls with all your pushes!

Recognizing the many benefits of pulling

Although nothing on it classifies it as a "mirror muscle," a strong, muscular back is sure to grab the gaze of onlookers at the beach. A muscly posterior makes for a very aesthetically pleasing physique and a functional one, too!

Strengthening the musculature of the back — particularly the musculature that surrounds and supports the spine — improves your posture and invariably wards off back problems later in life. Pulling naturally balances out the shoulders as well and helps to protect them from injuries brought on from imbalances.

And, yes, pulling makes you strong, too — very strong, if you follow the progressions in this book. Everyone (both male and female) should be able to pull his or her own body weight up to a bar for multiple repetitions.

Beginner Pulls

To build up your pulling strength, start with rows and chin-ups. Don't worry if you don't have the chin-up down just yet; this section gives you a few variations to play with to help you along.

To work these exercises, you need something to hang from. For rows, a low bar or straps, such as a TRX suspension trainer, work nicely. For chin-ups, you need a high bar, a set of gymnastic rings, or maybe even a tree branch.

The bodyweight row

The bodyweight row is a horizontal pulling exercise. You can think of it almost as a reverse push-up. The row strengthens just about all the muscles of the back as well as the shoulders and biceps.

Furthermore, the row is easily scaled, like the push-up, simply by adjusting your angle. For an easier row, start more upright. To increase the difficulty, work your way into a more horizontal position.

Here's how to do the bodyweight row:

1. **Grab hold of a bar or a set of straps.**

   If using straps, tug on them to make sure they're secure before leaning back.

2. **While holding on to the bar or straps, lean back and adjust your stance until you find a challenging angle to work from (see Figure 2-8a).**

   Be sure to keep your back flat, your shoulders back (don't let them pitch forward), and your armpits tight like you would in a swing. There should be a straight line running from the back of your head down through your tailbone, just as if you were in a push-up.

3. **Start to row yourself up by driving your elbows down toward your hips (see Figure 2-8b).**

   At the finish, your hands should land in line with your sternum.

Book IV

Primal Power Moves for a Healthier Body

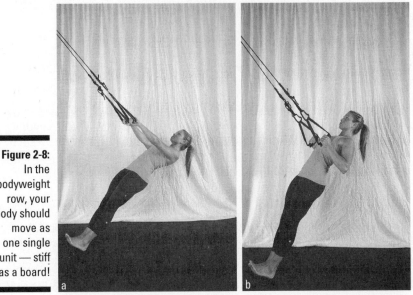

Figure 2-8:
In the bodyweight row, your body should move as one single unit — stiff as a board!

Photos courtesy of Rebekah Ulmer

The chin-up

The chin-up is a pull-up with your palms facing toward you. Because most people find the chin-up easier than a standard pull-up, it's a good place to start when working toward your first full pull-up.

The chin-up puts a greater emphasis on the biceps than the pull-up, which explains in part why some find the movement slightly easier. Nevertheless, it develops all the posterior pulling muscles and remains one of the most effective full-body strengthening exercises.

Here's how to do it:

1. **Grab hold of a bar with your hands shoulder-width apart and palms facing you. When your grip is secure, assume a dead hang (see Figure 2-9a).**

2. **Start the chin-up by sucking your shoulders down (think opposite of a shrug), bracing your abs/core, squeezing your butt (try to flatten the arch out of your back), and driving your elbows down hard toward your sides (see Figure 2-9b).**

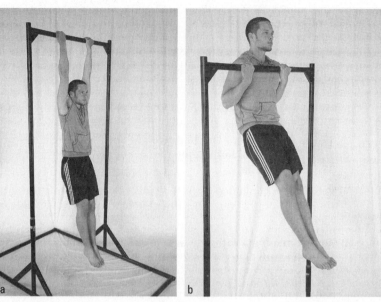

Figure 2-9:
Mastering
the chin-up
helps you
work toward
the pull-up.

a   b

Photos courtesy of Rebekah Ulmer

3. **Keep pulling until your throat reaches the bar — if you can get higher, great!**

   Don't try to complete a rep by reaching up with your chin. You either have it or you don't; you won't get any stronger trying to fake it.

4. **Pause momentarily at the top, and then control yourself back down to a full dead hang before starting the next rep.**

Intermediate Pulls

Book IV

Primal
Power
Moves for
a Healthier
Body

After you master the beginner pulls, it's time to move on to some more challenging variations: the one-arm row and the pull-up. The one-arm row, just like the one-arm push-up (see earlier section), is difficult because it adds in an additional core challenge (rotation stability) and limits the effort to only one arm! And the pull-up, a classic test of upper body strength, is the next logical step after the chin-up.

Take your time and work toward these intermediate pulls only after you feel like you have a very strong foundation with the beginner pulls. Attempting to progress too soon will result in delayed progress.

The one-arm row

The one-arm row, quite simply, is the bodyweight row performed with one arm. Expect many of the same challenges with the one-arm row that you would with the one-arm push-up.

1. **Set up precisely how you would for a two-arm row (the more narrow your stance, the more difficult this movement will be; see the earlier section "The bodyweight row"). Release one arm from the bar or straps, but keep your shoulders and your hips square (see Figure 2-10a).**

   The biggest challenge with this movement is fighting the rotation. Adjust your stance until you find a position where you'll be challenged but successful.

2. **Row yourself up with one arm. Your fist should finish in line with your sternum (see Figure 2-10b).**

   The difficulty of this movement also depends on the angle of your body in relation to the floor: More upright = less difficult; more horizontal = more difficult. Keep your shoulder pulled down and back by tensing your "armpit muscles;" don't allow it to be yanked forward.

3. **Control yourself back down to the starting position and repeat.**

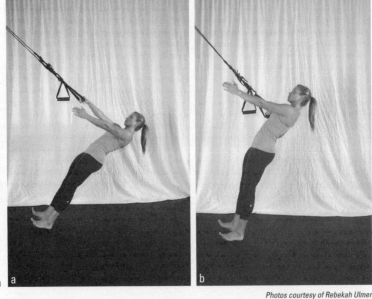

Figure 2-10: Change your angle to make the one-arm row more or less difficult.

a   b

Photos courtesy of Rebekah Ulmer

The pull-up

Everyone should be able to do pull-ups, with very few exceptions. The pull-up is by all accounts one of the best back and upper body strengthening exercises. It is an exercise of the ages, if there ever was such a thing.

The pull-up punishes those with excessive body fat, and, interestingly enough, it may even be used as a sort of body fat analysis tool. For example, if you gain weight and your number of pull-ups stays the same, chances are the weight you've gained is muscle. But if you gain weight and your pull-ups go down, well, you've likely gained fat. The reverse also holds true when you lose weight.

If you can't do a pull-up, make it a priority and be diligent in your pursuit. This section shows you how to get there; you just have to put in the legwork — or armwork.

1. **Take a shoulder-width grip on the bar with palms facing away from you and assume a full dead-hang position (see Figure 2-11a).**

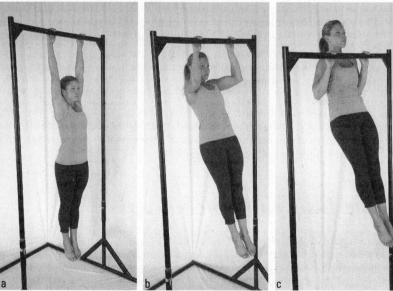

Figure 2-11: Start and finish the pull-up in a dead hang.

a   b   c

Photos courtesy of Rebekah Ulmer

2. **Initiate the pull-up by sucking your shoulders down, bracing your abs/ core, squeezing your butt (try to flatten the arch out of your back), and driving your elbows down hard to your sides (see Figure 2-11b).**

   You may find it easier to engage your back if you imagine you're trying to "rip the bar apart" or "bend the bar in half" (like the bench press) while performing a pull-up.

3. **Continue to pull until your throat is against the bar, as shown in Figure 2-11c.**

4. **Control back down to a full dead-hang position and repeat.**

   Don't just drop back into a dead hang because you may injure yourself. Control the descent.

Pull-ups make for a great exercise to practice intermittently throughout the day. Hang an easily removable pull-up bar, such as the Iron Gym brand, in your bathroom door. Every time you go to the bathroom, do five pull-ups.

Advanced Pulls

The exercises in this section are heinous, plain and simple. To get to this level, you need raw strength, total body control, and technical proficiency. Oh, and a lot of patience, too. These movements sometimes take years to develop. If you think you're going to get to this point overnight, you're in for a disappointing morning.

The L-sit pull-up/chin-up is a fantastic exercise for the front and the backside. The muscle-up really combines pulling and pushing; it's essentially a pull-up into a dip. And the one-arm chin-up is very close to a circus act. All these exercises build tremendous strength.

The L-sit pull-up/chin-up

The L-sit turns a chin-up or a pull-up into a brutalizing core exercise. The entire body must maintain an adequate amount of tension; otherwise, the L-sit won't hold. This movement requires a strong core and a strong back; it's surely one of the finest full-body movements anywhere.

Here are the steps for the L-sit pull-up/chin-up:

1. **Assume a pull-up or chin-up position (see the earlier sections on these exercises).**

2. **Raise your legs up to 90 degrees so your body forms an *L*. Lock your knees and point your toes (see Figure 2-12a).**

3. **While holding the L-sit, perform a full pull-up/chin-up (see Figure 2-12b).**

   To gain control and to increase its effectiveness, work this movement slowly.

The muscle-up

The muscle-up is a movement that comes from gymnastics and is best performed on a set of gymnastic rings. However, if you have only a bar to work with, you may use that instead.

The muscle-up is a pull-up into a dip. The most difficult part of this movement is the transition between the pull-up and the dip, where your elbows go from pointing down to pointing up. This transition requires strength through a range of motion that few people train.

The best ways to develop the strength for the muscle-up is to first get really strong at pull-ups and dips, and then begin working the muscle-up slowly in reverse. Nobody's first muscle-up is ever pretty. Just keep practicing.

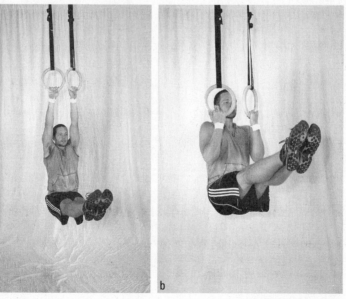

Figure 2-12: You must keep your abs under constant tension during the L-sit pull-up/ chin-up.

a   b

Photos courtesy of Rebekah Ulmer

The muscle-up can be quite stressful on unconditioned elbows and shoulders, so don't do too much too quickly. Your joints need time to toughen up.

Here are the steps for the muscle-up:

1. **Set up on the rings with a false grip (where the wrists are positioned over the rings, and the rings cut a diagonal across the bottom of the palm; see Figure 2-13a).**

   Developing the strength to hold a false grip takes a while. The best way to develop this strength is to start hanging with a false grip and practice pull-ups with a false grip as much as possible.

2. **Initiate a forceful pull-up, driving the rings down hard toward your sternum (see Figure 2-13b).**

   Imagine that you're trying to pull the rings through your sternum. Starting out, it may help to lean slightly back (almost like you would with a row) during the pull-up portion. Also, be sure to accelerate through the entire movement to avoid getting stuck.

3. **After you've gained enough height, push your chest through the rings and pop your elbows up so you land in the bottom of a dip position (see Figure 2-13c).**

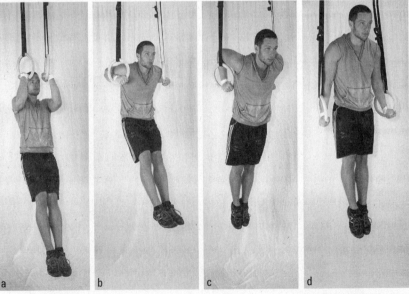

Figure 2-13:
The most difficult part of the muscle-up is the transition.

a   b   c   d

Photos courtesy of Rebekah Ulmer

4. **Finish the movement by locking out the dip (see Figure 2-13d).**

   A full lockout on the muscle-up means your elbows are extended fully and shoulders are shrugged down.

The one-arm chin-up

The one-arm chin-up is a feat very few achieve. It's perhaps the ultimate test of upper body pulling strength. There are no tricks to the one-arm chin-up; it's a product of hard work and practice. If you want it, you have to work for it. Here are the steps:

1. **Assume a dead-hang position from one arm from a bar or a set of rings. Keep the shoulders sucked down.**

   As you can see in Figure 2-14a, your body will naturally rotate sideways after you release one arm from the bar/ring.

2. **Tighten everything up like you would with a normal chin-up (see the earlier section), drive your elbow down hard, and pull yourself up until your throat reaches the bar or rings (see Figure 2-14b).**

3. **Control back down to a full dead hang and repeat.**

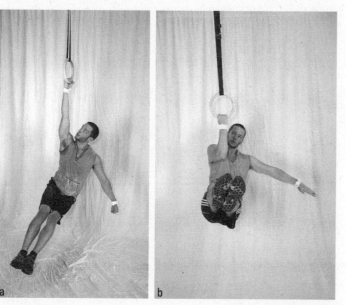

Figure 2-14:
The one-arm chin-up is the ultimate upper body pull.

a

b

Photos courtesy of Rebekah Ulmer

TIP

Ease yourself into the one-arm chin-up practice. Elbow tendonitis is common with this movement from overuse.

One way to start developing the strength for the one-arm chin-up is to practice holding positions throughout the movement for time. For example, practice holding just the top position for a few seconds, then the middle, and everywhere in between.

Chapter 3

Carrying Heavy Things and Ab Exercises That Don't Suck

- -

In This Chapter

▶ Carrying heavy things without hurting yourself

▶ Strengthening the grip, shoulders, forearms, and torso

▶ Mastering functional core training

▶ Developing indestructible abs

- -

Carrying is perhaps the most primitive exercise of all and also perhaps the least performed in the gym. However, you see carrying regularly in many other places: the grocery store, the Laundromat, or the playground. When people carry, they rarely do it with any true purpose or intent. It's simply the transportation of an object from one location to another through the means of human locomotion (that's movement).

Can you think of a more functional movement than carrying? People carry in some form every day without exception. Many of the other movements in this book, as marvelous as they are, are avoidable. Not every day demands a push-up, a pull-up, or a squat, but carrying is nearly inevitable, and you explore different types of carries in this chapter.

The cave man surely carried many heavy things and carried them quite often. Carrying heavy things is referred to as *loaded carries,* a term coined by strength and conditioning coach Dan John. Loaded carries train everything all at once — the shoulders, the core, the legs. That's the simplest way to look at them at least. The loaded carry has jurisdiction over all the major muscle groups and punishes them all equally.

In this chapter, you find a prime selection of movements to strengthen, firm, and slenderize the midsection — "ab exercises that don't suck." You discover how to train your core in a functional manner — one that's in line with the core's true purpose — and ultimately how to carve out abs that will have you looking for opportunities to take your shirt off.

Mastering the Art of the Loaded Carry

Carrying is far from a fine art. It's an art of the simplest nature, really, kind of like finger painting. Out of all the movements in this book, loaded carries are probably the quickest skill to acquire. In fact, they're very hard to do wrong, but don't think this makes them easy. Although the skill is low, the effort often climbs to a very high altitude.

How a movement looks and how it feels are often two different things. Just because a movement or an exercise looks easy doesn't mean it will be easy to perform. Often, the very fine nuances are imperceptible to the untrained eye. A gymnast makes his routine on the rings look easy, but it'd be foolish to assume anything about the movements of a high-level gymnast are easy to perform.

The following sections explore the art of carrying things, from fine-tuning everyday activities to developing strength and fitness with heavy loads.

Focusing on an everyday activity

Try to get through a day without carrying something. If you're an able-bodied individual, not carrying *something* at some point in the day would be a difficult task. Whether it's a baby, a bag of groceries, or a backpack, people carry on almost all occasions, so you may as well do it right.

Every now and then you run into the mom (or dad) who tells the story of how carrying her baby — for all those *very long years* — ruined her back. Well, this book clears the baby's name. The truth is that the baby was never at fault for any back injury or pain. In fact, it's very unlikely that any baby ever had any intentions of purposefully wrecking his or her parent's back. It wasn't the carrying of the baby that led to back problems; it was *how* the parent carried the baby.

Lifting doesn't cause injury; how you lift causes injury.

Carrying heavy things for strength and fitness

Loaded carries strengthen the grip, improve posture, and peel away body fat. You can perform loaded carries anywhere and with just about anything. And we do mean anything — dumbbells, kettlebells, sandbags, logs, boulders, or even a small child, so long as the tyke is permitting.

The carryover from loaded carries into real life is likely higher than that of any other exercise in this book and is as equally beneficial to the layperson as it is to the elite athlete. Loaded carries show you how to safely lift and transport heavy objects. If you've ever thrown out your back or tweaked this or strained that from lifting furniture, luggage, or whatever, then you can immediately see why carrying is a valuable skill to master.

From here on out, be conscious of how you lift and carry things. Whether it be as light as a notebook or as heavy as a couch, you should get into the habit of lifting and carrying it all in the same manner — with good form and proper body alignment. This is how you develop the habit of a safe lifting and carrying technique.

Beginner Carries

The two movements in this section, the farmer's carry and the waiter's carry, are as basic as it gets. But remember: You don't become elite because you move beyond the basics; you become elite when you move deeper into the basic movements — when you master them, perfect them, and own them.

No matter how strong you are now or will be, you'll never move beyond the basics. Yes, you'll begin to practice more "advanced" movements, but the basics will always be there, and you should continuously rehearse them, because the more you practice something, the more it becomes second nature.

Strength is a skill, and a skill is a habit of operation. If you want to be strong, move well, and perform optimally, you must get into the habit of rehearsing and strengthening your movement patterns with the utmost meticulousness — no matter how basic or simple they appear to be.

The farmer's carry

The farmer's carry is a classic strongman type of exercise. It's evident where the name comes from; what's not evident, however, is just how comprehensive this seemingly modest exercise is.

The farmer's carry is one of the finest exercises for strengthening the grip and forearms. If Popeye had a favorite exercise, it'd likely be the farmer's carry. The farmer's carry also reinforces good posture and core stability.

The farmer's carry is most easily performed with a set of dumbbells or kettlebells, but really, you can perform it with just about anything you can hold

Book IV

Primal Power Moves for a Healthier Body

on to — try a pail of water or a few buckets of sand if you really want to pay homage to the movement.

Here's how to do the farmer's carry:

1. **Dead lift one or two weights off the ground so they hang down by your sides. (See Book IV, Chapter 1, if necessary to review proper dead lift technique.)**

   To prep for this exercise, set up the weights for the dead lift so they're outside of your feet, as shown in Figure 3-1a. This way, when you lift them, they're right where you need them.

2. **Stand as tall as you can (imagine that you're trying to balance a set of books on your head), keep your shoulders "on the shelf" (that is, keep them back and don't let them hunch forward), and your core engaged (see Figure 3-1b).**

   The only way you can do this exercise wrong is to execute it with poor posture. Don't slouch or lean backward; stand as upright as possible. Think "long, tall spine" while you're holding the weight.

3. **Start walking, keeping your steps relatively small.**

   When you feel like you can't hold on with good form anymore, set the weights back down just how you picked them up.

Figure 3-1: Focus on good posture and a flat back for the farmer's carry.

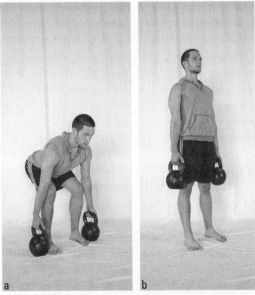

a   b

Photos courtesy of Rebekah Ulmer

The waiter's carry

The waiter's carry is an overhead carry. This type of carry is slightly more demanding than the farmer's carry because it requires additional shoulder strength and mobility and core stability. Don't expect to be able to do this carry with as much weight as the farmer's carry; it just isn't going to happen.

The waiter's carry strengthens the shoulders in a unique way, and aside from the Turkish get-up (later in this chapter), it's one of the best ways to make your shoulders indestructible. This carry is best performed with either a kettlebell or a dumbbell. The following steps walk you through the waiter's carry.

WARNING!

If you can't achieve a full, stable lockout, don't do this movement. Simply perform the farmer's carry in place of it until your shoulder mobility and stability improves.

1. **Clean a weight up (see Book IV, Chapter 1, for details on the clean) into the rack position, press it overhead, and hold it there (see Figure 3-2a).**

   Take a few seconds to make sure everything feels okay before you start walking. Your elbow should be locked and your bicep should be next to your ear. Keep everything in line to support the weight. There should be a straight line down from the bell to the floor.

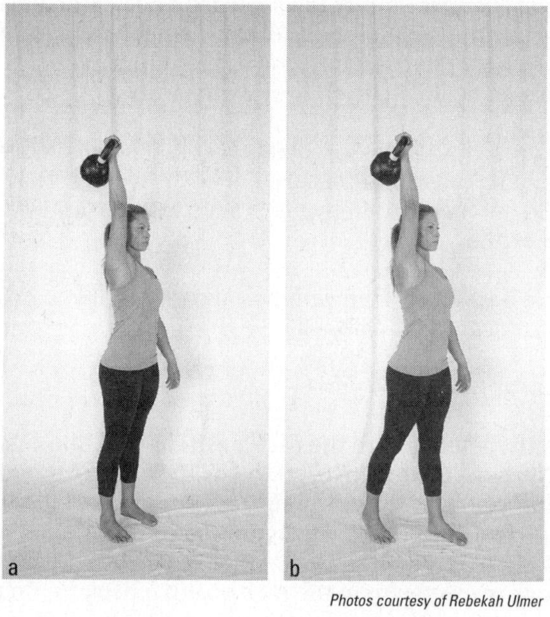

Figure 3-2: The waiter's carry is a great shoulder workout.

a   b

Photos courtesy of Rebekah Ulmer

Book IV

Primal Power Moves for a Healthier Body

2. **Slowly start to walk around (see Figure 3-2b).**

   For an additional challenge, try walking on a slightly uneven surface outdoors.

Don't take any chances when you're holding weight overhead. If you don't feel like you can keep the weight up there or if something feels wrong, don't force it! Set the weight down, rest, and continue only when you feel confident.

Intermediate Carries

In this section, you start to increase the load by moving from one-arm carries to two-arm carries. As you may expect, all the effects of the beginner carries will now be amplified. But don't rush into these intermediate carries too quickly; spend plenty of time building your foundation with the farmer's carry and waiter's carry in the previous section before venturing into the racked carry and two-arm waiter's carry.

The racked carry

The racked carry, and even just the rack hold for that matter, is one of the most boring-looking exercises but at the same time one of the most intense. Anyone who's spent time holding a considerable amount of weight in the rack position will quickly describe it to you as the direct opposite of a comfortable feeling, like an ever-constricting straight jacket.

The racked carry presents a colossal total-body stability challenge. The primary aim is to maintain poise and posture under the weight. That's it. The end result is a solid and nearly unmovable frame, with the added benefit of an impervious set of abs.

The racked carry is best performed with two kettlebells. If you don't have a set of kettlebells, you can use dumbbells.

Follow these steps for the racked carry:

1. **Clean two kettlebells up into the rack position (see Book IV, Chapter 1, for details). Be sure to keep everything as tight as you possibly can — bracing your abs/core, squeezing your glutes, and engaging your quads — and stand tall (see Figure 3-3a).**

   Don't lean back while you're in the rack position because doing so will immediately compromise your back. If at any time you catch yourself leaning back, set the weights down immediately.

2. **When you've gained a stable position, start to walk around in any direction you want (see Figure 3-3b).**

When performing rack holds and racked carries, breathe shallow and into your belly. When the weight gets heavy, you'll find it nearly impossible to take a deep breath anyhow, so taking shallow breaths in this manner will help you keep your back safe and control the stress level.

The two-arm waiter's carry

Walking while holding weight overhead, especially two weights — two heavy weights — is an immense challenge. Everything in the body must be working together to make this happen. The core needs to be engaged, the shoulders need to be alert, and the legs need to be limber. All muscles are put to work in this movement.

Don't even think about trying this movement until you feel super confident with the regular waiter's carry (see earlier section). Supporting weight overhead yields a high return, but don't assume any more risk with this movement than necessary. Take your time and gain stability through the one-arm version first.

Figure 3-3: Maintain your pose and posture in the racked carry.

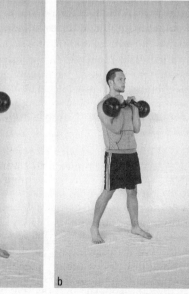

Photos courtesy of Rebekah Ulmer

Book IV

Primal Power Moves for a Healthier Body

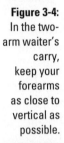

Figure 3-4:
In the two-
arm waiter's
carry,
keep your
forearms
as close to
vertical as
possible.

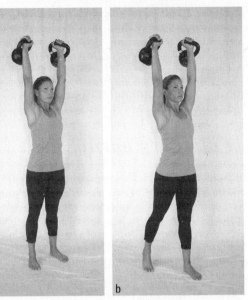

a   b

Photos courtesy of Rebekah Ulmer

Here's how to do the two-arm waiter's carry:

1. **Clean two weights up to the rack position, press them overhead, and hold (see Book IV, Chapter 1, for details on the clean, and check out Figure 3-4a).**

   Make sure all your body parts are neatly stacked. Make sure you aren't overarching your back or flaring out your rib cage; squeeze the abs and keep everything in proper alignment.

2. **When you feel ready, begin to slowly walk around, taking small steps (see Figure 3-4b).**

Always err on the side of caution with overhead holds. Push yourself to a comfortable challenge but never into too much fatigue. Never let form deteriorate.

Advanced Carries: The Bottoms-Up Carry

The advanced carries — or *carry* — is of a different sort entirely. It isn't necessarily more difficult from the perspective of loading or mobility. What makes this movement "advanced" is the high degree of concentration and tension that you must maintain throughout. Also, the bottoms-up carry pulls a balancing component into the mix.

The bottoms-up carry can really only be performed with a kettlebell because it's one of the very few weight-training devices with an offset center of gravity. The bottoms-up carry, as the name implies, involves carrying the kettlebell in an inverted position — that is, with the handle below the actual weight. As you may expect, this position presents a colossal challenge for the grip, the abs/core, and the shoulders.

Don't expect to walk with this position at first. It will take you some time to be able to "catch" the kettlebell in the bottoms-up position from the clean and hold it there. It will take you double the time to get the hang of it on your non-dominant side.

Be sure to work with a kettlebell that's heavy enough; it must be a challenge to hold it in the bottoms-up position. If you choose too light of a weight, this profitable task becomes a joke.

Here's how to do the bottoms-up carry:

1. **Start to clean a kettlebell but, as the kettlebell begins to roll over onto your forearm, stop it halfway and hold it in the bottoms-up position (with the bottom of the kettlebell facing up toward the ceiling; see Figure 3-5).**

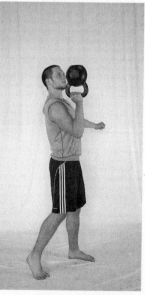

Figure 3-5:
The bottoms-up carry requires strength, balance, and coordination.

Photo courtesy of Rebekah Ulmer

To maintain the bottoms-up position, you have to squeeze everything — your abs, your butt, and, of course, the handle of the kettlebell!

2. **Stabilize your position. Keep your forearm perfectly vertical (otherwise, the bell will topple), and let the handle of the bell rest deep in the base of your palm.**

3. **When you've owned the position standing, start walking with it.**

To get better at the bottoms-up carry, you may want to start by practicing bottoms-up cleans for a while. The bottoms-up clean is simply performing a clean (see Book IV, Chapter 1) but catching the kettlebell in the inverted or "bottoms-up" position rather than the rack position.

Getting the Abs of Your Dreams

Here we are at last. The section everyone has been waiting for. Just about everyone, at one time or another, has longed for a sleek, sexy set of abs.

Nothing is wrong with wanting six-pack abs. Just know that there are many ways to go about forging an indestructible midsection, some of them healthy, some of them not so healthy; some of them effective, and others not so effective.

Six-pack abs aren't always a reflection of good health. People often use extremely unhealthy methods to reduce body fat to a nearly nonexistent percentile. But with Paleo fitness, we take the opposite approach and guarantee your six-pack abs to be the result of vibrant health.

The following ab sections instruct you on how to perform the highest-yield ab exercises on the planet. That means using functional core training that offers the highest return on your time and effort.

Functional training is a term that gets thrown around loosely and often without any true meaning. In this book, functional core training must address the three primary functions of the core. The first of which is stability — that is, to maintain spinal position in the presence of change. The second is flexion and extension (think bend and unbend). The third involves rotation. The movements in the following sections cover all three.

Beginner Ab Exercises

In this section, you discover three exercises: the four-point plank, which develops core stability and is a clear demonstration thereof; the V-up, which is the preferred alternative to the classic crunch or sit-up because it punishes the abs and teaches valuable alignment drills that you don't get with the crunch or the sit-up; and the windmill, which blasts your obliques.

The four-point plank

Most likely, you're familiar with the plank. If not, think of the plank as the top of the push-up position (see Book IV, Chapter 2). The name is symbolic of the looked-for body position, which should be flat; the hips shouldn't sag or pike up and neither should the belly.

The plank helps to develop linear core stability, or the ability to resist extension of the spine, which is the major function of your abs.

Here's how to do a perfect plank:

1. **Set up at the top of a push-up position; place your feet together and your hands directly under your shoulders (see Figure 3-6).**

   Keep your back flat at all times — no rounding or overarching — and keep everything in line, from head to tailbone.

2. **Hold the plank position for at least 20 seconds.**

3. **To get even more out of the plank, throw in some isometric contractions: Simultaneously squeeze your butt, abs, quads, triceps — every possible muscle that you can.**

   Adding in these contractions not only makes the plank more challenging but also serves to keep your body parts properly and neatly ordered.

The V-up

The V-up is a wonderful ab exercise to strengthen the abdominal wall, and it's typically much easier on the back than traditional sit-ups (which often aggravate or initiate back issues). The V-up is a useful progression toward the more challenging ab exercises, such as the hanging leg raise, which you find later in this chapter.

Book IV

Primal Power Moves for a Healthier Body

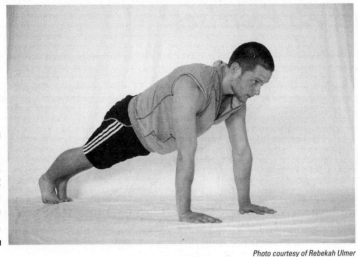

Figure 3-6:
The plank
looks a lot
like the top
of a push-up
position.

Photo courtesy of Rebekah Ulmer

Perform the V-up on a relatively soft surface and follow these steps:

1. **Lie down flat on your back with your legs fully extended and your arms next to your side.**

2. **Squeeze your abs as hard as you can, trying to take the arch out of your lower back (imagine you're trying to push your lower back hard into the ground).**

   This step results in what's often referred to as a *hollow position,* which looks sort of like a human banana. It's an excellent ab exercise by itself. Be sure to own this position before progressing forward.

3. **Slowly begin to raise your legs and torso simultaneously, trying to fold yourself in half while balancing on your buttocks (see Figure 3-7a).**

   Keep your legs straight the entire time. Go slowly; it will take some time before you're able to maintain your balance. You may rest your hands on the ground for balance when starting out, but eventually the goal is to perform this step without any "kickstands."

   For a more challenging variation, extend your arms up overhead, as shown in Figure 3-7b.

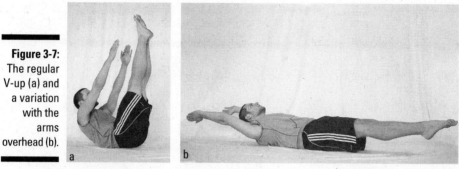

Figure 3-7: The regular V-up (a) and a variation with the arms overhead (b).

Photos courtesy of Rebekah Ulmer

The windmill

Although many mistake the windmill for a side bend, it isn't. This movement blends hip flexion and thoracic rotation, which means the hips support the load, not the lower back. The windmill is a heavy-hitting rotational core exercise, but you must approach it with caution. Don't rush weight onto this movement. First, practice the windmill without weight, and then after you perfect the movement pattern, try the windmill with a kettlebell or dumbbell. Here are the steps:

1. **Press the weight overhead and lock it. Then assume a shoulder-width stance, but point your feet at a 45-degree angle away from the weight (see Figure 3-8a).**

   The stance setup is critically important. You must angle your feet away from the weight; otherwise, you won't be able to properly push your hips back and perform the movement.

2. **Start the windmill by pushing your hips back and shifting most of your weight onto your rear leg (the leg under the weight; see Figure 3-8b).**

   You should displace approximately 75 percent or more of your weight to your hind leg. If this isn't the case, you need to work on pushing your hips back farther.

3. **As you start to bend at the hips, look up at the bell, slightly rotate your torso, and use your free arm to guide you into the windmill by tracking it down your front leg (on the inside of your thigh; see Figure 3-8c).**

   Only go as low as you're comfortable with the windmill, and be sure to keep your eye on the weight at all times.

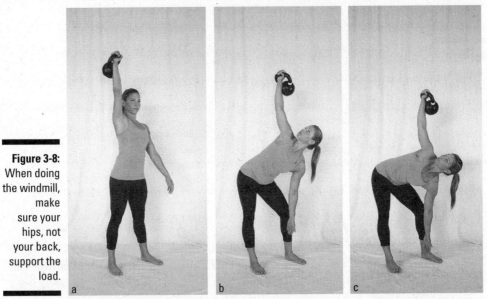

Figure 3-8:
When doing
the windmill,
make
sure your
hips, not
your back,
support the
load.

Photos courtesy of Rebekah Ulmer

   4. **To come out of the windmill, squeeze your butt, drive your hips for-
      ward, and follow the same path in reverse.**

The windmill offers the added benefit of stretching the lower back. Light
windmills are a great way to loosen up a tight back.

Intermediate Ab Exercises

The hanging knee raise is the next step in the progression toward what is perhaps the most effective and brutalizing ab exercise in existence, the hanging
leg raise (see the later section for this exercise).

This section also introduces you to two challenging plank variations that
incorporate a rotary stability challenge (the ability to resist rotation). Be sure
you master all the beginner exercises before moving on to the intermediate
section.

The hanging knee raise

For this movement, you need something to hang off of. A pull-up bar is the obvious first choice, but a set of gymnastic rings or any other sort of hanging device will work well.

The hanging knee raise works the entire abdominal wall — the upper, the middle, and the lower. It's easy on the back and really helps develop the strength needed to complete a full hanging leg raise. The following steps walk you through the hanging knee raise:

1. **Assume a dead-hang position (see Book IV, Chapter 2) from a pull-up bar or rings. Brace your abs and flatten the arch out of your back — think about trying to mimic the "hollow position" from the V-up (see earlier section and check out Figure 3-9a).**

   Try not to use any momentum when performing the hanging knee raise — that means no swinging or kipping! Keep space between your shoulders and your ears while hanging.

2. **Slowly raise your knees up toward your chest, but don't lean back. Instead, try to keep your torso as vertical as possible throughout the entire movement (see Figure 3-9b).**

   This step is often what makes the hanging knee raise and hanging leg raise so difficult but so effective for strengthening the abs.

Figure 3-9: The hanging knee raise helps you progress to the hanging leg raise.

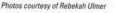

Photos courtesy of Rebekah Ulmer

Book IV

Primal Power Moves for a Healthier Body

At the top of the hanging knee raise, your shoulders should still be positioned close to your ears. If they've gotten too far away, you're probably leaning back too much.

3. **Slowly lower your knees all the way back down and repeat.**

The two-point plank

The two-point plank brings in an anti-rotational component as well as a balance challenge. For this movement to happen, you must keep everything tight, so expect a full-body challenge as well as an ample burn in the midsection.

Here's how to do the two-point plank:

1. **Assume a four-point plank position (see earlier section), but start with your feet approximately shoulder-width apart.**

2. **Lift one leg a couple inches off the ground. Keep the leg straight.**

   Your alignment shouldn't change when you lift your leg off the ground. If something changes, reset and try again.

3. **When you feel stable with a leg off the ground, slowly raise the opposite arm, placing it behind your back or straight up overhead (see Figure 3-10).**

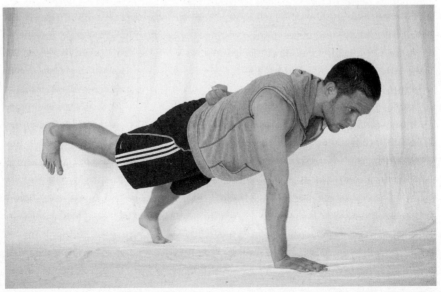

Figure 3-10: A two-point plank works the full body.

Photo courtesy of Rebekah Ulmer

The torso and the hips shouldn't rotate when you enter into a two-point plank. Ideally, everything is aligned precisely how it would be if you had all four limbs on the ground.

It's best to work into the two-point plank by first mastering a three-point plank off of each limb. For example, hold a four-point plank and slowly raise each limb off the ground, one at a time, for a count of five.

Advanced Ab Exercises

Both movements in this section are hanging ab exercises. And unless you're a practiced gymnast, you'll likely find both of these movements exceptionally difficult at first. The effort to master these movements is intense, but the rewards that follow are great. Most people who can perform either of these two movements have a strong, hard-hitting, and functional set of abs.

The exercises in the beginner and intermediate sections earlier in this chapter are designed to prepare you for the advanced ab exercises: the hanging leg raise and the windshield wiper. But don't think — even after training extensively with all the preceding exercises — that your first attempt at either of these two movements will be easy.

The hanging leg raise

Almost nobody's first hanging leg raise looks even remotely passable, and that's okay. Over time, as the abdominal wall thickens and strengthens as well as the hip flexors, this movement will start to take on a sort of elegance that few other exercises exhibit.

The hanging leg raise is a staple in gymnastics training, which should give you an idea as to the kind of strength it builds. It blasts the entire abdominal wall — nothing escapes it. Not to mention, it strengthens the hip flexors, the back, and the grip. It really is the ultimate ab exercise.

The hanging leg raise is the ability to hang from a bar and fold yourself in half. This movement requires not only a great deal of strength but also a lot of flexibility. When most people first attempt this movement, they have a tendency to lean back or swing their legs up to compensate for their lack of strength, flexibility, or both. Although both of these options make the movement easier, you should try to avoid them.

Book IV

Primal Power Moves for a Healthier Body

Here's how to do the hanging leg raise:

1. **Hang from a pull-up bar (or a set of gymnastic rings) with a shoulder-width grip. Tighten everything up as if you're in a plank position and flatten the arch out of your back (see Figure 3-11a).**

   Flattening your back will help prevent using sway or momentum to complete the movement.

   From time to time, you may want to experiment with various grip positions. Occasionally, you can try the hanging leg raise with a narrower grip (hands together) or a wider grip (outside shoulder-width).

2. **Without leaning back or bending your elbows, raise your toes up toward the bar (see Figure 3-11b).**

   Think of trying to "pull the bar to your feet" throughout the movement. Doing so will help engage your lats (armpit/back muscles) and supercharge your abs.

3. **When your feet reach eye level, lean slightly back if you have to but only as much as you need to (see Figure 3-11c).**

   The hanging leg raise is complete when your feet reach your hands. It should almost look like you're performing a toe-touch stretch.

4. **Lower your legs back down in a slow and controlled manner and repeat.**

Figure 3-11:
The hanging leg raise builds strength like you wouldn't believe.

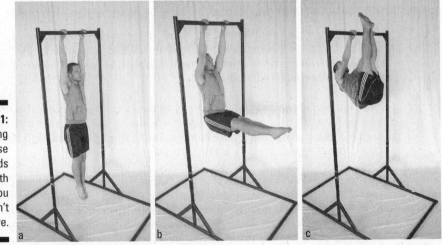

a   b   c

Photos courtesy of Rebekah Ulmer

To make this movement easier, first bend your knees before using momentum or leaning back. The more knee bend, the easier the movement, which is why the hanging knee raise is the first step toward the full hanging leg raise. So to progress toward the full hanging leg raise, slowly start to extend your knees farther and farther until you have achieved full extension. This may take a while, but it works.

The windshield wiper

The windshield wiper is a pseudo hanging leg raise, adding in a fierce rotational component. (*Note:* You must achieve the hanging leg raise in the previous section before you can do the windshield wiper.) The benefits of the windshield wiper are vast, especially for those seeking rotation power and a ripped midsection. You'll feel this movement across your entire abdominal wall, and we say *across* purposefully because you'll specifically feel its effects around the finger-like muscles of the rib cage (the *serratus anterior*).

Follow these steps for the windshield wiper:

1. **Perform a full hanging leg raise (see previous section), bringing your feet all the way up to the bar.**

2. **Lean back so your torso is horizontal to the ground and your legs are pointed straight up (see Figure 3-12a).**

   Ideally, your legs and your torso should be at a 90-degree angle at the start of the windshield wiper. Do your best to keep your elbows locked throughout this movement.

3. **Slowly lower your legs to one side while keeping your torso facing upward (see Figure 3-12b).**

   Take the movement slow at first! If you throw your legs around too quickly, before you're conditioned for the movement, you may injure your shoulders or back.

4. **Raise your legs back up to the starting position and then lower them to the other side. Bring them back up to the starting position once more to complete the movement.**

Book IV

Primal Power Moves for a Healthier Body

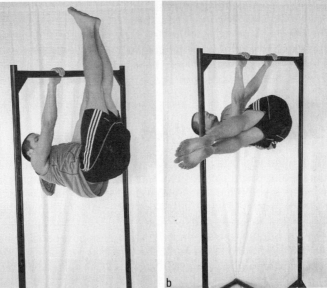

Figure 3-12:
The windshield wiper starts with a full hanging leg raise and then rotates.

a   b

Photos courtesy of Rebekah Ulmer

An All-Around Paleo Exercise: The Turkish Get-Up

If you're ever exiled and allowed to take with you only one exercise to preserve yourself, take the Turkish get-up. This primitive exercise has you moving from just about every joint in your body, forcing you to stabilize where you need to stabilize and mobilize where you need to mobilize. Its primary purpose is to get you up off the ground safely.

Furthermore, this movement is the most comprehensive of all primal warm-ups. Five minutes of consecutive Turkish get-ups will prep the body for any and all rigors of vigorous exercise.

You can perform the Turkish get-up anywhere, anytime. To keep on the move and to reap the maximum benefit of this exercise, set yourself a daily Turkish get-up quota. Try working even just one unweighted Turkish get-up every hour you're awake. You'll be amazed at how refreshing it feels!

The Turkish get-up — or *get-up* for the sake of brevity — toughens the shoulders, hardens the abs, and loosens the hips through an exhibition of litheness. It's a graceful movement with many nuances.

Don't rush the get-up. In fact, the slower you go, the better. Take time to master each position and enjoy the ride.

A proper setup for the get-up is essential; an improper setup impedes the crusade downstream, which is to say that any get-up is only as good as any setup. *Note:* When first performing the get-up, don't use any weight. After you're proficient at the movement, you may then use a kettlebell (preferred), a dumbbell (second best), or a barbell (most awkward but doable).

Here are the steps for the Turkish get-up:

1. **Start by lying on your back (prone position).**

   Your arms and legs should be fully extended and angled out away from your body at roughly 45 degrees. Your right arm should run parallel to your right leg and your left arm parallel to your left leg. Think of the bottom of a snow angel position.

2. **Pick a side to start with, follow these steps, and refer to Figure 3-13 to continue the setup:**

   a. To work the right side of your body, press your right arm directly up in line with your sternum (midchest) as if you're performing a one-arm bench press.

   b. Bend your right knee and plant your right heel relatively (not directly) close to your butt.

   Note: To work on the left side, follow the steps with your left arm and left leg.

3. **Perform a roll by pushing hard into your planted heel, pulling hard from your planted elbow, driving your chest upward, and propping yourself up onto your planted forearm (see Figure 3-14a).**

   Keep your other arm extended straight overhead (imagine you're balancing a half cup of water on your fist at all times — don't let it spill!).

   This step is to be a roll, not a crunch or a sit-up. If you lead with your head and round your back, then you're doing it wrong. Lead with a proud chest, and keep your back flat.

4. **Move from your forearm up to your hand by extending the elbow (see Figure 3-14b).**

   Don't lift your hand to do this step; instead, simply pivot on it. An effective, but somewhat crude, cue is to pretend you're squishing a beetle. Also, don't let your shoulders shrug up in this position. Keep as much distance between your shoulders and ears as possible.

Book IV

Primal Power Moves for a Healthier Body

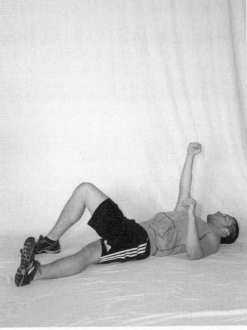

Figure 3-13:
A proper setup is crucial for an effective execution of the Turkish get-up.

Photo courtesy of Rebekah Ulmer

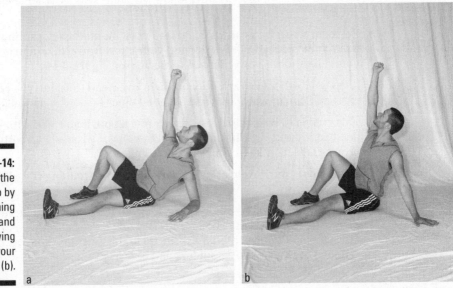

Figure 3-14:
Start the get-up by performing a roll (a) and then moving to your hand (b).

a

b

Photos courtesy of Rebekah Ulmer

5. **Complete a bridge by pushing your heel into the ground, squeezing your butt, and driving your hips up into the air (see Figure 3-15a).**

   Try your very best to come into a full bridge, but don't overextend. You should be able to freely lift your straight leg off the ground in the bridge position. If you can't, you need to shift your weight onto the heel of your bent leg.

6. **Sweep your straight leg back under your hips, planting your knee directly in line with your planted hand (see Figure 3-15b).**

   When done right, your legs should form an *L* with one knee facing forward and the other knee facing outward.

   Don't try to sweep your leg back in such a manner that both knees face forward, like they would in a lunge position. Doing so feels awkward and will put you into a bad position.

7. **Simultaneously lift your planted hand and rotate your back leg to come up off the ground and into an overhead lunge position (see Figure 3-16a).**

   The movement of your back leg should look similar to a windshield wiper as your back calf swings outward until both knees are pointed in the same direction.

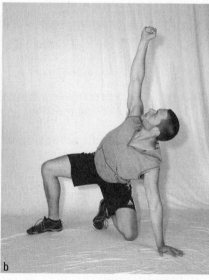

Figure 3-15: Push into the bridge (a) and then do the sweep (b).

a

b

Photos courtesy of Rebekah Ulmer

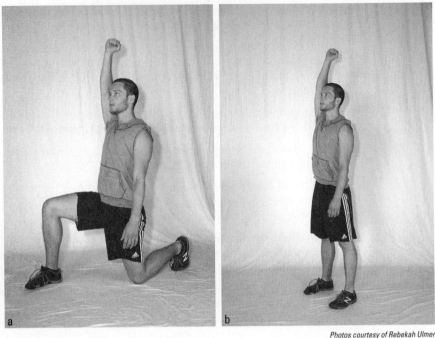

Photos courtesy of Rebekah Ulmer

Figure 3-16:
Move to
a lunge
position (a)
and then
stand up (b).

8. **Stand up out of the lunge, as shown in Figure 3-16b.**

   Note that in the lunge position (Step 7), you want your back toes to be firmly planted on the ground (not pointed behind you) so you can push off your back leg just as much as your front leg to stand up.

9. **Reverse everything you just did — step by step — and return to the starting position.**

Practice the get-up as often as you can and get comfortable with it because you'll use it in other movements throughout this book. Eventually, you'll load the get-up and execute it with a considerable amount of weight overhead, enhancing your strength, stability, mobility, and coordination.

Chapter 4

Primal Power Moves for Explosive Athleticism

In This Chapter

▶ Discovering what power training is and how you can benefit from it

▶ Forging dense, durable muscle with the primal power moves

▶ Developing raw, explosive power

The benefits of power training are humungous. Power moves rely on a highly efficient nervous system and perfectly coordinated movement. To express force rapidly is to exhibit movement efficiency, which is a marker of natural athleticism. Power training makes you stronger, leaner, faster, and more robust. It gives you the edge.

That said, precision should always precede power. That's why the movements in this chapter are the last in the series of the primal exercise progressions. They're the true power movements — *power* meaning the ability to rapidly exert force. Previous chapters cover explosive movements, such as the swing, the clean, and the snatch, but the movements in this chapter require a higher degree of technical proficiency and take the most skill.

All the movements in this chapter are extremely explosive, high-velocity exercises. They build on the skills in Book IV, Chapters 1, 2, and 3. For example, the swing shows you how to produce and reduce force with your hips, a necessary skill before attempting the broad jump or the box jump, which you find in this chapter. The military press (Book IV, Chapter 2) and the Turkish get-up (Book IV, Chapter 3) prepare your shoulders for the overhead demands of the jerk.

If you haven't mastered with confidence all the skills leading up to this chapter, be sure to get comfortable with those skills before proceeding. If you try the movements in this chapter too soon, you may increase the risk of injury.

Understanding Primal Power

You develop primal power by pushing around heavy things, by jumping, and by sprinting. You don't need any fancy technical equipment. The good old-fashioned moves work just fine — actually, they work the best.

As you find in this chapter's introduction, power is the ability to exert force rapidly. In other words, power is the amount of work you perform in a certain amount of time. So you can increase power in only three ways:

✔ Increasing the amount of work you perform over a certain amount of time

✔ Performing the same amount of work but decreasing the amount of time it takes you to do it

✔ Performing more work in less time

Although power should be your priority when seeking strength, leanness, and athleticism, it shouldn't necessarily come first. You need a solid foundation of mobility, stability, and strength before you start to add in power training. If you train power without the proper foundation, injury isn't a matter of if but when. See Book IV, Chapters 1, 2, and 3, for exercises to build this foundation.

Your need for speed

The cave man likely engaged in power-based movements on a regular basis. These types of movements were essential to his survival, after all. If he wanted to eat, he likely had to sprint to catch his food and even more likely had to spear it (or stone it) and then throw it up over his shoulder and haul it back to camp. He couldn't perform these tasks sluggishly.

Humans aren't meant to be slow-moving creatures, at least not all the time. We're designed to sprint, run, jump, throw, and everything in between. For this reason, our muscles are made up of both slow-twitch fibers (for endurance endeavors) and fast-twitch fibers (for short, explosive bouts).

The benefits of power training

Training the fast-twitch fibers, or training in an explosive manner, is quite taxing on the nervous system, especially when you train with weight; therefore, power training offers a very high strength return. Many of the power training movements we explore throughout the rest of the chapter become a blend of heavy strength efforts and elevated cardiovascular stress — meaning you get more work done and burn more calories in less time.

Fast-twitch fibers are also the "look good" muscle fibers, the kind that grow the quickest and offer the most definition. You can think of them as the mirror muscles because they stand out most vividly when you look in a mirror.

Those who benefit most frequently from power training are athletes. The power moves help them move faster, hit harder, jump higher, and so on. But you don't have to be an athlete to reap these rewards. In other words, you don't have to be an athlete to train like an athlete. Now, that's not to say that everyone should train exactly like an athlete, but everyone can benefit from some elements of training like high-level athletes — power training is one of them.

When training the power movements, you want to minimize fatigue as much as possible. Fatigue slows you down and saps your power. The easiest way to minimize fatigue is to allow as much rest as you need between sets.

Beginner Power Moves

The push press and the broad jump are fairly low-skill movements, but they each have their little nuances. Often, the nuances make up movement quality.

With that being said, go easy on yourself with these two movements. They're a starting point, intended to give you the framework needed for the more technical lifts later in this chapter, such as the jerk and the box jump.

The push press

The push press is what people tend to do naturally when attempting to press a weight that's too heavy for them — they use their legs to help drive it up. The difference with this power movement is that you do the leg drive intentionally, not out of desperation.

The push press shows you how to generate force from the ground and transfer it through your body and up overhead. You often see movements similar to the push press, such as the Viking push press, in strongman competitions because it's a clear demonstration of upper body power and work capacity as well as a developer of both.

The *groove,* or path of the weight, with the push press is slightly different from the military press (see Book IV, Chapter 2). Because you're driving the weight up more from your lower body than your upper body, the path should be more vertical, or straight up and down, instead of arcing slightly outward.

Other than that, if you have a solid military press, you should be able to master the push press in no time. Simply follow these steps:

1. **Clean a weight (either a kettlebell or dumbbell) up into the rack position (see Book IV, Chapter 1, for cleaning techniques and check out Figure 4-1a).**

   Keep your forearm vertical in the rack position, not angled, to ensure a smooth transition into the overhead lockout.

2. **Dip down, slightly bending your knees (see Figure 4-1b).**

   It's okay if your knees come forward here because you're performing a dip, not a squat; just be sure you don't dip too low — dip just enough but not a smidgeon more. Doing so will diminish your power and fatigue your quads prematurely.

3. **Immediately reverse the dip, driving your heel hard into the ground and imagine that you're trying to jump the weight up overhead. Catch the weight overhead in a full lockout position (see Figure 4-1c).**

   The bell should float up overhead from the drive of your lower body. The arm assists, but the legs do most of the work.

4. **Let the weight drop back down into the rack quickly (don't resist it) and catch it softly by re-entering the dip.**

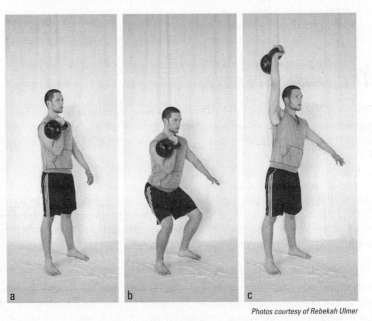

Figure 4-1:
The push press develops upper body power and work capacity.

a   b   c

Photos courtesy of Rebekah Ulmer

The broad jump

WARNING!

If, for any reason, you have issues with jumping — whether in your knees, back, or hips — don't jump! And if you have prominent movement restrictions or dysfunction, especially with your squatting or hinging, then jumping probably isn't the best option for you. Stick with the lower-impact variations until your movement quality improves. If you don't have any issues with jumping and want to keep it that way, then pay very close attention to everything we say in this section.

Jumping is a necessary endeavor in almost all sports and many other recreational activities, so it's important to know how to jump properly. Jumping is a tremendous tool for developing explosive lower body power and improving the rate of force production.

The broad jump is an outward jump, or a distance jump (think jumping across a stream); it's not a vertical leap. The movement that most closely mimics the broad jump is the kettlebell swing because you direct the force outward. In fact, you can think of your kettlebell swing almost like a broad jump where you don't leave the ground. See Book IV, Chapter 1, for details on the kettlebell swing.

Here are the steps to the broad jump:

1. **Assume a shoulder-width stance; initiate the jump by hinging at your hips, just like you would a kettlebell swing, and throwing your arms back behind you (see Figure 4-2a).**

2. **Explode forward (don't forget to swing your arms!) and spring off the balls of your feet; let the sway of your arms guide the movement (see Figure 4-2b).**

   Be sure to synchronize your arm swing with your hip hinge. You'll have to experiment a little with the amount of torso lean in your jump to find that "just right" position.

3. **When you land, make contact first with the balls of your feet (your feet should land slightly apart) and roll gently back onto your heels and into a partial position to disperse the impact (see Figure 4-2c).**

   Whatever you do, *don't* lock your knees because they act as natural shock absorbers.

WARNING!

If anything feels wrong with the broad jump, stop immediately. Pain is your body's way of telling you that you're doing something wrong.

Book IV

Primal Power Moves for a Healthier Body

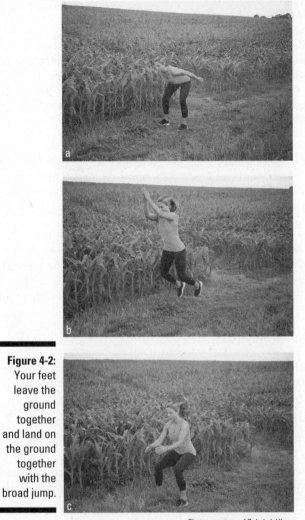

Photos courtesy of Rebekah Ulmer

Figure 4-2:
Your feet
leave the
ground
together
and land on
the ground
together
with the
broad jump.

Intermediate Power Moves

You can expect to spend a considerable amount of time working out the
technical nuances of the two movements in this section: the jerk and the
box jump. These two colossal power and speed exercises are both technical
and delicate. Even the most minor infraction, or incongruence, impedes
performance.

These two movements develop much more than force production. They show you how to move rapidly and how to do so with eloquence. Think of an Olympic lifter who snatches or jerks a barbell; the movement is so fluid it could almost be described as romantic.

The jerk

The jerk was originally intended for a single purpose: to heave the most weight overhead as humanly possible. And although that's still a commendable purpose, the jerk has since taken on many other useful functions. When performed with a lighter load and for higher repetitions, the jerk not only remains a great power developer but also challenges the cardiovascular system.

Kettlebell sport (called *Girevoy sport*), which is much more popular in European culture than in the United States, features high-repetition jerks (often performed for ten minutes at a time) as a competitive event. The power, muscularity, and fluid movement of these competitors are a testament to the effectiveness of high-repetition jerks for building a truly remarkable physique.

With that being said, a kettlebell lends itself perfectly for the movement. But if you don't have a kettlebell handy, a dumbbell will work fine as well.

The jerk starts out as a push press (see the earlier section in this chapter) but adds in a second dip (or quarter squat) where the lifter attempts to "sneak under the weight." The idea here is that by moving your body under the weight, you shorten the distance the weight has to travel; the less distance the weight has to travel, the more weight you should be able to lift. Makes sense, right?

Follow these steps to do the jerk:

1. **Clean the weight up into the rack position and assume a shoulder-width stance. Start the jerk the same way you would a push press, by taking a shallow dip (see Figure 4-3a).**

   Don't take long to get into the dip. Think "quick down, quick up," like a spring!

2. **Explode out of the dip exactly how you would a push press. As the weight is accelerating upward, shoot your hips back and land your weight back onto your heels (see Figure 4-3b), coming into a quarter squat position to "sneak under the weight" and catching the weight overhead in a full lockout position (see Figure 4-3c).**

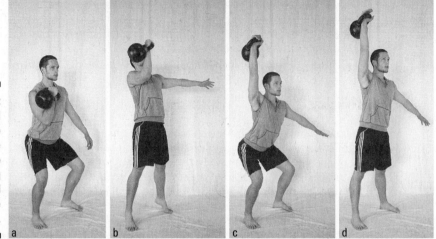

Photos courtesy of Rebekah Ulmer

Figure 4-3:
You need patience to learn the jerk. Keep practicing and you'll find the groove.

It's okay if your heels leave the ground during the upward portion of the jerk, but they should be planted when you shoot your hips back to catch the weight.

3. **Stand up out of the quarter squat with the weight locked out overhead to complete the repetition (see Figure 4-3d). Let the weight fall quickly back into the rack position (catch it softly with a dip if you need to) and repeat.**

The box jump

The box jump takes some of the impact out of jumping because you're landing on an elevated surface. So then why is the box jump in the intermediate section and the broad jump in the beginner section, you ask? Because you need to develop proper landing mechanics before anything else, and the broad jump is a great way to do that.

Although the box jump is a bit more forgiving than the broad jump, it's equally challenging and offers its own unique benefits. For one, the box jump helps you develop *stand-still explosiveness* — the ability to rapidly "turn it on." Like the broad jump, the box jump helps you increase your natural rate of force production. The box jump is more of a vertical leap, whereas the broad jump is horizontal. Simply put, you jump *up* with the box jump, and you jump *out* with the broad jump. The projection of force with the box jump is more like the snatch, while the broad jump is more like the swing.

TIP

When working the box jump, keep the box you're using at or under 36 inches. Higher box jumps ultimately become more of a function of hip mobility than actual explosiveness, and the marginal benefits to be had from leaping to such heights don't merit the additional risks.

The following steps walk you through the box jump:

1. **Set up slightly behind the box or surface you're leaping onto, and assume your natural jumping stance. Initiate the jump by squatting slightly downward, taking a shallow dip (see Figure 4-4a).**

   Here's one way the movement differs from the broad jump. When leaping upward, your takeoff comes out of something more like a shallow dip than a hinge.

2. **Explode out of the dip, leaping up onto the box (see Figure 4-4b).**

   The goal is to stick the landing softly, like a cat, with some knee bend and both feet landing simultaneously. Essentially, you should land in almost the exact same position you took off from. If you're landing in a very deep squat, you're probably using too high of a box.

3. **Step — don't jump — down from the box.**

   Jumping down from the box has little benefit and can cause injury.

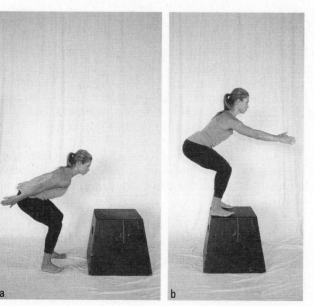

Figure 4-4: Use a box under 36 inches when performing the box jump.

a   b

Photos courtesy of Rebekah Ulmer

Advanced Power Moves

In this section, you discover the double jerk and the double snatch. Both of these movements ultimately land the weight in the same overhead position as the jerk or military press, but each of them takes a distinctly different method of getting it there.

What's great about these double techniques is that they're nearly identical to their single technique counterparts, save a few minor tweaks here and there. All you really need to do is add more power. So if you master techniques in progression of difficulty/power, you should be able to pick up these advanced movements more quickly and easily. That said, don't hesitate to review the single techniques before jumping into the advanced moves in this section.

For as explosive as the double jerk and double snatch are, they're both relatively low impact. Neither movement — which is best performed with either a set of kettlebells or dumbbells, by the way — has you leaving the ground. So although these movements are advanced, chances are they're still viable options to develop power for those who haven't been cleared for high-impact exercises.

The double jerk

The double jerk basically involves cleaning two weights up into the rack position and then blasting them up overhead. Like the jerk, which you find earlier in this chapter, the double jerk may serve multiple purposes. You can use it for pure power and strength generation (lifting the most possible weight overhead), or you can use it for strength endurance and metabolic purposes (lifting weight overhead for multiple repetitions).

What makes the double jerk so special is that when you combine it with the clean (which you'll do most of the time), it works just about every single pushing and pulling muscle in the entire body. It's as comprehensive as an exercise can possibly get.

When you perform the jerk consecutively (without cleaning the weight between each repetition), it's referred to as *short-cycle*. When you perform a clean between each repetition of the jerk, it's referred to as *long-cycle*.

Here's how to do the double jerk:

1. **Clean two kettlebells or dumbbells up into the rack position (see Figure 4-5a) and initiate the double jerk the same way you would the single jerk by taking a shallow dip (see earlier section and check out Figure 4-5b).**

   Don't waste any more time down in the dip than you have to. The more time you spend in the dip, the more fatigued your legs will become, and the less power you'll have.

2. **Explode out of the dip, launching the bells upward.**

   As you explode out of the dip, think "jump the weight up."

3. **As the weight soars upward, shoot your hips back to "sneak under it," achieving a full lockout overhead and landing in a quarter squat position (see Figure 4-5c).**

   Be explosive when shooting your hips back into the quarter squat and shift the majority of your weight onto your heels.

4. **Stand up out of the quarter squat while keeping the weight locked out overhead to complete the movement, as shown in Figure 4-5d.**

5. **Rise up onto your tippy toes to meet the weight halfway as you let it drop back down into the rack position.**

   You may want to further cushion the impact by landing again in a shallow dip.

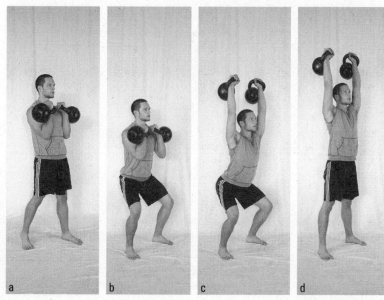

Figure 4-5:
The double jerk works multiple pushing and pulling muscles.

a   b   c   d

Photos courtesy of Rebekah Ulmer

The double snatch

The double snatch is identical to the single snatch with the exception of stance width (just wide enough to accommodate the weight).

Simply put, the double snatch is a power bomb. You rip the weight off the ground, swing it between your legs, and explode it up overhead in one smooth, uninterrupted fashion. Completing this movement is a commendable effort to say the least.

The double snatch develops hip drive (an athlete's engine) like nothing before it. Except for high-level Olympic lifting, the double snatch is perhaps the ultimate exercise for developing explosive power. It's quite a heinous conditioning tool as well. Think you're ready to give it a go? Follow these steps:

1. **Set up precisely how you would for a kettlebell swing (see Book IV, Chapter 1) with a stance just wide enough to accommodate both weights (either two kettlebells or two dumbbells).**

2. **Start with a forceful hike back.**

   This movement isn't a dead snatch, where you rip the weight straight from the ground, so be sure to start each rep with a strong hike back.

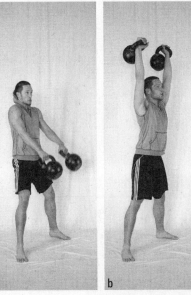

Figure 4-6: The hips power the double snatch entirely; the arms simply guide the weights where they need to go.

a   b

Photos courtesy of Rebekah Ulmer

3. Explode out of the hinge, standing up as quickly as possible (think "jump," but keep your heels on the ground).

4. Let your elbows bend slightly to guide the path of the weight upward, but don't let the weight arc out too wildly (see Figure 4-6a).

5. As the bells approach eye level, begin to "punch through" into the overhead lockout position (see Figure 4-6b). Bring the weights back down into the rack position before throwing them into another backswing and repeating the movement.

Chapter 5

Beyond Strength Training and Cardio to Metabolic Conditioning

In This Chapter

▶ Finding good reasons to pick up heavy things

▶ Preventing weight gain while building strength

▶ Avoiding an excess of cardio training

▶ Putting together a smart and effective exercise program

▶ Discovering an efficient way to burn fat and improve fitness

▶ Using combinations of exercises to get great physical gains

Most exercise programs fail because they try to accomplish everything and, by doing so, accomplish nothing. People have the most success when they focus intently on the pursuit of a major goal and put all other minor goals in maintenance mode.

For example, if muscle gain is your goal, pursue muscle gain. Don't attempt to pursue both muscle gain and fat loss at the same time because they are, to a degree, mutually exclusive goals (one requires calorie surplus; the other, a deficit) and will get you nowhere when you chase them simultaneously. Instead, put fat loss on maintenance — that is, keep your body fat levels where they are — while putting on muscle. After you reach your muscle-building goals and are willing to put that into maintenance mode, then you're in a better condition to pursue fat loss.

REMEMBER

Make strength a priority. No matter what your goals are — whether they be fat loss, muscle gain, or athletic enhancement — strength assists in all endeavors.

This chapter explains why many fitness programs fail to get you the results you want and introduces some key concepts that are necessary in any successful exercise program. It also looks at common questions or concerns when it comes to exercise — whether you're training for strength or fat loss — such as whether you're doing too little or too much and fears about "bulking up."

Paleo fitness is about doing the least amount of work you need to do to get the job done, but that work won't be easy. To be frank, this chapter discusses what may very well be the most intense form of exercise you've ever experienced.

Heinous, diabolical, merciless, inhumane, and monstrous are just a few of the adjectives used to describe *metabolic conditioning* — the practice of taxing multiple muscle groups and energy systems simultaneously. Get ready to add your own adjectives as you dive into metabolic conditioning in this chapter.

Introducing Primal Strength Training

Plainly, this chapter is about making you strong(er). This section demystifies the domain of strength training and trots out the primal strength-training philosophy, which may be couched conveniently in the following sentence: To get strong, lift heavy.

You find out what *heavy* means shortly, but for now, just know that rarely is it anything pink or rubbery. Don't let this intimidate you. Heavy lifting is by no means a dangerous endeavor — assuming you're a healthy individual — unless you go about it unwisely. As with anything else, proper execution is key, which is why Chapters 1 through 4 in Book IV drive proper form into your head like railway spikes.

The following sections outline the different types of strength training, give you the benefits of following the primal strength-training approach, and explain how heavy is heavy enough.

Defining strength training

Strength comes in many forms and extends far beyond the realm of hoisting weight overhead. Although working against resistance is a true test and demonstration of strength, strength is much more than that and serves a much greater purpose than simply allowing you to "lift weights."

Here are a few of the many types of strength:

- ✔ **Limit** or **absolute strength** measures the most force you can exert for a single repetition. A one-rep maximum dead lift is an example of limit strength.

- ✔ **Strength endurance** is your ability to exert a submaximal force over a prolonged period of time. An example of strength endurance is performing push-ups for 30 to 60 seconds.

- ✔ **Power** is your ability to exert force rapidly, such as in the jerk or the snatch (see Book IV, Chapter 4).

You need to know the difference between these strength qualities. You also need to understand that increasing your limit strength will almost invariably increase your strength endurance and power output as well.

The cave man likely didn't have any sort of planned heavy lifting routine, but he probably engaged in some heavy lifting almost every day. And that's what sets apart the primal strength-training approach from most others. Following the primal strength approach, you do a little heavy lifting *almost* every day. That's just enough to get the job done, not a smidgen more.

Strength is cumulative. Strength is more a function of volume (the total amount of work you perform) rather than a function of density (how much work you perform in a fixed period of time, such as a day, an hour, or a set). Therefore, you'll likely get just as strong — if not the teensiest bit stronger — by performing ten reps a day spread out over seven days than by performing 70 reps all in one day.

Acknowledging the benefits of lifting heavy things

No endeavor is more profitable to the body than the effort of lifting heavy things. We just can't overstate this. And make no mistake about it: Strength training *is* lifting heavy things. Just because you're lifting weights doesn't necessarily mean you're strength training. In fact, you really don't need any weights to train strength, as you find out through the challenging bodyweight exercises found in Book IV, Chapters 1 and 2.

Book IV

Primal Power Moves for a Healthier Body

Aside from the more obvious benefits of looking good with your clothes off and enhanced athletic performance, strength training may also help prevent, reverse, or ward off the symptoms of the following malaises:

- Arthritis
- Back problems
- Depression
- Diabetes
- Obesity
- Osteoporosis

Being strong fixes just about everything. If you struggle with weight issues, getting stronger will help you lean out. If your athletic performance isn't quite where you want it to be, getting stronger will certainly help you with that, too. And if you suffer frequently from injuries, additional strength will amplify your resilience.

Determining how heavy is heavy enough

To get strong, you have to lift heavy, but what exactly is *heavy?* Well, unfortunately, no definite number or weight can define heavy, because *heavy* is a relative term. What may be heavy to you may not be heavy to someone else, such as a gymnast or power lifter.

You have to define your own definition of heavy, and that definition will change as you grow stronger and stronger. The goal, therefore, should always be to make your current heavy light.

To answer the question "what is heavy?" as simply as possible, if you can lift something for more than five repetitions, it's not heavy. So you could say that a "heavy" weight is any weight that you can move one to five times, but no more than that. If you go over five reps throughout any of the strength exercises, then you're training something other than limit strength. For example, the push-up may start out as a heavy strength effort, but as you become proficient at it and can perform multiple repetitions, it becomes a strength endurance effort.

The lighter the weight, the more reps you add, and the more you start venturing into strength endurance training.

Gaining Strength Without Gaining Weight

This section could also be called "Gaining Strength *with the Option of* Gaining Weight," because for those of you who want to add some muscle mass, your ability to do so increases in direct proportion to your absolute strength. To say it another way, the stronger you are, the more potential you have to add muscle mass.

The reverse is also true to a large extent; that is, the stronger you are, the more potential you have for total body leanness. Either way, it pays to be strong.

The key to gaining strength isn't found in gaining muscle, although the key to gaining muscle is found in gaining strength. Really, the key to gaining strength is found in gaining movement efficiency, or to put it more succinctly, fine-tuning your nervous system.

Your nervous system is your operations manager; it dictates how hard your muscles are allowed to tense. And tension is strength, loosely speaking. So the harder you can tense a muscle, the more strength you can display.

The following sections explore how to build tension, strength, and relaxation into your normal routine to get the results you want.

Tensing (and relaxing) muscles to develop strength

There are really only two ways to go about generating more tension. The first is to lift more weight. The second is to lift the same weight faster. Both of these options are viable for gaining strength. But there's more to it than that.

The body will allow only so much tension to be generated at any given time. This is a safety mechanism, to be sure, designed mostly to protect your joints. But, unfortunately, this mechanism typically kicks in far too soon — long before you're in any real danger of harming yourself from tensing too hard. So you have to teach the nervous system that it's okay to generate more tension, to push back the tension threshold. That is strength.

Flexibility is achieved in much the same way, but instead of teaching the nervous system that it's okay to tense up, you must teach the nervous system that it's okay to relax. And it's between these two spectrums (tension and relaxation) that all human movement lies. It's important to practice both because too much of either one (tension or relaxation) isn't a desirable thing. Ideally, you want to be tense only when you have to be.

While tension is strength, relaxation is speed. Most athletic movements, such as a punch or a jump, are a blend of tension and relaxation.

Combining heavy weight and low reps

The secret to building strength is heavy weight and low reps. If you can work high reps, then the weight you're using isn't heavy enough. Simple as that. You pick a lift — any lift you want — then find a weight you can lift for no more than five repetitions at a time, and then you work multiple sets, resting as much as you need to between each set.

So here's the strength equation you should use to focus your workouts:

$$\text{Strength} = \text{Heavy weight} + \text{Low reps} + \text{Multiple sets}$$

- ✔ *Heavy weight* is relative to you, but you shouldn't be able to lift it for more than five repetitions.
- ✔ A *low rep* range indicates sets of five repetitions or less.
- ✔ *Multiple sets* may be anywhere from 2 to 12 sets, depending on the structure of the program.

This formula is at the heart of primal fitness programs, and with a solid understanding of this equation, you can design your own strength program. But don't worry about that, because this book has you covered.

Deciding on your training frequency

Training frequency answers the question, "How often should I train?" The answer is, if you want to get stronger, train pretty often.

Strength is acquired through practice, so wouldn't it make sense to practice as often as possible? Well, sort of, but not entirely. The human body needs rest. It needs time to recover and to adapt. Rest is done outside of the gym, so more isn't always better in this regard.

Furthermore, you must keep in mind the Paleo fitness principle of doing the absolute least amount to reach your goals. So what's the least amount of practice you need to hit your strength goals? The answer varies for each individual, but you'll likely need somewhere between three and five days a week of strength-training practice.

If you're new to weight lifting, gains will come quickly, and you may be able to get away with a little more. If you're a veteran, then you'll likely need more recovery time to get to the next level and would probably do better with less. Either way, the goal should be to practice as much as you have to but as little as you need to.

Working the best strength-building exercises

Are some exercises better suited for building total body strength than others? Most likely, yes. Typically, the bigger the movement, the higher the strength return.

For example, the squat is often hailed as the king of all strength-building exercises, with the dead lift trailing close behind. Both of these movements allow for a tremendous amount of stress (weight) to be put on the system. No other lift allows you to move as much weight as the squat or dead lift.

A classic starter strength-building program may typically be comprised of the following lifts:

- ✔ Dead lift
- ✔ Squat
- ✔ Bench press
- ✔ Pull-up
- ✔ Loaded carry

This list is fairly simple but somewhat lacking. Humans are meant to move in all ways, so don't think you should restrict your strength training to just these five exercises. In fact, you don't even have to worry about selecting the best strength-training exercises because this book has done it for you. All the movements in Book IV, Chapters 1–4, are the choicest selection of total body strength-building exercises. They're the movements that offer the biggest bang for your buck (the vital few). There's nothing superfluous.

But constructing a good exercise program is a lot like building a delicious recipe. The ingredients (exercises) are only part of what makes it successful. The success of a recipe depends largely on the ordering, the pairing, and the preparation of the ingredients. So, too, does the success of an exercise program depend on how you mix, match, and serve the exercises. An exercise program can be overdone and collapse in on itself like an overcooked soufflé, or it can be underdone and fall flat as a biscuit. It's a delicate art.

But you need not concern yourself with any of that, really, because the recipes are in Book IV, Chapter 6. All you need do is follow them and make sure you master the form.

Moving Past Chronic Cardio Syndrome

Chronic cardio is the nefarious condition of overtraining brought about by an unjustified abundance of steady-state cardiovascular activities. The most common culprit is the treadmill. This condition is communicable, as you can see for yourself should you ever feel the need to walk into a big-box gym again. The treadmills are always *occupado,* swarmed like Porta-potties at a tailgate, but for no really good reason.

Steady-state cardiovascular efforts, such as trudging for hours at a time on a treadmill, offer very poor metabolic return. To put it as delicately as possible, it's just not worth your time, and it's not a coincidence that those who lift weights and engage in short, intense bouts of exercise almost always look and perform better than those who commit themselves solely to the treadmill, elliptical, or bicycle.

It's been proven again and again in scientific circles that short bouts of intense exercise are far more effective for fat loss and overall vitality than long bouts of moderate-intensity exercise have ever been. So throw out the idea that you need to run on a treadmill to lose weight. It's a garbage idea and a wholly ineffective way to go about weight loss and cardiovascular conditioning. The cave man never did this type of exercise and neither should you.

Excessive moderate- to high-intensity cardiovascular activities — often referred to as *steady-state cardio* — creates a *hormonal nightmare* — the result of chronically elevated cortisol levels (or natural stress hormone) that may lead to a plethora of ailments linked to overtraining, such as poor sleep quality, mood swings, loss of libido, joint problems, and injury.

In the following sections, you dig a little deeper into the side effects of excessive cardio and explore ways you can use cardio to your benefit, alongside strength training.

Facing the little-known drawbacks of excessive cardio

Excessive steady-state cardio — or excessive moderate-intensity exercise, such as running on a treadmill — is at best a shoddy investment of time that could be better spent lifting heavy things or engaging in shorter, more intense forms of exercise (such as metabolic conditioning). At worst (and more likely), it's an investment in your destruction!

Here are some of the drawbacks of excessive cardio:

✔ Chronic levels of inflammation

✔ Decreased ability to recover

✔ Increased free radical production (oxidative damage)

✔ Increased likelihood of injury

✔ Joint problems

✔ Persistently elevated levels of cortisol (stress hormone)

Chances are the definition of *excessive* is probably less than you think. An hour or two of steady-state cardio a day is often more than enough to trigger the harmful conditions of chronic cardio. Sometimes it takes even less than that.

Really, all of this should come with a great sigh of relief, because who really enjoys long, trudging runs on the treadmill anyway? Very few.

Don't take all this wrong: A light, springy jog every now and then is all very well and good. Just do it outdoors and enjoy it! Moderate-intensity exercise is best performed in as relaxed a state as possible. But rarely do you see people on the treadmill in this state. What takes form on the treadmill can hardly be described as proper running form; it's more of a continuously falling motion. The mechanics are heavily distorted, and force isn't properly transmitted. This form wreaks havoc on the joints, so it's no wonder joint pain and other ailments, such as shin splints, are so prevalent among those who run on a treadmill.

Doing what you love

The best recommendation for light- to moderate-intensity cardiovascular efforts is simply to do what you love, so long as the activity is relatively light and joyful. If you truly love to run, then run. Just monitor for the signs of chronic cardio, and scale back as needed. Again, take your running outdoors and spend plenty of time on mastering proper running mechanics.

If you like basketball, play basketball; if tennis is more your thing, then tennis it is! Maybe you enjoy Frisbee, which is great because Frisbee is a perfect low-intensity cardiovascular activity. And if you like to cycle, then go cycle (again, just don't overdo it).

The possibilities here are endless, and you're encouraged to experiment, change it up, and try new things. The mind and body thrive on variety (to an extent). And when you begin something new, the excitement of developing new skills often helps motivate you and gets you moving when you otherwise wouldn't. So if you've never tried dancing before, well, now's your chance!

Hiking is a marvelous endeavor, as well as a potent fat burner. Fasted hiking — such as hiking first thing in the morning — is a sneaky little way to shed stubborn body fat. (See the next section for more on fasting.) Hiking is also a relaxing endeavor, offering a sense of tranquility.

Getting more out of your cardio with fasting

Your body is naturally in a fat-burning state when you wake up, so why not take advantage of this and perform your low-intensity exercise first thing in the morning, right before breakfast!

Even just a brisk, 20-minute walk in a fasted state can yield some seriously impressive fat-loss results, especially when combined with all the other strategies outlined in this book. And don't worry about losing your precious muscle; low-intensity cardiovascular training first thing in the morning, while fasted, selectively destroys body fat, leaving your lean muscle practically untouched. Just be sure to keep the intensity low enough — that is, at a level of exertion where you can comfortably hold a conversation.

When performed in a fasted state, all the positive effects of exercise are amplified (both low-intensity and high-intensity). This combination is potent not only for fat loss but also brain function, cellular cleansing, and immune support. Fasting and exercise are perhaps nature's ultimate tonic for longevity.

While fasted cardio is a good option for most people, it's not always the best option for people with blood sugar regulation issues or diabetes. You should never feel faint, light-headed, or like you're going to pass out while doing fasted exercise. If you do, stop immediately.

Developing the Recipe for a Good Exercise Program

A good exercise program comes from a well-developed recipe. As long as you understand the ingredients needed for the recipe, you can produce, with a fair amount of consistency, an exercise program that produces predictable and repeatable results.

A fitness program is like a recipe in more than one way. For example, even a cook with very little experience can prepare a decent dish as long as he accurately follows a recipe. And so, too, can a person with very little fitness experience have great results as long as he accurately follows a well-thought-out program.

To construct a successful exercise program, you need ingredients that are simple, sensible, and reasonable. You find out about these ingredients in the following sections.

Simple

Simplicity is the key ingredient. The secret to a good exercise program is to strip it down to the fundamentals and leave it at that. The more clutter an exercise program accumulates, the less potent it becomes. Don't let your exercise program look like a teenager's bedroom. Keep it clean.

A good exercise program is neat, tidy, and organized. It's uncluttered. It's not busy solely for the sake of being busy. It focuses on the vital few efforts that produce the biggest results. It ignores the trivial things.

Simplicity also aids in sanity. A cluttered exercise program can feel, and often is, overwhelming, which is no doubt why many people quit. But a simple exercise program is efficient and tidy. It includes only the exercises that allow you to derive the greatest benefit (depending on your goals) and that require the least amount of time necessary for you to reach those goals.

An exercise program improves in direct proportion to the number of things you can keep out of it that don't need to be there.

Sensible

Sensible means the program is designed to directly assist you in hitting your goals. It makes sense. It's logical. It has progressions, and, if necessary, regressions.

If your goal is to gain strength, the exercise program should provide a clear, uncluttered path toward that goal. A series of proven progressions should take you from where you are to where you want to be in the quickest time possible.

Many fitness programs aren't designed with an end goal in mind and are too often a hodgepodge of various exercises and modalities, strung together with no apparent rhyme or reason — and so you wind up with a sort of tapioca.

An exercise program shouldn't have in it variety solely for the sake of having variety, any more than it should be busy solely for the sake of being busy. It should, instead, feature the least number of components necessary to get you to your goals. That's efficiency. That's sensibility.

Reasonable

Reasonable means it's something you can handle, especially in the long term. Too many programs burn you out too quickly because they're unsustainable.

The popularity of "insane" fitness programs is surging. Although the idea of working out until you're blue in the face may sound enticing, it's not necessarily such a wise idea, nor is it necessary.

Intense exercise is best served in small to moderate doses. Cellular recovery happens on its own accord and can't be rushed. Not naturally, at least. When you put too much stress on the system for too long — when recovery can't keep up with stress — then you suffer burnout, overtraining, and failure. The problem with unreasonable exercise programs is that although they may work in the short term, they do just as much, if not more, harm than good in the long run due to their unsustainable and insensible practices that put too much strain on both the body and the mind.

You must approach a fitness program thinking of the long term. Doing so isn't such an easy task, because people want results, and they want them quickly. But take a step back before beginning any fitness program and honestly ask yourself, "Do I see myself doing this program six months from now? A year? Ten years?" If the answer to any of these questions is no, it's time to pause and reconsider what you're doing.

Introducing Metabolic Conditioning

The human body relies on a substance known as ATP (adenosine triphosphate) to supply energy, commonly referred to as the body's "energy currency." The human body can use carbohydrates, fats, and protein to supply itself with this energy currency. *Metabolic conditioning* is any form of exercise aimed to increase your body's efficiency for storing and delivering energy (ATP).

To further understand this process, you must also know that three energy systems, or *metabolic pathways,* in the human body supply ATP:

- **Phosphagen:** The phosphagen energy system fuels the high-intensity and shortest-lived bouts of movement (typically ten seconds or less), such as the swinging of a baseball bat, a jump over a creek, or the first couple of seconds of a sprint. This system is *anaerobic,* meaning it doesn't require oxygen to fuel metabolism.

- **Glycolytic:** The glycolytic pathway is the traditional carb pathway that fuels moderately intense and relatively short-lived exercise (lasting only a few minutes). It takes over after the phosphagen system. Also, the conversion of carbs into ATP results in the production of lactate, which leads to that burning sensation in your muscles. This system is also anaerobic.

- **Oxidative:** The oxidative energy system is the primary endurance system that supports long-term, low-intensity forms of exercise, such as jogging, hiking, and so on. This system is *aerobic,* meaning it uses oxygen to fuel metabolism.

In short, when you increase the efficiency of the various metabolic pathways, you increase your overall work capacity, which in turn leads to the ability to perform a broad range of physical tasks with general competency.

The body responds to stress by becoming more efficient. Strength is a form of efficiency and so is conditioning.

You can use a number of fitness methods for metabolic conditioning. As long as the multiple pathways are all appropriately taxed, you'll achieve the desired effect. A few of the more common approaches include interval training, cross-training, and circuit training. Although these approaches are all very well and good, we prefer an entirely different method altogether. You can explore this method in the section "Turbocharging Fat Loss with Complexes," later in this chapter.

Metabolic conditioning, commonly referred to as *metcon,* has been around formally since the 1970s. The name was originally coined by Arthur Jones

Book IV

Primal Power Moves for a Healthier Body

(the inventor of the Nautilus), who wrote about the amazing benefits of shortening the rest between exercises performed in a circuit (back to back). The following sections go into detail about those benefits and explain why metabolic conditioning is far more effective than traditional cardio for burning fat and building muscle.

Discovering the benefits of metabolic conditioning

Work capacity is your ability to produce and maintain work of various intensities and durations. It's a desirable trait for any type of athlete because when your sport-specific skills match your opponent's, the sheer ability to outwork your opponent often leads to victory.

And because the direct result of metabolic conditioning is an increase in work capacity, it can literally help you defeat your opponents. Through metabolic conditioning, you'll be able to go harder, go farther, and go longer. Now *that* is a competitive advantage. Moreover, short and intense metcon sessions have a profoundly positive hormonal impact, surging the production of natural growth hormone (that's a good thing).

Too much intense exercise is *not* a good thing, though. In fact, almost all the positive hormonal benefits of intense exercise may be reversed if you push it for too long or too often. In this case, less truly is more.

The miraculous fat-loss effects brought about by metabolic conditioning are likely to interest you the most. Nothing cuts through fat quicker than short, intense metabolic conditioning sessions. And here's why: Short, intense metcon workouts create a huge oxygen debt, also known as *exercise post oxygen consumption* (EPOC) or, informally, the *after-burn effect*. EPOC brings about an elevated and prolonged consumption of fuel — that fuel being calories. It also results in the breakdown of fatty acids into the bloodstream, where, if your body takes proper advantage of it (see the section "Getting results in just 15 minutes"), the fatty acids may then be oxidized (burned off).

So metabolic conditioning results not only in a long-term calorie burn — that is, your metabolism may stay elevated for up to 48 hours post workout, not something you can get through traditional cardiovascular efforts! — but also in the immediate breakdown of stored body fat. In this vulnerable state, fat burning may be swiftly executed by following up your short and intense metcon sessions with low-intensity cardiovascular efforts.

Switching on your fat-burning furnace

If there's an ultimate exercise formula for fat loss, here it is:

High-intensity metabolic conditioning (short duration) + Low-intensity cardiovascular efforts (moderate to long duration)

The simplest example of this combination is to pair 15 minutes of sprints (a high-intensity form of metabolic work) with 30 to 60 minutes of walking (a low-intensity cardiovascular activity). The goal is to use the power of high-intensity metcon work to drive the fatty acids into the bloodstream and then switch over to the low-intensity cardiovascular efforts to oxidize (burn off) those fatty acids.

Metabolic conditioning alone is primarily an anaerobic endeavor (without oxygen) and doesn't rely heavily on fatty acids for fuel as much as low-intensity aerobics do. The down side to just working aerobics, however, is that you miss out on all the positive hormonal benefits of high-intensity work as well as the huge caloric after-burn. When you combine these efforts — the high and the low — you're truly able to switch on your natural fat-burning furnace.

Instead of eating after a high-intensity workout, go for a brisk 20-minute walk, and then eat. This little tweak can really make a difference in your fat-loss results.

Getting results in just 15 minutes

When you're cooking something, say, a piece of chicken, you typically cook it only until it's done, right? You don't continue to cook it after it's done, because then it's overdone, and that's bad.

You need to approach exercise the very same way. You want to apply just the right amount you need to get the job done and no more. You can easily overdo exercise with metabolic conditioning. And in this case, less is better.

In other words, metabolic conditioning imparts a considerable amount of stress on the system; therefore, you must apply it judiciously. So how much do you need exactly? Well, the answer is, as any good coach will tell you, it depends. And mostly it depends on what you want to achieve.

You can typically achieve the best results with as little as 15 minutes of metabolic conditioning! Yes, believe it or not, this stuff is so potent that 15 minutes is usually the most you'll ever need at any one time.

Book IV

Primal Power Moves for a Healthier Body

A good exercise program shouldn't be designed to destroy you and leave you feeling crushed, dismantled, or obliterated. A good exercise program should challenge you but leave you feeling charged, confident, and successful. So even if you feel like you can do a lot more, rarely does that mean you should.

Turbocharging Fat Loss with Complexes

Complexes are a series of exercises you perform successively — flowing from exercise to exercise with little to no rest in between. Complexes are different from circuit training because you typically perform them with a single modality, such as a barbell, dumbbells, a sandbag, your own body weight, or a set of kettlebells.

Complex design is a delicate art. It must be constructed in such a way that it allows you to cycle through various muscle groups and energy systems. This way, the system as a whole may be kept under a prolonged period of stress, and no one muscle group is fatigued to the point of failure.

Like most other forms of metabolic conditioning, complexes combine moderate to heavy strength efforts with elevated cardiovascular stress. Complexes keep the kidneys, the heart, and the lungs working hard while stressing various muscle groups and doing so in a super time-efficient manner — very rarely will a complex take more than three minutes to complete.

To keep the body adapting, you'll do some complexes for time and some for reps. You'll do some heavy complexes and some light. You'll do some long complexes and some short. When you get into the primal programs in Book IV, Chapter 6, you'll quickly see that there's no shortage of complexes to choose from to keep your metabolic conditioning varied and exciting.

Complexes are best performed with either your own body weight or with kettlebells because they both allow for "flow." Dumbbells are clunky and sometimes hard to handle with the ballistic movements, such as swings, cleans, and snatches, and barbells are far too large, impossible to swing between the legs, and bring with them the added inconvenience of having to load and unload weight plates. However, you *can* do complex work with barbells or dumbbells. And you can adapt any complex throughout this book to dumbbells or barbells, but the top pick remains kettlebells.

Although barbell complexes are possible and can be quite effective, we don't recommend starting out with them. The barbell is a large instrument and commands respect. Poor form with a barbell isn't as easily forgiven as poor form with your own body weight — and the punishments are far more severe.

In the following sections, you find out how to put together beginner complexes that work for you, using just your body weight or stepping it up with a kettlebell.

Starting with basic bodyweight complexes

Think for a moment what a bodyweight complex may look like. A complex combines strength and cardiovascular efforts, taxing multiple muscle groups and various energy systems. And a complex combines two or more exercises into a series.

Start by taking a minimalistic approach: What two exercises can you combine to form a bodyweight complex? The answer is limitless. Some combinations may be more worthwhile than others, for sure, but the possibilities are limited only by your imagination.

A simple pairing of push-ups and pull-ups — which you'll see more than occasionally in the primal exercise programs in Book IV, Chapter 6 — is a fantastic "starter" complex. Although not the most strenuous complex ever devised, a pairing of five to ten push-ups with five to ten pull-ups will impose a metabolic demand, even more so when you work in the higher repetition range.

Now, what if you added a set of bodyweight squats in there, making the complex five push-ups, five squats, and five pull-ups performed in a row? In this complex, you switch from upper body to lower body and then back to upper body — the prolonged stress of this complex will quickly elevate your heart rate.

Could you add in another five squats after the pull-ups to round out the work ratio between upper body and lower body? Certainly! Or better yet, you could add lunges instead or any other lower body exercise. The complex then becomes five push-ups, five squats, five pull-ups, and ten lunges (five for each leg). Go ahead and give this complex a try. A taxing effort, is it not?

As you can see, complexes are perhaps the ultimate conditioning tool because they allow you to perform an incredible amount of work in a very short time. You find a number of ways to construct an effective complex in Book IV, Chapter 6.

Book IV

Primal Power Moves for a Healthier Body

The following lists provide a couple of example bodyweight complexes, using six simple exercises: push-ups, pull-ups (perform rows if you're not able to do a pull-up), planks, squats, lunges, and V-ups. These workouts are a shallow sampling of bodyweight complexes but should give you an even greater idea of the true power of complexes.

When training a complex, never go to failure. If at any time your form starts to deteriorate, take a break and start up again when you can resume with good form.

Here's the first example of a beginner bodyweight complex. (***Note:*** When a time is given for an exercise, perform as many reps as possible with good form within that time.)

- Exercise 1: Plank for 15 seconds (see Book IV, Chapter 3)
- Exercise 2: Squats for 15 seconds (see Book IV, Chapter 1)
- Exercise 3: Plank for 15 seconds
- Exercise 4: Push-ups for 15 seconds (see Book IV, Chapter 2)
- Exercise 5: Plank for 15 seconds
- Exercise 6: Mountain climber for 15 seconds

    Note: A mountain climber is a plank where you drive your knees one at a time up to your chest as quickly as you can (see Figure 5-1).

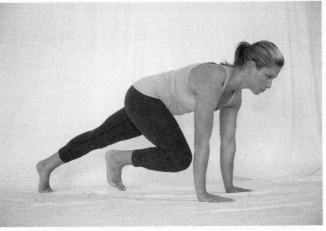

Figure 5-1:
The mountain climber.

Photo courtesy of Rebekah Ulmer

The following beginner bodyweight complex combines exercises for time and some for reps:

- Exercise 1: Five push-ups
- Exercise 2: Plank for 15 seconds
- Exercise 3: Five pull-ups (see Book IV, Chapter 2)
- Exercise 4: V-ups for 15 seconds (see Book IV, Chapter 3)
- Exercise 5: Five bodyweight squats (see Book IV, Chapter 1)
- Exercise 6: Plank for 15 seconds
- Exercise 7: Ten lunges (five reps each leg; see Book IV, Chapter 1)
- Exercise 8: V-ups for 15 seconds

Taking it up a notch with kettlebell complexes

The best device for complex work, from the power moves to the heavy strength efforts, is the kettlebell, hands down. The kettlebell allows for "flow" — that is, seamless execution, the ability to hop from exercise to exercise without any hiccups, stumbling, or delay. The compact design of the kettlebell also allows you to swing it between your legs with great ease.

Even though you can select a number of tools to get the same job done, you should always strive to choose the best tool for the job. When it comes to complexes, the kettlebell is king. However, you can adapt any complex to dumbbells or barbells if that's all you have.

Kettlebell complexes typically combine a variety of power movements, such as swings, cleans, snatches, and jerks, and grinding strength movements, such as squats, presses, lunges, and loaded carries. Because the key to metabolic conditioning is found in inefficiency — meaning, variety is your friend — you want to keep the body guessing, or keep it responding to different forms of stress.

The following lists provide a few workouts to play around with. For these complexes, men should use one 16- to 24-kilogram kettlebell and women should use one 8- to 12-kilogram kettlebell.

Book IV

Primal Power Moves for a Healthier Body

Here's a look at a beginner kettlebell complex:

- Exercise 1: Two two-arm swings (see Book IV, Chapter 1)
- Exercise 2: One goblet squat (see Book IV, Chapter 1)
- Exercise 3: Four two-arm swings
- Exercise 4: Two goblet squats
- Exercise 5: Six two-arm swings
- Exercise 6: Three goblet squats
- Exercise 7: Eight two-arm swings
- Exercise 8: Four goblet squats
- Exercise 9: Ten two-arm swings
- Exercise 10: Five goblet squats

For the next beginner kettlebell complex, perform the complex entirely on your right side first and then switch and repeat immediately on your left:

- Exercise 1: Five one-arm swings (see Book IV, Chapter 1)
- Exercise 2: Five one-arm cleans (see Book IV, Chapter 1)
- Exercise 3: Five one-arm military presses (see Book IV, Chapter 2)
- Exercise 4: Five reverse lunges (see Book IV, Chapter 1)

The next beginner kettlebell complex adds in the *thruster:* Do a squat and then use the momentum out of the squat to go into a press (see Figure 5-2). And, no, using the momentum from the squat here isn't cheating, at least not for metabolic purposes.

- Exercise 1: Two two-arm swings (see Book IV, Chapter 1)
- Exercise 2: Two thrusters
- Exercise 3: Four two-arm swings
- Exercise 4: Four thrusters
- Exercise 5: Six two-arm swings
- Exercise 6: Six thrusters
- Exercise 7: Eight two-arm swings
- Exercise 8: Eight thrusters
- Exercise 9: Ten two-arm swings
- Exercise 10: Ten thrusters

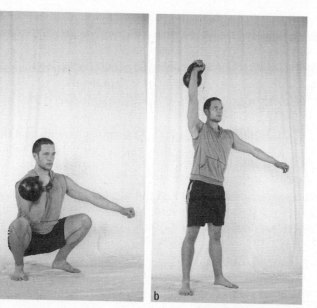

Figure 5-2:
The
thruster.

Photos courtesy of Rebekah Ulmer

✔ Exercise 11: Eight two-arm swings

✔ Exercise 12: Eight thrusters

✔ Exercise 13: Six two-arm swings

✔ Exercise 14: Six thrusters

✔ Exercise 15: Four two-arm swings

✔ Exercise 16: Four thrusters

✔ Exercise 17: Two two-arm swings

✔ Exercise 18: Two thrusters

Here's another complex where you simply alternate between two
movements. (***Note:*** To complete this complex, you do a reverse lunge
directly into a strict military press, making sure not to use momentum
from the lunge.)

✔ Exercise 1: Ten alternating lunges (five reps each leg; see Book IV,
Chapter 1)

✔ Exercise 2: Ten military presses (see Book IV, Chapter 2)

Book IV

**Primal
Power
Moves for
a Healthier
Body**

To perform the following beginner kettlebell complex, cycle through the three exercises for five rounds without putting the kettlebell down:

- ✔ Exercise 1: One one-arm clean (see Book IV, Chapter 2)
- ✔ Exercise 2: One squat (see Book IV, Chapter 1)
- ✔ Exercise 3: One press (see Book IV, Chapter 2)

So now you have a general idea of what to expect on your metabolic conditioning days. And as you can see, they can be pretty brutal, which again is why less is more!

And don't forget that this is still just the beginning of the beginning; in Book IV, Chapter 6, you'll progress toward double kettlebell complexes using some of the more advanced kettlebell movements, such as the double snatch, the double jerk, and the double front squat.

Chapter 6

Programs for Getting Started — and for Pushing Forward

. . . .

In This Chapter

▶ Diving into your first primal fitness program

▶ Building baseline strength, conditioning, mobility, and stability

▶ Taking your fitness to a new level

. . . .

*Y*our work begins now.

You *must* be comfortable with all the movements and exercises outlined in Book IV, Chapters 1 through 4, before moving on to the 21-Day Primal Quick Start program or the 90-Day Primal Body Transformation. You don't need to be a master at the one-arm push-up, but you should have a solid understanding of proper technique for all of the beginner and most of the intermediate exercises. If you don't, take a couple of extra weeks, or as long as you need, to continue practicing these movements.

The 21-Day Primal Quick Start sets you on your way to primal fitness, and the 90-Day Primal Body Transformation program is the pinnacle program of this book. And, yes, you need to start with the 21-Day Quick Start, even if you don't think you have to. If you progress too quickly before building a strong foundation, you run the risk of acquiring bad habits that may ultimately lead to injury.

The one elementary truth about fitness is that when people fully commit themselves, success is inevitable. So give your all, commit fully, and work the programs with unswerving enthusiasm. Success, like strength, is a habit that you must practice every day.

Beginning at the Beginning: The 21-Day Primal Quick Start

If you're new to exercise, you can experience enormous and wonderful changes in just 21 days on the Primal Quick Start program. And even if you're a veteran, 21 days is a fair amount of time to realize substantial gains.

If you stick to the program and the nutrition strategies in Book I with unflagging enthusiasm, you can expect some truly tremendous results over the next 21 days. For starters, you can expect an increase in strength, conditioning, and movement quality and a decrease in body fat. You can also expect the following:

✔ Greater awareness of your body and a deeper understanding of how all the parts work together as a whole

✔ A boost in confidence as you monitor your progress (and see results!)

✔ Workouts that leave you feeling energized, not depleted or beaten

✔ A challenge that leads to success

Gearing Up for the 21-Day Program

On the 21-Day Primal Quick Start program, you work out two days, rest for one day, work out two days, and then rest for two days, and repeat (for three weeks total). Another way to think of it is you work out on Monday, Tuesday, Thursday, and Friday, and rest on the other days. Although the actual days you choose are flexible — you can start Day 1 on Sunday or even Tuesday — you need to maintain the work-to-rest schedule. Broken up into 21 days, this schedule amounts to 12 total days of training and 9 days of rest.

Each workout session contains strength training and metabolic conditioning, starting with a warm-up — mostly comprised of Turkish get-ups (see Book IV, Chapter 3), crawling, and rolling. Metabolic conditioning should always come *after* your strength training — never before it. Most strength-training sessions take no longer than 20 minutes to complete, and most metabolic conditioning sessions take no longer than 15 minutes. So on average, you'll be done with your workout in less than 40 minutes.

Don't forget to add low-intensity cardiovascular activity throughout your week as much as possible, both on work days and rest days. You can do anything you want for cardio as long as it's lower intensity. Shoot for six to seven hours a week of low-intensity cardio, spread out however you want.

Start with a warm-up

Each work day of the 21-Day Quick Start begins with a warm-up — usually five minutes of unweighted Turkish get-ups and five minutes of crawling and rolling. Here are some tips on doing these warm-ups:

✔ To make the most of the Turkish get-up practice, alternate sides with each repetition and go as slow as you possibly can with every repetition. Focus on the integrity of each position of the get-up and don't rush it. See Book IV, Chapter 3, for more on the Turkish get-up.

✔ When crawling and rolling, take your time and have fun. Explore the crawling and rolling patterns described in the following sections. Mix it up and take as long as you need. Five minutes is just a starting point.

The combination of Turkish get-ups, crawling, and rolling is the go-to warm-up before any workout. If you feel like you need additional time warming up or stretching, take as long as you need.

Rolling

Proprioception, or the awareness of your body position, ties all the senses together. High proprioception enables you to move skillfully without thinking about it. Low proprioception, however, results in awkward and often dysfunctional movement.

Proprioception is supported partly by the vestibular system, which coordinates your movement through changes in head position. You garner information about your position through all your senses — seeing, feeling, hearing, smelling, and so forth.

Those with low proprioception are often undersensitized to changes in position; hence, their body doesn't react accordingly, and they move clumsily, putting them at a higher risk for injury.

Because skin is the largest sensory organ on the body, movements designed to increase the surface area contact between skin and the ground — like rolling — will likely improve proprioception. In other words, the more time you spend on the ground, the better your movement will be off the ground. Rolling is one of the best movements to improve proprioception and to prep the body for the rigors of exercise.

Here we describe four types of simple rolling:

✔ **Rolling from your back onto your stomach from your upper body:**
  • Lie flat on your back with your legs and arms fully extended.

- To roll to one side, slowly reach across and down your body with your opposite arm almost as if you're trying to reach something in your opposite pocket (see Figure 6-1). Move nothing from the waist down.

   For example, to roll to your right side, reach across with your left arm. To roll to your left, reach with your right arm.

- Continue to reach with your arm, head, and shoulders until you achieve lift and can flip yourself onto your stomach without any assistance from the lower body.

✔ **Rolling from your stomach onto your back from your upper body:**

- Lie flat on your stomach with your legs and arms fully extended.

- To roll to one side, slowly turn your head to your opposite side and attempt to look behind you as far as you can. Simultaneously reach your arm up and as far back behind you as possible. Move nothing from your waist down.

   For example, to roll to your right side, turn your head to the left and reach your left arm up. To roll to your left, turn to the right and reach up with your right arm.

- Continue to lead with your head and reach back with your arm until you can flip yourself onto your back without any assistance from your lower body.

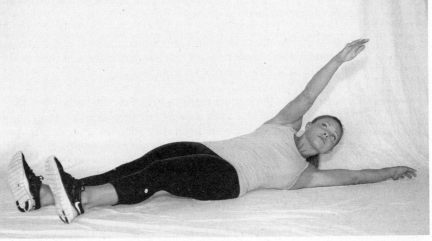

Figure 6-1:
When rolling from your top half, let your head and arm guide the motion.

Photo courtesy of Rebekah Ulmer

In this case, the body follows the head. If you get stuck when attempting to roll from your upper body, you may not be looking or leading enough with the head.

✔ **Rolling from your back onto your stomach from your lower body:**

- Lie flat on your back with your arms and legs fully extended.

- To roll to one side, reach your knee up and across your body until your hips begin to lift and you can flip yourself onto your stomach without any assistance from your upper body (see Figure 6-2).

   For example, to roll to your right side, reach up with your left knee. To roll to your left, reach up with your right knee.

✔ **Rolling from your stomach onto your back from your lower body:**

- Lie flat on your stomach with your arms and legs fully extended.

- To roll to one side, reach your leg back and across your body until your hips begin to lift and you can flip yourself onto your back without any assistance from your upper body.

   For example, to roll to your right side, reach your left leg back. To roll to your left, reach your right knee back.

You shouldn't have to use any momentum when rolling. Perform this movement in a slow-reaching manner, like how a baby would do it.

Crawling

Simple crawling movements loosen the hips, prime the core, and warm up the shoulders. Crawling also ties your movement together; it syncs the right

Figure 6-2:
When rolling from your bottom half, let your leg and hips control the movement.

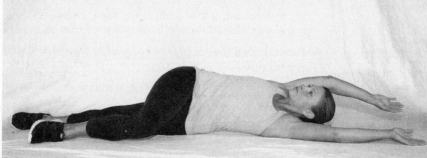

Photo courtesy of Rebekah Ulmer

and left hemispheres of your brain through *contralateral movement* — the movement of corresponding body parts on opposite sides, such as moving your right arm and left leg together and vice versa.

Humans are naturally contralateral movers. This means that when you walk, you ought to move your left arm with your right leg and your right arm with your left leg. Crawling can help reset these natural contralateral patterns, which, in turn, reduces your risk of injury.

And depending on how you serve it, crawling, just like the Turkish get-up (see Book IV, Chapter 3), makes for a great workout in and of itself. In fact, it's a marvelous cardiovascular and metabolic conditioning exercise.

The two variations of crawling are as follows:

✓ **Crawling on your hands, knees, and feet (creeping):**

- Get down on your hands and knees, and place your arms directly under your shoulders and your knees directly under your hips. Your feet should be planted, not pointed — meaning your toes are tucked.

    Keep your back flat at all times. Refer to Figure 6-3.

- Move forward by moving your opposite arm and leg together. Your right arm should move with your left leg, and your left arm should move with your left leg.

    Move backward by simply reversing the movement of Step 2.

    Creep laterally, or sideways, by matching the movement of your right arm to your left leg and vice versa.

✓ **Crawling on just your hands and feet (also known as *bear crawls*):**

- Get down on your hands and knees, and place your hands directly under your shoulders and your knees directly under your hips.

- Lift your knees slightly off the ground and turn your hands and feet slightly outward if that feels more comfortable. (See Figure 6-4.) Your knees should remain bent and your butt relatively low.

- Move forward the same way you would with creeping, by matching up your opposite arm and leg.

    Reverse the movement from Step 3 to crawl backward.

    Move to your left and right, following the instructions for the creeping exercise.

Take five minutes right now to get down on the ground and crawl around. Try crawling forward, backward, left and right. It may seem tricky or awkward at first, but keep practicing. Over time, crawling will feel more and more fluid.

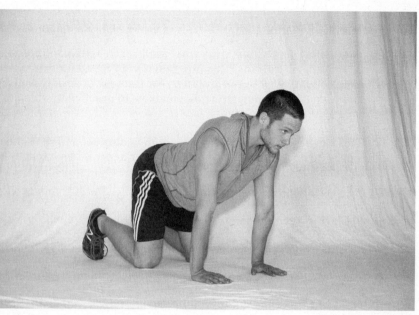

Figure 6-3:
Getting into
crawling
position
means
arms under
shoulders
and a flat
back.

Photo courtesy of Rebekah Ulmer

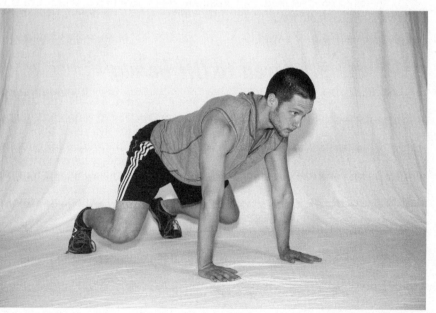

Figure 6-4:
You set up
for bear
crawls as
you would
for creeping
but then
bring your
knees off
the ground.

Book IV

**Primal
Power
Moves for
a Healthier
Body**

Photo courtesy of Rebekah Ulmer

Get ready for some repetition

This 21-Day Quick Start gives you baseline strength in a series of fundamental movement patterns. This program is your foundation. It may seem very simple, but that's the point. Variety for the sake of variety isn't a good thing. If you want to develop strength, you have to practice it, which means lots of repetition and little variety.

This simple approach is a low-rep, high-quality set-and-rep scheme and is similar to how a gymnast or a power lifter approaches strength training (arguably the two strongest types of people in the world). When training strength, you rarely do more than five reps in any given set. Instead, you use ladders, or escalating sets — where you add reps with each set. A ladder allows you to sensibly accumulate *volume* (the amount of time you spend under stress or load) without getting too fatigued.

A ladder is comprised of rungs, and each rung has a number of repetitions. For example, most ladders in this book follow either a 1-2-3-1-2-3- or a 1-2-3-4-5-1-2-3-4-5-rep structure. The former is a three-rung ladder; the latter is five-rung. The first rung is one rep, the second rung is two reps, the third rung is three reps, and so on, after which the ladder repeats itself. When working ladders, you rest as long as you need to in between each rung — that is, until you feel fresh and confident that you can perform the next rung with impeccable form.

Be prepared to lift heavy

And now you may be asking, "What weight do I use?" The answer: a heavy one! The weight you use varies from exercise to exercise, but in general, you want to find a weight that challenges you for five repetitions in any given movement. You shouldn't be able to move the weight for more than five repetitions. If five reps is easy for you for the bodyweight movements, such as the push-up or pull-up, seek out one of the more challenging variations from Book IV, Chapter 2, such as the one-arm push up. And if any of the prescribed bodyweight movements are too difficult, regress to an easier variation. For example, if you can't perform pull-ups, do rows.

Don't be so quick to shrug off the basic push-up as "easy" and move on to the more challenging variations. Most people who can bang out 20 reps or more of sloppy push-ups can rarely handle even 5 done properly. Use this 21-Day Primal Quick Start program to dial in your technique and establish quality movement.

The goal is to start the 21-day program with a heavy weight (heavy to you) and to continue to use that exact same weight throughout the entire 21 days. So don't bump up the weight even once over the course of this quick start program, even if it starts to feel light. Only *after* the 21 days should you bump up the weight. You want to finish these 21 days with the weight you're using starting to feel light.

Expect to improve your conditioning

The metabolic conditioning is constantly varied, using complexes, interval training, and sprinting. In this part of the program, you begin pushing the reps into the higher reaches, start feeling the burn, and really start sweating.

As for what weight to use for metabolic conditioning, the general rule is to find a challenging weight for whatever regimen you're doing. Sometimes you'll need a lighter weight and sometimes a heavier one. Don't be afraid to experiment, and don't feel like you have to go heavy all the time, either — mix it up and wave the load.

Your 21-Day Primal Quick Start

Time to start sweating. Here is your daily workout and rest schedule for the next 21 days.

Day 1

Warm-up

5 minutes of unweighted Turkish get-up practice
5 minutes of crawling and rolling

Strength training

Push-ups: 1-2-3-1-2-3 ladder
Dead lifts: 1-2-3-1-2-3 ladder
Turkish get-ups: 1-2-3-1-2-3 ladder
(perform one ladder for each side)

Metabolic conditioning

Four rounds of the following Tabata interval sequence with the two-arm swing:

20 seconds of two-arm swings
10 seconds of rest
20 seconds of two-arm swings
10 seconds of rest
20 seconds of two-arm swings
10 seconds of rest

Note: Tabata intervals are 20 seconds of work followed by 10 seconds of rest. Repeat for four minutes.

Day 2

Warm-up

5 minutes of unweighted Turkish get-up practice
5 minutes of crawling and rolling

Strength training

Pull-ups: 1-2-3-1-2-3 ladder (perform rows if you lack the strength for pull-ups)
Dead lifts: 1-2-3-1-2-3 ladder
Hanging knee raises: 1-2-3-1-2-3 ladder

Metabolic conditioning

Three to five rounds of the following complex:

5 two-arm swings
5 one-arm swings (5 each arm)
5 goblet squats
5 push-ups
30 seconds plank

Day 3 — Off

Day 4

Warm-up

5 minutes of unweighted Turkish get-up practice
5 minutes of crawling and rolling

Strength training

Push-ups: 1-2-3-1-2-3 ladder
Goblet squats: 1-2-3-1-2-3 ladder
V-ups: 1-2-3-1-2-3 ladder

Metabolic conditioning

15 minutes of sprints

Tip: Select a sprinting distance that's challenging but that you can complete — 50 to 75 meters is a fair starting point for most. Run as many rounds with good form as you can in 15 minutes. Be sure to rest as much as you need to between rounds so your sprint doesn't turn into a jog.

Warning: Sprinting is a super high-velocity movement. Take a few extra minutes to run a few strides and do warm-up rounds before running a full sprint.

Day 5

Warm-up

5 minutes of unweighted Turkish get-up practice
5 minutes of crawling and rolling

Strength training

Pull-ups: 1-2-3-1-2-3 ladder
Dead lifts: 1-2-3-1-2-3 ladder
Hanging knee raises: 1-2-3-1-2-3 ladder

Metabolic conditioning

300 two-arm swings

Tip: Perform these swings as quickly as possible with good form. Divide the sets and reps however you want, and be sure to rest if form starts to sour. We recommend that men use a 16- to 24-kilogram (35- to 52-pound) weight and women use an 8- to 16-kilogram (17- to 35-pound) weight.

Day 6 — Off

Day 7 — Off

Day 8

Warm-up

5 minutes of unweighted Turkish get-up practice
5 minutes of crawling and rolling

Strength training

Turkish get-ups: 1-2-3-1-2-3 ladder
Goblet squats: 1-2-3-4-5-1-2-3-4-5 ladder
Push-ups: 1-2-3-4-5-1-2-3-4-5 ladder

Metabolic conditioning

Three to five rounds of the following complex:

5 one-arm swings (5 each arm)
5 cleans
5 snatches
5 military presses
5 reverse lunges

Tip: Perform the entire complex on your right side first and then immediately on your left. Rest as long as you need to but as little as you have to between rounds.

Day 9

Warm-up

5 minutes of unweighted Turkish get-up practice
5 minutes of crawling and rolling

Strength training

Dead lifts: 1-2-3-4-5-1-2-3-4-5 ladder
Pull-ups: 1-2-3-4-5-1-2-3-4-5 ladder
Hanging knee raises: 1-2-3-4-5-1-2-3-4-5 ladder

Metabolic conditioning

Two rounds of the following exercises:

1 minute of one-arm swings (30 seconds each arm)
1 minute of one-arm cleans (30 seconds each arm)
30 seconds of military presses
1 minute of reverse lunges (alternating legs)
30 seconds of military presses
1 minute of single-leg dead lifts (30 seconds each leg)
30 seconds of two-arm swings
30 seconds of goblet squats
1 minute four-point plank

Tip: Metabolic conditioning isn't just a time to "feel the burn;" it's also a time to work on your technique, or more specifically, to see how your technique holds up under stress. Keep your focus first and foremost on form, and always be sure to maintain poise while under pressure (fatigue).

Day 10 — Off

Day 11

Warm-up

5 minutes of unweighted Turkish get-up practice
5 minutes of crawling and rolling

Book IV

Primal Power Moves for a Healthier Body

Strength training

Push-ups: 1-2-3-4-5-1-2-3-4-5 ladder
Goblet squats: 1-2-3-4-5-1-2-3-4-5 ladder
Turkish get-ups: 1-2-3-1-2-3 ladder
120 seconds three-point plank
(30 seconds each limb; lift a different limb off the ground each set)

Metabolic conditioning

15 minutes of sprints

Day 12

Warm-up

5 minutes of unweighted Turkish get-up practice
5 minutes of crawling and rolling

Strength training

Pull-ups: 1-2-3-4-5-1-2-3-4-5 ladder
Dead lifts: 1-2-3-4-5-1-2-3-4-5 ladder
Hanging knee raises: 1-2-3-4-5-1-2-3-4-5 ladder

Metabolic conditioning

15 minutes of bear crawl sprints

Tip: Find a long and relatively flat stretch of ground. Pick a distance that provides a good challenge — 25 to 50 meters is a good start — and then work bear crawls (see the earlier "Crawling" section) as fast as you can for 15 minutes. Rest as long as you need between rounds.

Day 13 — Off

Day 14 — Off

Day 15

Warm-up

5 minutes of unweighted Turkish get-up practice
5 minutes of crawling and rolling

Strength training

Turkish get-ups: 1-2-3-1-2-3 ladder
Goblet squats: 1-2-3-4-5-1-2-3-4-5 ladder
Push-ups: 1-2-3-4-5-1-2-3-4-5 ladder
V-ups: 1-2-3-4-5-1-2-3-4-5 ladder

Metabolic conditioning

Two rounds of the following complex:

2 two-arm swings
2 one-arm swings
2 thrusters (2 reps each side)
4 two-arm swings
4 one-arm swings
4 thrusters
6 two-arm swings
6 one-arm swings
6 thrusters
8 two-arm swings
8 one-arm swings
8 thrusters

Tip: Try to get all the way through the complex without setting the weight down. If form starts to deteriorate, rest immediately.

Day 16

Warm-up

5 minutes of unweighted Turkish get-up practice
5 minutes of crawling and rolling

Strength training

Dead lifts: 1-2-3-1-2-3 ladder
Pull-ups: 1-2-3-1-2-3 ladder
Hanging leg raises: 1-2-3-1-2-3 ladder

Metabolic conditioning

Four rounds of thruster Tabata intervals:

20 seconds of thrusters
10 seconds of rest
20 seconds of thrusters
10 seconds of rest
20 seconds of thrusters

Day 17 — Off

Day 18

Warm-up

5 minutes of unweighted Turkish get-up practice
5 minutes of crawling and rolling

Strength training

Push-ups: 1-2-3-1-2-3 ladder
Goblet squats: 1-2-3-1-2-3 ladder
Turkish get-ups: 1-2-3-1-2-3 ladder
V-ups: 1-2-3-1-2-3 ladder

Metabolic conditioning

20 snatches (10 each side), on the minute, every minute for 15 minutes

Day 19

Warm-up

5 minutes of unweighted Turkish get-up practice
5 minutes of crawling and rolling

Strength training

Pull-ups: 1-2-3-1-2-3 ladder
Dead lifts: 1-2-3-1-2-3 ladder
Hanging knee raises: 1-2-3-1-2-3 ladder

Metabolic conditioning

15 minutes of sprints

Day 20 — Off

Day 21 — Off

From Average to Elite: The 90-Day Primal Body Transformation

When you're feeling strong and the movements in the 21-Day Primal Quick Start have become second nature to you — and when your commitment to success is high — you're ready to push yourself with the 90-Day Primal

Book IV

Primal Power Moves for a Healthier Body

Body Transformation. It's a demanding and worthwhile program made up of exercises and workouts that challenge you but that you *can* complete. And it starts with you acknowledging where you are now and envisioning where you want to be after 90 days.

If you approach the program with unswerving enthusiasm, it will reward you with results.

Taking before pictures is a proven way to increase motivation and adherence, and taking after pictures, or *progress pictures,* is a great way to keep motivated and see the results you're looking for.

The best way to take before pictures is to wear a bathing suit or tight-fitting fitness apparel, and take one frontal picture (head on) and one profile picture (from the side). Take your before pictures on Day 1, and then take the same poses in your progress pictures every 30 days.

Building a Balanced 90-Day Program

Elite performers are the ones who've moved deeper into the basics. In this program, you'll find repetition, repetition, repetition. The strength training slowly increases in volume (total work performed) over the next 90 days, but the movements themselves won't change, nor will the weight you use.

You will, however, be offered the refreshment of variety with the metabolic conditioning routines. These routines vary from day to day, offering new and exciting challenges. This combination of purposeful, repetitive strength training and variable, high-intensity conditioning will make you a true physical specimen, upgraded in every regard, impervious to damage.

Elements of this program are very tough, so be sure to listen to your body. If you feel too beat to train on any one day, take an extra day off — no big deal. Just be sure it's due to legitimate fatigue and not laziness. There is a stark difference.

The ultimate goal of the 90-Day Primal Body Transformation program is to eventually progress through 90 days with the ability to perform all advanced level exercises found in Book IV, Chapter 4. No one, save the elite gymnast, is going to be able to do that right off the bat. So start with something that's challenging enough for your first 90 days, and then bump it up each time you do this 90-day program. You find out how to design this program for where you are now and how to progress further in the following sections.

Strength-training exercises

For strength training, you choose a series of exercises — one from each of the fundamental movements in Book IV, Chapters 1 through 3 — that are challenging but that also ensure success. In other words, you want to pick exercises that challenge you for five reps but that you *can* do for five reps. (***Note:*** For movements that you don't count by reps, such as planks and carries, consider 15 seconds equal to one rep.) You do these same exercises for 90 days.

After 90 days, you repeat the program with a more challenging set of exercises; however, don't progress onto a more challenging variation at any point *during* the 90 days, even when the variations or weights you've chosen start to feel easy or light. You want to finish this 90-day period with all the difficult movements you started out with starting to feel easy. The next sections walk you through exactly what that means and provide some example strength-training lineups.

Putting together your strength exercise routine

To build your strength-training routine, select two movements (an "A" movement and a "B" movement) from Book IV, Chapters 1 through 3, for each movement category (we've listed them here for easy reference):

- ✔ **Push:** Push-up, military press, one-arm push-up, bench press, dip, one-arm one-leg push-up, handstand push-up

- ✔ **Pull:** Bodyweight row, chin-up, one-arm row, pull-up, L-sit pull-up/chin-up, muscle-up, one-arm chin-up

- ✔ **Hinge:** Dead lift, single-leg dead lift, swing, one-arm swing, clean, snatch

- ✔ **Squat:** Goblet squat, bodyweight squat, goblet lunge, racked squat, racked lunge, front squat, pistol squat

- ✔ **Carry:** Farmer's carry, waiter's carry, racked carry, two-arm waiter's carry, bottoms-up carry, Turkish get-up

- ✔ **Core:** Four-point plank, V-up, windmill, hanging knee raise, three-point plank, two-point plank, hanging leg raise, windshield wiper

- ✔ **Power:** Push press, broad jump, jerk, box jump, double jerk, double snatch

Throughout this chapter, you'll see references to "double" exercises, like double jerk, double snatch, double front squat, and so on. The "double" simply means you're holding a weight in each hand.

You'll do most of the strength training in a ladder format, beginning with three-rung (1-2-3) ladders and ultimately ending with five-rung (1-2-3-4-5) ladders.

Book IV

Primal Power Moves for a Healthier Body

Every ladder is comprised of rungs, and each rung is comprised of a number of repetitions. For example, the first rung of a three-rung ladder is one rep, the second rung is two reps, and the third rung is three reps. Be sure to rest as long as you need to between each rung.

The order you do these exercises doesn't really matter, but generally, you should start with the movements or exercises that are most challenging to you. For example, in the daily workouts outlined in the section "Your 90-Day Primal Body Transformation," the power movements appear first because they tend to require a bit more concentration, but you may perform the exercises in any sequence you desire, as long as you do them all.

If you're a fitness veteran, you may pick an *advanced* lineup that looks something like this:

- Push A: One-arm push-up
- Push B: Handstand push-up
- Pull A: Muscle-up
- Pull B: One-arm chin-up
- Hinge A: Dead lift
- Hinge B: Single-leg dead lift
- Squat A: Front squat
- Squat B: Pistol squat
- Carry A: Turkish get-up
- Carry B: Bottoms-up carry
- Core A: Hanging leg raise
- Core B: Two-point plank
- Power A: Double snatch
- Power B: Double jerk

If you're somewhere in the middle, you may pick an *intermediate* lineup that looks something like this:

- Push A: Dip
- Push B: Bench press
- Pull A: Pull-up
- Pull B: One-arm row
- Hinge A: Dead lift

- Hinge B: Single-leg dead lift
- Squat A: Front squat
- Squat B: Racked lunge
- Core A: Hanging knee raise
- Core B: Three-point plank
- Power A: Jerk
- Power B: Box jump

And if you're relatively new to fitness or are still working on building strength, a *beginner* lineup may look something like this:

- Push A: Push-up
- Push B: Military press
- Pull A: Bodyweight row
- Pull B: Flexed arm hang
- Hinge A: Dead lift
- Hinge B: Single-leg dead lift
- Squat A: Goblet squat
- Squat B: Goblet lunge
- Core A: Four-point plank
- Core B: V-up
- Power A: Push press
- Power B: Broad jump

Did you notice that the hinges stay consistent with the dead lift and single-leg dead lift for each level? That's because these two movements allow you to move the most weight. You'll get plenty of the other hinges, such as swings, cleans, and snatches, with your metabolic conditioning.

Now you may very well just take one of these lineups and run with it, or you may design one of your own. The key is to select an exercise or a weight that challenges you for five reps. If you can perform a bodyweight exercise, such as the push-up, for more than 10 to 15 reps, then it's probably time to move on to a one-arm push-up variation. For the weighted exercises, such as the bench press or front squat, be sure to work with a heavy-enough weight. The dead lift by itself isn't necessarily "advanced," but a 500-pound dead lift probably is.

Book IV

Primal Power Moves for a Healthier Body

Choosing a weight that challenges you

The weight you choose for strength training should be something with which you can perform for five reps. If you can move it much more than that, it's likely not heavy enough. Because you do most of the strength-training work in sets of five repetitions or fewer, it's imperative that you work with a significant load; otherwise, you'll find it difficult to make any significant strength gains.

Like the 21-Day Primal Quick Start program, you won't increase the weight or move on to a more difficult bodyweight exercise until the 90 days are up. The goal is to start the program with a weight that feels heavy and to finish with that same weight feeling light. Then, after the 90 days are up, you bump the weight up or move on to a more difficult bodyweight exercise, and do 90 days with that weight. This progression takes patience because people are always anxious to progress faster than they should. ***Remember:*** You can't rush strength or cellular recovery. It occurs on its own accord. When it comes to strength, patience is a virtue.

Metabolic conditioning

You don't need to worry about building your metabolic conditioning routine; this book has you covered. For each work day of the 90-day program, you find a unique metabolic conditioning routine. All you have to do is select a challenging weight for whatever is prescribed that day (naturally, you'll go lighter on higher-rep complexes and heavier on lower-rep complexes). Other than that, it's all laid out for you.

For the double movements — the double swing, double clean, double (military) press, double front squat, and double snatch — follow the techniques for the single movements but use two kettlebells instead of one. For the double swing, clean, and snatch, adjust your stance so it's wide enough to accommodate the extra bell, but stand only as wide as you need to fit both bells between your legs.

Your daily warm-up

So now that you know what exercises you'll be doing in this 90-day program, you don't want to forget about warming up before each workout. Your daily warm-up consists of five minutes of unweighted Turkish get-ups and five minutes of crawling and rolling (see the related sections earlier in this chapter). The point of the warm-up is to wake the system up, to warm the muscles, and to have fun! Crawl and roll around as much as you need to until you feel limber and energized.

One of the simplest but most effective warm-ups is to perform a few light sets of whatever exercises you're going to be working that day.

Your weekly schedule

This program follows a workout-rest pattern just like the 21-Day Primal Quick Start. You work out for two days, rest for one day, work out for two days, and then rest for two days. Work this pattern into your week however you can, such as the following:

- ✔ Monday: Work out
- ✔ Tuesday: Work out
- ✔ Wednesday: Rest
- ✔ Thursday: Work out
- ✔ Friday: Work out
- ✔ Saturday: Rest
- ✔ Sunday: Rest

Your 90-Day Primal Body Transformation

This is it. You're about to go from zero to awesome in 90 days. You're mentally prepared, and you've made the commitment. Now dive in and have fun!

Day 1

Warm-up

5 minutes of unweighted Turkish get-ups
5 minutes of crawling and rolling

Strength training

Power A: 1-2-3-1-2-3 ladder
Push A: 1-2-3-1-2-3 ladder
Pull A: 1-2-3-1-2-3 ladder
Carry A: 1-2-3 ladder

Remember: Because you don't count carries by reps, consider 15 seconds equal to one rep. So for the three-rung ladder here, you do 15 seconds for the first rung, 30 seconds for the second rung, and 45 seconds for the third rung. The exception to this rule is the Turkish get-up, which you do count in reps.

Book IV

Primal Power Moves for a Healthier Body

Metabolic conditioning

Two rounds of the following complex:

2 two-arm swings
1 goblet squat
4 two-arm swings
2 goblet squats
6 two-arm swings
3 goblet squats
8 two-arm swings
4 goblet squats
10 two-arm swings
5 goblet squats

Day 2

Warm-up

5 minutes of unweighted Turkish get-ups
5 minutes of crawling and rolling

Strength training

Power B: 1-2-3-1-2-3 ladder
Push B: 1-2-3-1-2-3 ladder
Pull B: 1-2-3-1-2-3 ladder
Carry B: 1-2-3 ladder

Metabolic conditioning

Four rounds of the following two-arm swing Tabata interval:

20 seconds of two-arm swings
10 seconds of rest
20 seconds of two-arm swings
10 seconds of rest
20 seconds of two-arm swings
10 seconds of rest

Day 3 — Off

Day 4

Warm-up

5 minutes of unweighted Turkish get-ups
5 minutes of crawling and rolling

Strength training

Hinge A: 1-2-3-1-2-3 ladder
Squat A: 1-2-3-1-2-3 ladder
Core A: 1-2-3-1-2-3 ladder

Metabolic conditioning

Three to five rounds of the following complex (perform entirely on your right side first and then immediately repeat on your left):

5 one-arm swings
5 one-arm cleans
5 one-arm snatches
5 one-arm push presses
5 reverse lunges

Day 5

Warm-up

5 minutes of unweighted Turkish get-ups
5 minutes of crawling and rolling

Strength training

Hinge B: 1-2-3-1-2-3 ladder
Squat B: 1-2-3-1-2-3 ladder
Core B: 1-2-3-1-2-3 ladder

Metabolic conditioning

15 minutes of sprints

Day 6 — Off

Day 7 — Off

Day 8

Warm-up

5 minutes of unweighted Turkish get-ups
5 minutes of crawling and rolling

Strength training

Power A: 1-2-3-1-2-3 ladder
Push A: 1-2-3-1-2-3 ladder
Pull A: 1-2-3-1-2-3 ladder
Carry A: 1-2-3 ladder

Metabolic conditioning

100 two-arm swings as quickly as possible with good form

Day 9

Warm-up

5 minutes of unweighted Turkish get-ups
5 minutes of crawling and rolling

Strength training

Power B: 1-2-3-1-2-3 ladder
Push B: 1-2-3-1-2-3 ladder
Pull B: 1-2-3-1-2-3 ladder
Carry B: 1-2-3 ladder

Metabolic conditioning

Three to five rounds of the following complex:

5 double swings
5 double cleans

5 double military presses
5 double front squats

Day 10 — Off

Day 11

Warm-up

5 minutes of unweighted Turkish get-ups
5 minutes of crawling and rolling

Strength training

Hinge A: 1-2-3-1-2-3 ladder
Squat A: 1-2-3-1-2-3 ladder
Core A: 1-2-3-1-2-3 ladder

Metabolic conditioning

15 minutes of bear crawl sprints

Tip: After you're comfortable with the forward bear crawl, try sprinting in various directions — backward, to the left, and to the right.

Day 12

Warm-up

5 minutes of unweighted Turkish get-ups
5 minutes of crawling and rolling

Strength training

Hinge B: 1-2-3-1-2-3 ladder
Squat B: 1-2-3-1-2-3 ladder
Core B: 1-2-3-1-2-3 ladder

Book IV

Primal Power Moves for a Healthier Body

Metabolic conditioning

Ten rounds of the following one-arm snatch interval (rest as little as needed between rounds):

*15 seconds of one-arm snatches
(right arm)
15 seconds of rest
15 seconds of one-arm snatches
(left arm)
15 seconds of rest*

Remember: When working interval training, the goal is to get in as many reps with good form as possible in the allotted work period. Again, we emphasize *with good form.*

Day 13 — Off

Day 14 — Off

Day 15

Warm-up

*5 minutes of unweighted Turkish get-ups
5 minutes of crawling and rolling*

Strength training

*Power A: 1-2-3-1-2-3-4 ladder
Push A: 1-2-3-1-2-3-4 ladder
Pull A: 1-2-3-1-2-3-4 ladder
Carry A: 1-2-3 ladder*

Metabolic conditioning

Two rounds of the following complex (perform each movement on your right side and then

immediately on your left before moving to the next exercise):

*8 one-arm cleans
5 one-arm racked squats
5 one-arm cleans
3 one-arm racked squats
3 one-arm cleans
2 one-arm racked squats
2 one-arm cleans
1 one-arm racked squat*

Day 16

Warm-up

*5 minutes of unweighted Turkish get-ups
5 minutes of crawling and rolling*

Strength training

*Power B: 1-2-3-1-2-3-4 ladder
Push B: 1-2-3-1-2-3-4 ladder
Pull B: 1-2-3-1-2-3-4 ladder
Carry B: 1-2-3 ladder*

Metabolic conditioning

5 double kettlebell cleans and 5 double kettlebell front squats on the minute, every minute, for ten minutes

Day 17 — Off

Day 18

Warm-up

*5 minutes of unweighted Turkish get-ups
5 minutes of crawling and rolling*

Strength training

Hinge A: 1-2-3-1-2-3-4 ladder
Squat A: 1-2-3-1-2-3-4 ladder
Core A: 1-2-3-1-2-3-4 ladder

Metabolic conditioning

5 double cleans and double military presses (that's one double clean between each double press) on the minute, every minute, for 15 minutes

Day 19

Warm-up

5 minutes of unweighted Turkish get-ups
5 minutes of crawling and rolling

Strength training

Hinge B: 1-2-3-1-2-3-4 ladder
Squat B: 1-2-3-1-2-3-4 ladder
Core B: 1-2-3-1-2-3-4 ladder

Metabolic conditioning

20 minutes of interval running (15- to 30-second sprint, 1-minute walk, and then 1-minute jog)

Tip: Interval running is a mix of jogging, sprinting, and walking. The key here is to keep moving but vary the intensity. We recommend the schedule of 1 minute of walking and 1 minute of jogging for every 30 seconds of sprinting. Simply repeat this sequence for whatever amount of time is prescribed.

Day 20 — Off

Day 21 — Off

Day 22

Warm-up

5 minutes of unweighted Turkish get-ups
5 minutes of crawling and rolling

Strength training

Power A: 1-2-3-1-2-3-4 ladder
Push A: 1-2-3-1-2-3-4 ladder
Pull A: 1-2-3-1-2-3-4 ladder
Carry A: 1-2-3 ladder

Metabolic conditioning

Two to three rounds of the following complex:

5 double swings
5 double snatches
5 front squats
5 double military presses
5 double swings

Day 23

Warm-up

5 minutes of unweighted Turkish get-ups
5 minutes of crawling and rolling

Strength training

Power B: 1-2-3-1-2-3-4 ladder
Push B: 1-2-3-1-2-3-4 ladder
Pull B: 1-2-3-1-2-3-4 ladder
Carry B: 1-2-3 ladder

Book IV

Primal Power Moves for a Healthier Body

Metabolic conditioning

Four rounds of thruster Tabata intervals (switch sides each working set):

20 seconds of thrusters
10 seconds of rest
20 seconds of thrusters
10 seconds of rest
20 seconds of thrusters

Day 24 — Off

Day 25

Warm-up

5 minutes of unweighted Turkish get-ups
5 minutes of crawling and rolling

Strength training

Hinge A: 1-2-3-4-1-2-3-4 ladder
Squat A: 1-2-3-4-1-2-3-4 ladder
Core A: 1-2-3-4-1-2-3-4 ladder

Metabolic conditioning

Two to three rounds of the following complex (complete entirely on your right side and then immediately on your left):

5 one-arm swings
5 one-arm cleans
5 one-arm snatches
5 one-arm jerks
5 reverse lunges

Day 26

Warm-up

5 minutes of unweighted Turkish get-ups
5 minutes of crawling and rolling

Strength training

Hinge B: 1-2-3-4-1-2-3-4 ladder
Squat B: 1-2-3-4-1-2-3-4 ladder
Core B: 1-2-3-4-1-2-3-4 ladder

Metabolic conditioning

15 minutes of sprints

Day 27 — Off

Day 28 — Off

Day 29

Warm-up

5 minutes of unweighted Turkish get-ups
5 minutes of crawling and rolling

Strength training

Power A: 1-2-3-4-1-2-3-4 ladder
Push A: 1-2-3-4-1-2-3-4 ladder
Pull A: 1-2-3-4-1-2-3-4 ladder
Carry A: 1-2-3-4 ladder

Metabolic conditioning

100 snatches (50 each arm) as quickly as possible with good form

Day 30

Warm-up

5 minutes of unweighted Turkish get-ups
5 minutes of crawling and rolling

Strength training

Power B: 1-2-3-4-1-2-3-4 ladder
Push B: 1-2-3-4-1-2-3-4 ladder
Pull B: 1-2-3-4-1-2-3-4 ladder
Carry B: 1-2-3-4 ladder

Metabolic conditioning

15 minutes of sprints

Day 31 — Off
Day 32

Warm-up

5 minutes of unweighted Turkish get-ups
5 minutes of crawling and rolling

Strength training

Hinge A: 1-2-3-4-1-2-3-4 ladder
Squat A: 1-2-3-4-1-2-3-4 ladder
Core A: 1-2-3-4-1-2-3-4 ladder

Metabolic conditioning

15 minutes of bear crawl sprints

Day 33

Warm-up

5 minutes of unweighted Turkish get-ups
5 minutes of crawling and rolling

Strength training

Hinge B: 1-2-3-4-1-2-3-4 ladder
Squat B: 1-2-3-4-1-2-3-4 ladder
Core B: 1-2-3-4-1-2-3-4 ladder

Metabolic conditioning

Two rounds of the following complex:
8 double cleans
5 double kettlebell front squats
5 double cleans
3 double kettlebell front squats
3 double cleans
2 double kettlebell front squats
2 double cleans
1 double kettlebell front squat

Day 34 — Off
Day 35 — Off
Day 36

Warm-up

5 minutes of unweighted Turkish get-ups
5 minutes of crawling and rolling

Strength training

Power A: 1-2-3-4-1-2-3-4 ladder
Push A: 1-2-3-4-1-2-3-4 ladder
Pull A: 1-2-3-4-1-2-3-4 ladder
Carry A: 1-2-3-4 ladder

Metabolic conditioning

Line up three various weights for two-arm swings: a light weight, a medium weight, and a heavy weight. Perform five swings at each weight. Continue cycling through this chain for ten minutes.

Book IV

Primal
Power
Moves for
a Healthier
Body

Day 37

Warm-up

5 minutes of unweighted Turkish get-ups
5 minutes of crawling and rolling

Strength training

Power B: 1-2-3-4-1-2-3-4 ladder
Push B: 1-2-3-4-1-2-3-4 ladder
Pull B: 1-2-3-4-1-2-3-4 ladder
Carry B: 1-2-3-4 ladder

Metabolic conditioning

Perform the following four-round complex:

Round 1:
5 double swings
5 double military presses

Round 2:
5 double swings
5 double cleans
5 double military presses

Round 3:
5 double swings
5 double cleans
5 double snatches
5 double military presses

Round 4:
5 double swings
5 double cleans
5 double snatches
5 double kettlebell front squats
5 double military presses

Day 38 — Off

Day 39

Warm-up

5 minutes of unweighted Turkish get-ups
5 minutes of crawling and rolling

Strength training

Hinge A: 1-2-3-4-1-2-3-4 ladder
Squat A: 1-2-3-4-1-2-3-4 ladder
Core A: 1-2-3-4-1-2-3-4 ladder

Metabolic conditioning

Four rounds of double kettlebell front squat Tabata intervals:

20 seconds of double kettlebell front squats
10 seconds of rest
20 seconds of double kettlebell front squats
10 seconds of rest
20 seconds of double kettlebell front squats
10 seconds of rest

Day 40

Warm-up

5 minutes of unweighted Turkish get-ups
5 minutes of crawling and rolling

Strength training

Hinge B: 1-2-3-4-1-2-3-4 ladder
Squat B: 1-2-3-4-1-2-3-4 ladder
Core B: 1-2-3-4-1-2-3-4 ladder

Metabolic conditioning

20 minutes of interval running

Day 41 — Off

Day 42 — Off

Day 43

Warm-up

5 minutes of unweighted Turkish get-ups
5 minutes of crawling and rolling

Strength training

Power A: 1-2-3-4-1-2-3-4 ladder
Push A: 1-2-3-4-1-2-3-4 ladder
Pull A: 1-2-3-4-1-2-3-4 ladder
Carry A: 1-2-3-4 ladder

Metabolic conditioning

100 one-arm snatches (50 each arm) as quickly as possible with good form

Tip: A classic test of conditioning and muscular endurance is the ability to perform 100 snatches in less than five minutes while using a 24-kilogram kettlebell (males) or a 16-kilogram kettlebell (females). Keep this in mind when choosing a weight for this conditioning drill!

Day 44

Warm-up

5 minutes of unweighted Turkish get-ups
5 minutes of crawling and rolling

Strength training

Power B: 1-2-3-4-1-2-3-4 ladder
Push B: 1-2-3-4-1-2-3-4 ladder
Pull B: 1-2-3-4-1-2-3-4 ladder
Carry B: 1-2-3-4 ladder

Metabolic conditioning

15 minutes of bear crawl sprints

Day 45 — Off

Day 46

Warm-up

5 minutes of unweighted Turkish get-ups
5 minutes of crawling and rolling

Strength training

Hinge A: 1-2-3-4-1-2-3-4 ladder
Squat A: 1-2-3-4-1-2-3-4 ladder
Core A: 1-2-3-4-1-2-3-4 ladder

Metabolic conditioning

Three double cleans, two double kettlebell front squats, and two double military presses on the minute, every minute, for ten minutes

Day 47

Warm-up

5 minutes of unweighted Turkish get-ups
5 minutes of crawling and rolling

Strength training

Hinge B: 1-2-3-4-1-2-3-4 ladder
Squat B: 1-2-3-4-1-2-3-4 ladder
Core B: 1-2-3-4-1-2-3-4 ladder

Book IV

Primal Power Moves for a Healthier Body

Metabolic conditioning

Two rounds of the following complex:

10 double swings
10 double snatches
10 double kettlebell front squats
10 double military presses
10 double swings

Day 48 — Off

Day 49 — Off

Day 50

Warm-up

5 minutes of unweighted Turkish get-ups
5 minutes of crawling and rolling

Strength training

Power A: 1-2-3-4-1-2-3-4 ladder
Push A: 1-2-3-4-1-2-3-4 ladder
Pull A: 1-2-3-4-1-2-3-4 ladder
Carry A: 1-2-3-4 ladder

Metabolic conditioning

20 minutes of interval running

Day 51

Warm-up

5 minutes of unweighted Turkish get-ups
5 minutes of crawling and rolling

Strength training

Power B: 1-2-3-4-1-2-3-4 ladder
Push B: 1-2-3-4-1-2-3-4 ladder

Pull B: 1-2-3-4-1-2-3-4 ladder
Carry B: 1-2-3-4 ladder

Metabolic conditioning

One to two rounds of the following complex:

2 double cleans
1 double kettlebell front squat
4 double cleans
2 double kettlebell front squats
6 double cleans
3 double kettlebell front squats
8 double cleans
4 double kettlebell front squats
10 double cleans
5 double kettlebell front squats

Day 52 — Off

Day 53

Warm-up

5 minutes of unweighted Turkish get-ups
5 minutes of crawling and rolling

Strength training

Hinge A: 1-2-3-4-1-2-3-4 ladder
Squat A: 1-2-3-4-1-2-3-4 ladder
Core A: 1-2-3-4-1-2-3-4 ladder

Metabolic conditioning

Five rounds of the following complex (complete entirely on your right side and then immediately on your left):

6 one-arm swings
6 one-arm cleans
6 one-arm snatches
6 one-arm jerks
6 reverse lunges

Day 54

Warm-up

5 minutes of unweighted Turkish get-ups
5 minutes of crawling and rolling

Strength training

Hinge B: 1-2-3-4-1-2-3-4 ladder
Squat B: 1-2-3-4-1-2-3-4 ladder
Core B: 1-2-3-4-1-2-3-4 ladder

Metabolic conditioning

15 minutes of sprints

Day 55 — Off

Day 56 — Off

Day 57

Warm-up

5 minutes of unweighted Turkish get-ups
5 minutes of crawling and rolling

Strength training

Power A: 1-2-3-4-1-2-3-4-5 ladder
Push A: 1-2-3-4-1-2-3-4-5 ladder
Pull A: 1-2-3-4-1-2-3-4-5 ladder
Carry A: 1-2-3-4 ladder

Metabolic conditioning

Perform the following interval sequence of jerks for ten minutes:

15 seconds of one-arm jerks (right arm)
15 seconds of rest

15 seconds of one-arm jerks (left arm)
15 seconds of rest

Day 58

Warm-up

5 minutes of unweighted Turkish get-ups
5 minutes of crawling and rolling

Strength training

Power B: 1-2-3-4-1-2-3-4-5 ladder
Push B: 1-2-3-4-1-2-3-4-5 ladder
Pull B: 1-2-3-4-1-2-3-4-5 ladder
Carry B: 1-2-3-4 ladder

Metabolic conditioning

Four rounds of the following lunge to military press Tabata interval (alternate sides each working set):

20 seconds of lunges to military presses
10 seconds of rest
20 seconds of lunges to military presses
10 seconds of rest
20 seconds of lunges to military presses

Day 59 — Off

Day 60

Warm-up

5 minutes of unweighted Turkish get-ups
5 minutes of crawling and rolling

Strength training

Hinge A: 1-2-3-4-1-2-3-4-5 ladder
Squat A: 1-2-3-4-1-2-3-4-5 ladder
Core A: 1-2-3-4-1-2-3-4-5 ladder

Book IV

Primal Power Moves for a Healthier Body

Metabolic conditioning

200 two-arm swings as quickly as possible with good form

Day 61

Warm-up

5 minutes of unweighted Turkish get-ups
5 minutes of crawling and rolling

Strength training

Hinge B: 1-2-3-4-1-2-3-4-5 ladder
Squat B: 1-2-3-4-1-2-3-4-5 ladder
Core B: 1-2-3-4-1-2-3-4-5 ladder

Metabolic conditioning

Ten rounds of the following one-arm snatch interval (rest as little as needed between rounds):

15 seconds of one-arm snatches (right arm)
15 seconds of rest
15 seconds of one-arm snatches (left arm)
15 seconds of rest

Day 62 — Off

Day 63 — Off

Day 64

Warm-up

5 minutes of unweighted Turkish get-ups
5 minutes of crawling and rolling

Strength training

Power A: 1-2-3-4-1-2-3-4-5 ladder
Push A: 1-2-3-4-1-2-3-4-5 ladder
Pull A: 1-2-3-4-1-2-3-4-5 ladder
Carry A: 1-2-3-4 ladder

Metabolic conditioning

Five rounds of the following complex:

5 double swings
5 double cleans and military presses (one double clean between each double press)
5 double kettlebell front squats

Day 65

Warm-up

5 minutes of unweighted Turkish get-ups
5 minutes of crawling and rolling

Strength training

Power B: 1-2-3-4-1-2-3-4-5 ladder
Push B: 1-2-3-4-1-2-3-4-5 ladder
Pull B: 1-2-3-4-1-2-3-4-5 ladder
Carry B: 1-2-3-4 ladder

Metabolic conditioning

Ten double snatches on the minute, every minute, for ten minutes

Day 66 — Off

Day 67

Warm-up

5 minutes of unweighted Turkish get-ups
5 minutes of crawling and rolling

Strength training

Hinge A: 1-2-3-4-1-2-3-4-5 ladder
Squat A: 1-2-3-4-1-2-3-4-5 ladder
Core A: 1-2-3-4-1-2-3-4-5 ladder

Metabolic conditioning

15 minutes of sprints

Day 68

Warm-up

5 minutes of unweighted Turkish get-ups
5 minutes of crawling and rolling

Strength training

Hinge B: 1-2-3-4-1-2-3-4-5 ladder
Squat B: 1-2-3-4-1-2-3-4-5 ladder
Core B: 1-2-3-4-1-2-3-4-5 ladder

Metabolic conditioning

Five rounds of the following complex:

1 double clean
3 double military presses
2 front squats
10 double swings

Day 69 — Off
Day 70 — Off
Day 71

Warm-up

5 minutes of unweighted Turkish get-ups
5 minutes of crawling and rolling

Strength training

Power A: 1-2-3-4-1-2-3-4-5 ladder
Push A: 1-2-3-4-1-2-3-4-5 ladder
Pull A: 1-2-3-4-1-2-3-4-5 ladder
Carry A: 1-2-3-4 ladder

Metabolic conditioning

15 minutes of bear crawl sprints

Day 72

Warm-up

5 minutes of unweighted Turkish get-ups
5 minutes of crawling and rolling

Strength training

Power B: 1-2-3-4-1-2-3-4-5 ladder
Push B: 1-2-3-4-1-2-3-4-5 ladder
Pull B: 1-2-3-4-1-2-3-4-5 ladder
Carry B: 1-2-3-4 ladder

Metabolic conditioning

Two rounds of the following complex:

15 double swings
15 double snatches
15 double kettlebell front squats
15 double military presses
15 push-ups

Day 73 — Off
Day 74

Warm-up

5 minutes of unweighted Turkish get-ups
5 minutes of crawling and rolling

Book IV

Primal Power Moves for a Healthier Body

Strength training

Hinge A: 1-2-3-4-1-2-3-4-5 ladder
Squat A: 1-2-3-4-1-2-3-4-5 ladder
Core A: 1-2-3-4-1-2-3-4-5 ladder

Metabolic conditioning

20 minutes of interval running

Day 75

Warm-up

5 minutes of unweighted Turkish get-ups
5 minutes of crawling and rolling

Strength training

Hinge B: 1-2-3-4-1-2-3-4-5 ladder
Squat B: 1-2-3-4-1-2-3-4-5 ladder
Core B: 1-2-3-4-1-2-3-4-5 ladder

Metabolic conditioning

Five rounds of the following complex (complete entirely on your right side and then immediately on your left):

5 one-arm swings
5 one-arm cleans
5 one-arm snatches
5 racked squats
5 push presses
5 reverse lunges

Day 76 — Off
Day 77 — Off

Day 78

Warm-up

5 minutes of unweighted Turkish get-ups
5 minutes of crawling and rolling

Strength training

Power A: 1-2-3-4-5-1-2-3-4-5 ladder
Push A: 1-2-3-4-5-1-2-3-4-5 ladder
Pull A: 1-2-3-4-5-1-2-3-4-5 ladder
Carry A: 1-2-3-4 ladder

Metabolic conditioning

150 one-arm snatches (75 each arm) as quickly as possible with good form

Day 79

Warm-up

5 minutes of unweighted Turkish get-ups
5 minutes of crawling and rolling

Strength training

Power B: 1-2-3-4-5-1-2-3-4-5 ladder
Push B: 1-2-3-4-5-1-2-3-4-5 ladder
Pull B: 1-2-3-4-5-1-2-3-4-5 ladder
Carry B: 1-2-3-4 ladder

Metabolic conditioning

Two rounds of the following complex:

15 double swings
15 double snatches
15 double kettlebell front squats
15 double military presses
15 push-ups

Day 80 — Off

Day 81

Warm-up

5 minutes of unweighted Turkish get-ups
5 minutes of crawling and rolling

Strength training

Hinge A: 1-2-3-4-5-1-2-3-4-5 ladder
Squat A: 1-2-3-4-5-1-2-3-4-5 ladder
Core A: 1-2-3-4-5-1-2-3-4-5 ladder

Metabolic conditioning

20 minutes of interval running

Day 82

Warm-up

5 minutes of unweighted Turkish get-ups
5 minutes of crawling and rolling

Strength training

Hinge B: 1-2-3-4-5-1-2-3-4-5 ladder
Squat B: 1-2-3-4-5-1-2-3-4-5 ladder
Core B: 1-2-3-4-5-1-2-3-4-5 ladder

Metabolic conditioning

15 minutes of bear crawl sprints

Day 83 — Off

Day 84 — Off

Day 85

Warm-up

5 minutes of unweighted Turkish get-ups
5 minutes of crawling and rolling

Strength training

Power A: 1-2-3-4-5-1-2-3-4-5 ladder
Push A: 1-2-3-4-5-1-2-3-4-5 ladder
Pull A: 1-2-3-4-5-1-2-3-4-5 ladder
Carry A: 1-2-3-4 ladder

Metabolic conditioning

Four rounds of the following two-arm swing Tabata interval:

20 seconds of two-arm swings
10 seconds of rest
20 seconds of two-arm swings
10 seconds of rest
20 seconds of two-arm swings

Day 86

Warm-up

5 minutes of unweighted Turkish get-ups
5 minutes of crawling and rolling

Strength training

Power B: 1-2-3-4-5-1-2-3-4-5 ladder
Push B: 1-2-3-4-5-1-2-3-4-5 ladder
Pull B: 1-2-3-4-5-1-2-3-4-5 ladder
Carry B: 1-2-3-4 ladder

Book IV

Primal Power Moves for a Healthier Body

Metabolic conditioning

Two to three rounds of the following complex (perform entirely on your right side and then immediately on your left):

5 one-arm swings
5 one-arm cleans and military presses (one clean between each press)
5 one-arm push presses
5 reverse lunges
5 single-leg dead lifts

Day 87 — Off

Day 88

Warm-up

5 minutes of unweighted Turkish get-ups
5 minutes of crawling and rolling

Strength training

Hinge A: 1-2-3-4-5-1-2-3-4-5 ladder
Squat A: 1-2-3-4-5-1-2-3-4-5 ladder
Core A: 1-2-3-4-5-1-2-3-4-5 ladder

Metabolic conditioning

15 minutes of sprints

Day 89

Warm-up

5 minutes of unweighted Turkish get-ups
5 minutes of crawling and rolling

Strength training

Hinge B: 1-2-3-4-5-1-2-3-4-5 ladder
Squat B: 1-2-3-4-5-1-2-3-4-5 ladder
Core B: 1-2-3-4-5-1-2-3-4-5 ladder

Metabolic conditioning

Two to three rounds of the following complex:

15 double swings
15 double snatches
15 double cleans and military presses (one double clean between each double press)
15 front squats
15 push-ups

Day 90 — Off and Done!

Don't forget to take your final progress pictures!

Appendix

Metric Conversion Guide

· ·

*T*he first tables in this appendix show you metric conversions for volume, weight, and temperature. Use them if you need to convert a recipe, but remember that these are approximate, and results could vary.

Note: The recipes in this book weren't developed or tested using metric measurements. There may be some variation in quality when converting to metric units.

Volume		
U.S. Units	*Canadian Metric*	*Australian Metric*
¼ teaspoon	1 milliliter	1 milliliter
½ teaspoon	2 milliliters	2 milliliters
1 teaspoon	5 milliliters	5 milliliters
1 tablespoon	15 milliliters	20 milliliters
¼ cup	50 milliliters	60 milliliters
⅓ cup	75 milliliters	80 milliliters
½ cup	125 milliliters	125 milliliters
⅔ cup	150 milliliters	170 milliliters
¾ cup	175 milliliters	190 milliliters
1 cup	250 milliliters	250 milliliters
1 quart	1 liter	1 liter
1½ quarts	1.5 liters	1.5 liters
2 quarts	2 liters	2 liters
2½ quarts	2.5 liters	2.5 liters
3 quarts	3 liters	3 liters
4 quarts (1 gallon)	4 liters	4 liters

Weight

U.S. Units	Canadian Metric	Australian Metric
1 ounce	30 grams	30 grams
2 ounces	55 grams	60 grams
3 ounces	85 grams	90 grams
4 ounces (¼ pound)	115 grams	125 grams
8 ounces (½ pound)	225 grams	225 grams
16 ounces (1 pound)	455 grams	500 grams (½ kilogram)

Length

Inches	Centimeters
0.5	1.5
1	2.5
2	5.0
3	7.5
4	10.0
5	12.5
6	15.0
7	17.5
8	20.5
9	23.0
10	25.5
11	28.0
12	30.5

Temperature (Degrees)

Fahrenheit	Celsius
32	0
212	100
250	120
275	140

Fahrenheit	Celsius
300	150
325	160
350	180
375	190
400	200
425	220
450	230
475	240
500	260

Although we spell out measurements in this book, many cookbooks use abbreviations. The following table lists common abbreviations and what they stand for.

Common Abbreviations

Abbreviation(s)	What It Stands For
cm	Centimeter
C., c.	Cup
G, g	Gram
kg	Kilogram
L, l	Liter
lb.	Pound
mL, ml	Milliliter
oz.	Ounce
pt.	Pint
t., tsp.	Teaspoon
T., Tb., Tbsp.	Tablespoon

Index

Numerics

2-plus-1 rule, 132
21-Day Primal Quick Start Program
  day-by-day program, 455–459
  overview, 448
  warm-up for, 449–453
30-Day Reset
  body cleansing from, 55–56
  breaking habits, 55
  guidelines for, 60–61
  journaling, 61–62
  overview, 54
  planning for, 56–57
80/20 rule, 98
80-percent rule, 23
90-Day Primal Body Transformation
  day-by-day program, 465–480
  metabolic conditioning, 464
  overview, 459–460
  strength exercise routine, 461–463
  warm-up for, 464–465
  weekly schedule, 465

• A •

abbreviations, 483
abdominal exercises
  four-point plank, 397
  general discussion, 396
  hanging knee raise, 401–402
  hanging leg raise, 403–405
  two-point plank, 402–403
  V-up, 397–399
  windmill, 399–400
  windshield wiper, 405–406
acesulfame-K, 131
acid-base balance. *See* pH balance
acne, 15, 53
acorn squash, 35
acute inflammation, 17
adenosine triphosphate (ATP), 437
aerobics, 104, 437
after-burn effect, 438
agave, 41, 308
agriculture, 10, 12
albacore, 207
alcohol, 45–46, 127
allergies, 18, 52–53, 110
almond flour, 82
almond meal, 38
almond milk, 82
almonds
  Almond Banana Pancakes, 150
  Almond Cookies with Cinnamon Glaze, 310–311
  Brussels Sprouts with Cranberries and Almonds, 241
  omega-6 fatty acids in, 72
  Roasted Rosemary Almonds, 262
Alzheimer's disease
  C-reactive protein and, 110
  exercise and, 29
  turmeric and, 296
amaranth, 39
anaerobic, defined, 437
anaphylaxis, 52
ancestor diet, 9, 10
antidepressant, 29
antinutrient, 39, 69
antioxidant, 44, 80
Anytime Waffles, 152
apigenin, 296
apple
  Classic Apple Crisp, 315
  Nutty Fruit Stackers, 274
  Waldorf Tuna Salad, 183
  "yes" foods, 37
apricot, 37, 222
arrowroot powder, 82
arteriosclerosis, 110
arthritis, 18, 52, 53
artichoke, 26, 35, 82
artificial sweetener, 41, 76, 131, 308
arugula, 35
asparagus
  cellular damage protection, 26
  complex carbohydrates, 74
  "yes" foods, 35
aspartame, 41, 131, 308
asthma, 18, 29

ATP (adenosine triphosphate), 437

attention deficit disorder, 53

autoimmune disease, 18, 36, 53

avocado
  Avocado and Egg Salad, 177
  Avocado Chocolate Bread, 328
  Avocado Cups, 268
  Cucumber Avocado Salsa, 293
  Kale with a Kick Salad, 176
  monosaturated fat from, 81
  Smooth and Creamy Avocado Dressing, 283
  snacks, 122
  "yes" foods, 37

• B •

bacon
  Bacon Butternut Squash Soup, 169
  Chocolate Bacon Brownie Muffins, 323
  Club Sandwich Salad, 195
  Coconut Curry Chowder, 164–165
  healthy fats for kids, 134
  Kale with a Kick Salad, 176
  Kalua Shredded Pork, 216
  Maple Bacon Ice Cream, 329
  Meatloaf, 220
  Sautéed Kale with Bacon and Mushrooms, 252

baking, 84

banana
  Almond Banana Pancakes, 150
  Banana Cacao Muffins, 322
  fruit consumption considerations, 44
  Mini Cinnamon Pancakes, 149
  Morning Honey Muffins, 151
  "yes" foods, 37

barley, 39

Basil and Walnut Pesto, 292

BBQ
  Barbecue-Flavored Kale Chips, 248
  Slow Cooker BBQ Pulled Pork, 215
  Tangy BBQ Sauce, 290

beans, 40, 118

bear crawl (exercise), 452

beef
  Beef Bone Broth, 211
  cellular damage protection, 26
  choosing, 78
  Hearty Chili, 174
  jerky, 82, 123, 246
  Leafy Tacos, 192
  Machacado and Eggs, 148
  Meatball Poppers, 266
  Meatloaf, 220
  Orange Shrimp and Beef with Broccoli, 194
  quality of, 189–190
  "yes" foods, 35

beer, 46

beets, 35, 134

belief system, changing, 22

bell pepper, 35

bench press, 369–371, 431

BIA (bioelectrical impedance), 107

biotin, 45

bison, 35

Bisphenol A (BPA), 83

black beans, 40, 118

black pepper, 295

blackberries, 37

blind measurements, 54

bloat, 14, 53

blood pressure, 108, 296

blood sugar
  cinnamon and, 296
  as health marker, 108–109
  misconceptions, 22
  Paleo impact on, 16–17

blueberries
  Berries and Whipped Coconut Cream, 332–333
  Blueberry Espresso Brownies, 326
  cellular damage protection, 26
  Frozen Blueberry Breakfast Bars, 154–155
  fruit consumption considerations, 44
  Lime-Blueberry Poppy Seed Coffee Cake, 153
  "yes" foods, 37

body composition, 106–107

bodyweight complex (exercises), 441–443

bodyweight row (exercise), 377–378

bodyweight squat
    (exercise), 354–355
bok choy, 35
bottoms-up carry
    (exercise), 394–396
bourbon, 46
box jump, 418–419
BPA (Bisphenol A), 83
braising, 84–85, 121
brazil nuts, 72
bread
    Avocado Chocolate
        Bread, 328
    Chocolate Zucchini
        Bread, 327
    "no" foods, 76
breakfast
    Almond Banana
        Pancakes, 150
    Anytime Waffles, 152
    Breakfast Sausage
        Scramble, 143
    Eggs in Spicy Tomato
        Sauce, 145
    Frozen Blueberry
        Breakfast Bars,
        154–155
    general discussion,
        139–140
    Grilled Eggs with
        Homemade Chorizo,
        146–147
    Huevos Rancheros, 142
    Lime-Blueberry Poppy
        Seed Coffee Cake, 153
    Machacado and Eggs, 148
    Mini Cinnamon
        Pancakes, 149
    Morning Honey Muffins,
        151
    Pizza Frittata, 141
    Thai Rolled Omelet, 144
breathing, 94–95

broad beans, 40
broad jump (exercise),
    415–416
broccoli
    complex carbohydrates,
        74
    Creamy Spiced Broccoli,
        238
    Curried Cream of
        Broccoli Soup, 167
    Italian Broccoli, 239
    Orange Shrimp and Beef
        with Broccoli, 194
    "yes" foods, 35
broiling, 121
broth
    Beef Bone Broth, 211
    Chicken Fennel Soup, 168
    Coconut Curry Chowder,
        164–165
    Deep Healing Chicken
        Broth, 161
    Hearty Chili, 174
    Immune-Building
        Vegetable Broth,
        162–163
    Provençal Veggie Soup,
        170
    Teriyaki-Turkey Meatball
        Soup, 172
    Thai Butternut Squash
        Soup, 173
    Tomato Fennel Soup, 171
    Turkey Spinach Soup,
        166
    "yes" foods, 38, 82
brown sugar, 41, 308
brownies
    Blueberry Espresso
        Brownies, 326
    Lemon Brownies with
        Coconut Lemon Glaze,
        324–325

Brussels sprouts
    Brussels Sprouts with
        Cranberries and
        Almonds, 241
    complex carbohydrates,
        74
    "yes" foods, 35
buckwheat, 39
bulgur, 39
butter
    clarified, 2, 37, 41, 81, 277
    grass-fed, 2, 134
    substitutions for, 128
butternut squash
    Bacon Butternut Squash
        Soup, 169
    healthy carbs for kids,
        134
    Thai Butternut Squash
        Soup, 173
    "yes" foods, 35

● C ●

cabbage
    calcium sources, 68
    Classic Cole Slaw, 188
    complex carbohydrates,
        74
    Easy Chicken Curry with
        Cabbage, 223
    Kimchi, 242
    "yes" foods, 35
calcium, 68
calcium caseinate/
    glutamate, 159
calories, 47–48
cancer
    C-reactive protein and,
        110
    in hunter-gatherer
        societies, 13
    turmeric and, 296

canola oil, 42, 73
cantaloupe, 37
car cooler, 123–124
carbazole alkaloids, 296
carbohydrates
  effects of transformation, 58, 114
  foundational foods for Paleo and, 9
  for kids, 134
  macronutrient sufficiency, 51
  in Paleo Big Three, 70, 74–75
  possible pitfalls, 114
  science behind Paleo, 13
cardiovascular disease, 8, 18
cardiovascular exercise, 432–434, 439
carrageenan, 159
carrot
  Bacon Butternut Squash Soup, 169
  Classic Cole Slaw, 188
  healthy carbs for kids, 134
  Immune-Building Vegetable Broth, 162–163
  Provençal Veggie Soup, 170
  Tangy Carrot and Ginger Salad Dressing, 282
  Vegetable Latkes, 243
  Vietnamese Cucumber Salad, 185
  "yes" foods, 35
carrying exercises
  bottoms-up carry, 394–396
  farmer's carry, 389–390

overview, 101–102, 387–389
racked carry, 392–393
strength exercise routine, 461–463
strength training, 431
two-arm waiter's carry, 393–394
waiter's carry, 391–392
cashews, 72, 185, 278
cassava, 134
cauliflower
  Cauliflower Rice, 234
  Cocoa Cauliflower, 235
  complex carbohydrates, 74
  Mashed Cauliflower, 233
  "yes" foods, 35
cayenne
  healing powers of, 296
  Teriyaki-Turkey Meatball Soup, 172
celery
  Immune-Building Vegetable Broth, 162–163
  Provençal Veggie Soup, 170
  "yes" foods, 35
celiac disease, 18, 157
cells, healthy, 51
cereal, 76, 140
chaconine, 41
Champagne, 127
Cheater Pork Stew, 217
cheese, 40
cheesecake, 254–255
cherries, 37
chi, 28
chicken
  Chicken Cacciatora, 213
  Chicken Fennel Soup, 168

Chicken Fingers, 193
Chinese Chicken Salad, 186–187
choosing, 78
Club Sandwich Salad, 195
Curried Chicken Salad, 179
Deep Healing Chicken Broth, 161
Easy Chicken Curry with Cabbage, 223
Mango and Fennel Chicken Salad, 180
Mango Coconut Chipotle Chicken, 214
Pineapple and Mango Sweet Heat Chicken Wings, 219
Slow Cooker Moroccan Apricot Chicken, 222
Tandoori Chicken Thighs, 199
Thai Butternut Squash Soup, 173
Thai Green Curry Chicken, 198
"yes" foods, 35
chickpeas, 40
children
  packed lunches, 245–246
  portions for, 134–135
  teaching about Paleo, 129–130
  treats for, 130–132
children-friendly recipes
  Barbecue-Flavored Kale Chips, 248
  Lunchbox Stuffed Peppers, 250
  Parsnip Hash Browns, 251
  Raspberry Cheesecake Bites, 254–255

Raspberry Peppermint Sorbet, 253

Sautéed Kale with Bacon and Mushrooms, 252

Spiced Sweet Potato Fries, 247

Star Fruit Magic Wands, 256

chile pepper

Grilled Eggs with Homemade Chorizo, 146–147

Hearty Chili, 174

"yes" foods, 35

Chinese Chicken Salad, 186–187

chin-up, 378–379

chipotle, 214

chiropractic treatment

30-Day Reset and, 57

importance of, 31

stress relief through, 28

chocolate

Avocado Chocolate Bread, 328

Chocolate Bacon Brownie Muffins, 323

Chocolate Chip Cookie Dough Granola Bars, 314

Chocolate Ice Cream, 330

Chocolate Zucchini Bread, 327

Chocolate-Strawberry Crumble Bars, 316

Cinnamon Chocolate Chip Muffins with Honey Frosting, 320–321

Coconut Chocolate Chip Cookies, 313

OMG Chocolate Chip Cookies, 312

purchasing, 127

Raspberry Cheesecake Bites, 254–255

"yes" foods, 83

cholesterol

eggs and, 45

exercise and, 29

as health marker, 110–112

choline, 45

Chopped Salad with Tahini Dressing, 184

chronic disease, 8

chronic fatigue syndrome, 36

chronic inflammation, 17–18

Cilantro Vinaigrette, 286

cinnamon

Almond Cookies with Cinnamon Glaze, 310–311

Cinnamon Chocolate Chip Muffins with Honey Frosting, 320–321

Cocoa-Cinnamon Coconut Chips, 273

healing powers of, 26, 296

Mini Cinnamon Pancakes, 149

citrate, 159

citric acid, 159

Citrus Carnitas, 197

CLA (conjugated linoleic acid), 190

clarified butter

dairy products and, 41

overview, 81

recipe for, 277

smoke point for, 87

substitutions, 2

"yes" foods, 37

Classic Apple Crisp, 315

Classic Cole Slaw, 188

Classic Stir-Fry Sauce, 281

clean (exercise), 347–348

clean grip, 359

clementine, 37

Club Sandwich Salad, 195

cocktail, 127

Cocoa Cauliflower, 235

Cocoa-Cinnamon Coconut Chips, 273

coconut

Berries and Whipped Coconut Cream, 332–333

choosing fats, 81

Coco-Mango Ice Cream, 331

Coconut Chocolate Chip Cookies, 313

Coconut Curry Chowder, 164–165

Coconut Shrimp with Sweet and Spicy Sauce, 203

flavoring of, 38

Lemon Brownies with Coconut Lemon Glaze, 324–325

Orange Coconut Marinade, 291

"yes" foods, 37

coconut aminos, 38

coconut flour, 38, 82

coconut milk, 82, 134

coconut sugar, 41

coffee, 38, 83, 326

cole slaw, 188

colitis, 157

complex (exercise)

bodyweight complex, 441–443

complex (exercise)
  (continued)
  kettlebell complex,
    443–446
  overview, 440–441
complex carbohydrates,
    70, 74–75
condiments
  Cooked Olive Oil Mayo,
    288
  Cucumber Avocado
    Salsa, 293
  homemade, 275–276
  Mark's Daily Apple
    Ketchup, 289
  Olive Oil Mayo, 287
  Tangy BBQ Sauce, 290
conditioning, 103–104
conjugated linoleic acid
    (CLA), 190
contralateral movement,
    452
conversion tables, 481–483
Cooked Olive Oil Mayo,
    288
cookies
  Almond Cookies with
    Cinnamon Glaze,
    310–311
  Chocolate Chip Cookie
    Dough Granola Bars,
    314
  Coconut Chocolate Chip
    Cookies, 313
  Cranberry Ginger
    Cookies, 309
  OMG Chocolate Chip
    Cookies, 312
cooking
  lack of experience in, 118
  methods of, 84–86, 121
  smoke point and, 86–87

corn, 39
corn oil, 42, 73
corn syrup, 41, 308
cortisol, 27
cost of eating Paleo, 117
cottonseed oil, 42, 73
crab, 181
cramps, 52, 53
cranberries
  Brussels Sprouts with
    Cranberries and
    Almonds, 241
  Cranberry Ginger
    Cookies, 309
  fruit consumption
    considerations, 44
  Pumpkin Cranberry
    Scones, 317
  "yes" foods, 37
cravings
  food sensitivities and, 53
  indulgence versus, 129
  journaling, 61
  possible pitfalls, 114–115
  30-Day Reset and, 55
crawling warm-up
    (exercise), 451–453
C-reactive protein,
    109–110
cream, 40, 128
Creamy Baked Scallops,
    204
Creamy Red Shrimp and
    Tomato Curry, 224
Creamy Spiced Broccoli,
    238
Crispy Kale Chips, 261
crocodile breathing, 95
Crohn's disease, 18, 157
cucumber
  Cucumber Avocado
    Salsa, 293

  Lemon Cucumber
    Noodles with Cumin,
    244
  Vietnamese Cucumber
    Salad, 185
  "yes" foods, 35
curcumin, 296
curry
  Coconut Curry Chowder,
    164–165
  Creamy Red Shrimp and
    Tomato Curry, 224
  Curried Chicken Salad,
    179
  Curried Cream of
    Broccoli Soup, 167
  Easy Chicken Curry with
    Cabbage, 223
  healing powers of, 296
  Sri Lankan Curry Sauce,
    280
  Thai Green Curry
    Chicken, 198
  "yes" foods, 38

• D •

dairy products
  calcium and, 68
  misconceptions about, 22
  "no" foods, 40–41
  Paleo pyramid and, 69
date, fresh, 37
dead lift
  single-leg, 341–343
  standard, 339–341
  strength training, 431
Deep Healing Chicken
    Broth, 161
deli meat, 79, 122
depression
  exercise and, 29

food sensitivities and, 53
impact of diet, 8
overtraining and, 105
turmeric and, 296
detox organs, 55
deviled eggs, 263
dextrose, 41
diabetes
  chronic inflammation
    and, 18
  C-reactive protein and,
    110
  impact of diet, 8
  turmeric and, 296
diet
  ancestor, 10
  body design and, 10–11
  lifestyle versus, 8–9
dietary fat, 110
digestion
  exercise and, 29
  foods body is designed
    to eat, 9
  ginger and, 296
  impact of diet, 8
  intestinal changes from
    Paleo, 15
dip (exercise), 372
disease. See also names of
    specific diseases
  cancer, 13
  prevalence of, 13
  stress and, 26
double jerk (exercise),
    420–421
double snatch (exercise),
    422–423
dressings
  Cilantro Vinaigrette, 286
  Cooked Olive Oil Mayo,
    288
  general discussion,
    275–276

Mark's Daily Apple
    Ketchup, 289
Olive Oil Mayo, 287
Orange Coconut
    Marinade, 291
Paleo Ranch Dressing,
    284
Smooth and Creamy
    Avocado Dressing, 283
Sweet and Spicy
    Vinaigrette, 285
Tangy BBQ Sauce, 290
Tangy Carrot and Ginger
    Salad Dressing, 282
drinks, 83
duck, 35
Dukkah, 301
dynamometer, 108

• E •

eczema, 15
edamame, 40, 118
EFT (Emotional Freedom
    Techniques), 28
eggplant
  complex carbohydrates,
    74
  Spicy Stuffed Eggplant,
    201
  "yes" foods, 35
eggs
  Almond Banana
    Pancakes, 150
  Anytime Waffles, 152
  Avocado and Egg Salad,
    177
  Breakfast Sausage
    Scramble, 143
  cholesterol and, 45
  choosing, 71, 79
  Eggs in Spicy Tomato
    Sauce, 145

fats for kids, 134
food allergens, 53
Grilled Eggs with
    Homemade Chorizo,
    146–147
Huevos Rancheros, 142
Lime-Blueberry Poppy
    Seed Coffee Cake, 153
Machacado and Eggs,
    148
Mini Cinnamon
    Pancakes, 149
misconceptions about,
    22
Morning Honey Muffins,
    151
packed lunches, 246
Pizza Frittata, 141
portion size, 49
Southwest Deviled Eggs,
    263
Thai Rolled Omelet, 144
as travel snack, 122–123
Tuscan Spinach Salad,
    178
"yes" foods, 35
80/20 rule, 98
80-percent rule, 23
electrical charge of food,
    51
electrosmog, 25
elk, 35
EMFs (electromagnetic
    fields), 25–26
Emotional Freedom
    Techniques (EFT), 28
endive, 35
endorphins, 29
energy
  electrical, 51
  forces in body, 28
  sleep cycles and, 16
epigenetics, 20–21

EPOC (exercise post oxygen consumption), 438

Equal, 41, 131

escarole, 35

essential fat, 72

eustress, 26

Everything Seafood Seasoning, 299

exercise
 bench press, 369–371
 benefits of, 29
 blood pressure and, 108
 blood sugar and, 108–109
 bodyweight row, 377–378
 bodyweight squat, 354–355
 bottoms-up carry, 394–396
 box jump, 418–419
 breathing, 94–95
 broad jump, 415–416
 cardiovascular, 432–434
 carrying, 101–102, 387–389
 chin-up, 378–379
 chiropractic treatment and, 31
 cholesterol levels and, 110–112
 clean, 347–348
 conditioning, 103–104
 crawling warm-up, 451–453
 C-reactive protein and, 109–110
 dead lift, 339–341
 dip, 372
 double jerk, 420–421
 double snatch, 422–423
 efficiency versus effectiveness, 104–105

farmer's carry, 389–390

formula for burning fat, 439

four-point plank, 397

front squat, 359–360

goblet lunge, 355–356

goblet squat, 352–353

handstand push-up, 373–375

hanging knee raise, 401–402

hanging leg raise, 403–405

hinging, 99–100, 337–339

intensity of, 30–31

jerk, 417–418

journaling, 62

L-sit pull-up/chin-up, 382–383

military press, 367–368

modern-day living and, 30–31

movement versus, 94

muscle-up, 383–385

one-arm chin-up, 385–386

one-arm one-leg push-up, 373–374

one-arm push-up, 368–370

one-arm row, 380

one-arm swing, 345–346

overtraining, 105–106

pistol squat, 360–361

principles of Paleo, 19

pulling, 99, 375–376

pull-up, 381–382

push press, 413–414

pushing, 98–99, 363–365

push-up, 365–367

racked carry, 392–393

racked lunge, 358

racked squat, 356–357

rolling warm-up, 449–451

single-leg dead lift, 341–343

snatch, 349–350

squatting, 100–101, 350–352

strength, 90–93, 431–432

stress relief through, 28

swing, 343–345

30-Day Reset, 57, 59

thruster, 444

Turkish get-up, 406–410

two-arm waiter's carry, 393–394

two-point plank, 402–403

V-up, 397–399

waiter's carry, 391–392

walking and sprinting, 102

windmill, 399–400

windshield wiper, 405–406

exercise post oxygen consumption (EPOC), 438

exercise program
 body composition marker, 106–107
 bodyweight complex, 441–443
 complexes, 440–441
 developing, 435–436
 health markers for, 106
 heavy lifting, 454–455
 identifying motivators, 96
 kettlebell complex, 443–446
 90-Day Primal Body Transformation, 459–460, 465–480

repetitions, 454
setting goals, 97
simplicity of, 19–20
strength exercise
      routine, 461–463
strength marker, 107–108
21-Day Primal Quick Start
      Program, 448, 455–459
warm-up for, 449–453

• F •

family
   convincing significant
      other, 135
   lack of support from, 117
   managing meals, 132–135
   teaching kids, 129–130
   treats for kids, 130–132
farm to table, 120
farmer's carry (exercise),
      389–390
fasting, 434
fasting insulin test,
      108–109
fat
   calcium sources, 68
   choosing, 81
   considerations for, 43–44
   exercise formula for
      burning, 439
   for kids, 134
   macronutrient
      sufficiency, 51
   misconceptions about, 22
   naturally occurring, 9,
      73–74
   omega-6 to omega-3
      ratio, 72–73
   in Paleo Big Three, 70
   portion size, 50
   smoke point of, 86–87

stress and, 27
trans fats, 42
unhealthy, 73
weight loss and, 14
"yes" foods, 37
fatigue
   carb flu, 114
   food sensitivities and, 53
   impact of diet, 8
   overtraining and, 105
   pH of body, 52
fennel
   Chicken Fennel Soup,
      168
   Mango and Fennel
      Chicken Salad, 180
   Tomato Fennel Soup, 171
fertility, 8
fiber
   foundational foods for
      Paleo and, 9
   in Paleo pyramid, 67
   weight loss and, 15
fibromyalgia, 36
fig, fresh, 37
finger food, 126
fish
   choosing, 71, 79
   food allergens, 53
   Macadamia Nut Crusted
      Mahi-Mahi, 206
   Olive-Oil Braised
      Albacore, 207
   omega-6 to omega-3
      ratio, 72
   purchasing, 191
   Salmon a L'Afrique du
      Nord, 208
   slow cooking, 210
   "yes" foods, 35
fitness. See exercise
Flame Out Blend, 304

flavoring, 38
flax milk, 82, 134
flour, 38, 76, 82, 128
food
   allergies, 52–53
   effects of stress on
      choices, 27
   foundation for Paleo, 9
   portions, 47–50
   sensitivity to, 52–53
four-point plank, 397
frankenfoods, 77, 119, 191
French fries, 231, 247
Fried Sage Leaves, 265
frittata, 141
front squat, 359–360
Frozen Blueberry
      Breakfast Bars,
      154–155
fruit
   considerations for, 36, 44
   foundational foods for
      Paleo, 9
   misconceptions about, 22
   portion size, 49
   portion size for kids, 134
   as travel snack, 122–123
   "yes" foods, 36–37
Fudge Bombs, 272
functional movements, 30
functional training, 396

• G •

Garam Masala, 302
garbanzo beans, 40
garlic
   cellular damage
      protection, 26
   Immune-Building
      Vegetable Broth,
      162–163

garlic *(continued)*
  Provençal Veggie Soup, 170
  Thai Butternut Squash Soup, 173
  "yes" foods, 35
genetics
  change over time, 12
  epigenetics, 20–21
ghee. *See* clarified butter
gin, 46, 127
ginger
  Coconut Curry Chowder, 164–165
  Cranberry Ginger Cookies, 309
  Ginger-Fried Pears, 271
  healing powers of, 296
  Tangy Carrot and Ginger Salad Dressing, 282
  Watermelon Soup, 175
glucose, 70
glutamate, 159
gluten
  ingredients indicating presence of, 158–159
  "no" foods, 39
  restaurant eating, 120
glycolytic pathway, 437
goals, fitness, 97
goat, 35
goblet lunge (exercise), 355–356
goblet squat (exercise), 352–353
grain
  alcohol from, 46
  misconceptions, 22
  "no" foods, 39
  Paleo pyramid and, 69
  science behind Paleo, 13
granola, 76, 314
grapefruit, 37

grapes, 37
grass-fed meat, 78, 190
green beans, 35, 68
Gremolata, 304
grilling
  defined, 86
  eating in restaurant, 121
  Grilled Buffalo Shrimp, 202
  Grilled Eggs with Homemade Chorizo, 146–147
  Grilled Spiced Peaches, 270
  Grilling Spice Rub, 297
guacamole, 134
guava, 37

• *H* •

half-and-half, 40
handstand push-up (exercise), 373–375
hanging knee raise (exercise), 401–402
hanging leg raise (exercise), 403–405
hash browns, 251
hazelnuts, 72
HCAs (heterocyclic amines), 86
HDL (high-density lipoprotein), 111
headache
  carb flu, 114
  migraine, 53
  pH of body, 52
health
  diet plans lacking, 8
  impact of diet, 7
  weight loss through, 21
health markers
  blood pressure, 108

blood sugar, 108–109
body composition, 106–107
cholesterol levels, 110–112
C-reactive protein, 109–110
pH balance, 112
strength, 107–108
heart disease, 110, 296
Hearty Chili, 174
hemoglobin A1C test, 108–109
heterocyclic amines (HCAs), 86
high pull (exercise), 349
high-density lipoprotein (HDL), 111
high-fructose corn syrup, 41, 131, 308
hinging exercises
  benefits of, 339
  clean, 347–348
  dead lift, 339–341
  one-arm swing, 345–346
  overview, 99–100, 337–338
  single-leg dead lift, 341–343
  snatch, 349–350
  strength exercise routine, 461–463
  swing, 343–345
holiday eating
  alcohol, 127
  menu planning, 126–127
  recipe substitution, 128
hollow position, 398
honey
  Cinnamon Chocolate Chip Muffins with Honey Frosting, 320–321

Frozen Blueberry Breakfast Bars, 154–155
Morning Honey Muffins, 151
"no" foods, 41
honeydew melon, 37
HPP (hydrolyzed plant protein), 158
Huevos Rancheros, 142
hunter-gatherer, 10, 12, 13
HVP (hydrolyzed vegetable protein), 158
hypertension, 108
hyperventilation, 95

● I ●

IBD (inflammatory bowel disease), 157
IBS (irritable bowel syndrome), 53, 157
ice cream
  Chocolate Ice Cream, 330
  Coco-Mango Ice Cream, 331
  Maple Bacon Ice Cream, 329
  "no" foods, 40
Immune-Building Vegetable Broth, 162–163
immunity, 227
indulgence, 128–129
Industrial Revolution, 10, 12
inflammation
  C-reactive protein and, 109–110
  Paleo impact on, 17–18
  pH of body, 52

inflammatory bowel disease (IBD), 157
insulin
  complex carbohydrates and, 74
  fasting insulin test, 108–109
  sugar cycle and, 43
intensity, exercise, 30–31
intestines
  30-Day Reset and, 55
  Paleo impact on, 15
irritable bowel syndrome (IBS), 53, 157
Italian Broccoli, 239
Italian Seasoning, 300

● J ●

jalapeño pepper
  Coconut Shrimp with Sweet and Spicy Sauce, 203
  Hearty Chili, 174
  Pineapple and Mango Sweet Heat Chicken Wings, 219
  Vietnamese Cucumber Salad, 185
  "yes" foods, 35
jerk (exercise), 417–418
jerky, beef, 82, 246
jicama, 36, 134

● K ●

kale
  Barbecue-Flavored Kale Chips, 248
  calcium sources, 68
  complex carbohydrates, 74

Creamy Kale, 230
Crispy Kale Chips, 261
Kale with a Kick Salad, 176
Sautéed Kale with Bacon and Mushrooms, 252
Sesame Kale, 229
"yes" foods, 36
Kalua Shredded Pork, 216
kefir, 118
ketchup, 289
kettlebell complex, 443–446
kidneys, 55
Kimchi, 242
kitchen
  choosing fats, 81
  choosing proteins, 78–79
  choosing vegetables, 79–80
  cleaning out non-Paleo foods, 75–77
  spices, 80–81
  stocking pantry, 82–83
kiwi, 37
kohlrabi
  healthy carbs for kids, 134
  Sautéed Kohlrabi, 240
  "yes" foods, 36
kumquat, 37

● L ●

lamb
  purchasing, 78
  Slow-Roasted Rack of Lamb, 200
  "yes" foods, 35
LDL (low-density lipoprotein), 111
Leafy Tacos, 192

leaky gut, 15, 157
lecithin, 45
lectins, 65
leeks
  Curried Cream of
    Broccoli Soup, 167
  Provençal Veggie Soup,
    170
  "yes" foods, 36
leftovers, 246
legumes, 40
lemon, 37, 244, 324–325
lemongrass, 173
length conversion, 482
lentils, 40, 118
lettuce, 36, 192
lifestyle
  80-percent rule, 23
  body design and, 10–11
  diet versus, 8–9
  EMF exposure, 25–26
  exposure to outdoors,
    24
  mind-set, 24–25
  Paleo as, 21
  roadblocks to, 115–118
  sleep quality, 23
  socialization, 23–24
  stress, minimizing,
    26–28
lima beans, 40
lime, 37, 153
liver, 55
loaded carry (exercise),
    387
long-cycle jerk (exercise),
    420
low-density lipoprotein
    (LDL), 111
L-sit pull-up/chin-up
    (exercise), 382–383

Lunchbox Stuffed
    Peppers, 250
lunge exercises
  goblet lunge, 355–356
  racked lunge, 358
lungs, 55
lychee, 37

● *M* ●

macadamia nuts, 72, 206
Machacado and Eggs, 148
macronutrients
  foundational foods for
    Paleo and, 9
  Paleo Big Three, 69–70
mad cow disease (MCD),
    190
magnesium glutamate, 159
mahi-mahi, 206
main dishes. *See also* slow
    cooking
  Chicken Fingers, 193
  Citrus Carnitas, 197
  Club Sandwich Salad, 195
  Coconut Shrimp with
    Sweet and Spicy
    Sauce, 203
  Creamy Baked Scallops,
    204
  Grilled Buffalo Shrimp,
    202
  Leafy Tacos, 192
  Macadamia Nut Crusted
    Mahi-Mahi, 206
  Olive-Oil Braised
    Albacore, 207
  Orange Shrimp and Beef
    with Broccoli, 194
  Roasted Oysters, 205
  Salmon a L'Afrique du
    Nord, 208

Slow-Roasted Rack of
    Lamb, 200
  Spicy Stuffed Eggplant,
    201
  Tandoori Chicken
    Thighs, 199
  Thai Green Curry
    Chicken, 198
  Winter Squash and
    Sausage Hash, 196
maltodextrin, 41, 158, 159,
    308
mandarin orange, 37
mango
  Coco-Mango Ice Cream,
    331
  fruit consumption
    considerations, 44
  Mango and Fennel
    Chicken Salad, 180
  Mango Coconut Chipotle
    Chicken, 214
  Pineapple and Mango
    Sweet Heat Chicken
    Wings, 219
  Tropical Mango Parfait,
    269
  Watermelon Soup, 175
  "yes" foods, 37
maple syrup, 41, 83, 329
margarine, 42, 73
marinade, 291
Mark's Daily Apple
    Ketchup, 289
massage
  stress relief through, 28
  30-Day Reset and, 57
mayonnaise
  Cooked Olive Oil Mayo,
    288
  Olive Oil Mayo, 287

MCD (mad cow disease), 190

meat
  browning, 210
  cellular damage protection, 26
  choosing, 71
  foundational foods for Paleo, 9
  Grilling Spice Rub, 297
  Meatball Poppers, 266
  Meatloaf, 220
  misconceptions about, 22
  quality of, 189–190
  Succulent Steak Seasoning, 298
  "yes" foods, 35

MED (minimum effective dose), 106

medication, 17, 29

meditation
  stress relief through, 28
  30-Day Reset and, 57

melon, 37, 44

menstruation, 8

metabolic conditioning
  benefits of, 438
  complexes, 440
  defined, 426
  formula for burning fat, 439
  improving, 455
  90-Day Primal Body Transformation and, 464
  overview, 437–438
  results in first 15 minutes, 439–440

metabolic pathways, 437

metric measurements, 481–483

migraine headache, 53

military press, 367–368

milk
  almond, 82
  calcium and, 68
  coconut, 82, 134
  flax, 82, 134
  food allergens, 53
  "no" foods, 40
  soy, 119
  substitutions for, 128

millet, 39

mind-set, 24–25

Mini Cinnamon Pancakes, 149

minimum effective dose (MED), 106

mint, 175

miso, 40

modified food starch, 158

molasses, 41

monoammonium glutamate, 159

monopotassium glutamate, 159

monosodium glutamate (MSG), 158, 159–160

monounsaturated fat (MUFA), 73

Morning Honey Muffins, 151

Morning Spice, 303

Moroccan Dipping Sauce, 279

movement, 93–94

MSG (monosodium glutamate), 158, 159–160

MUFA (monounsaturated fat), 73

muffins
  Banana Cacao Muffins, 322
  Chocolate Bacon Brownie Muffins, 323
  Cinnamon Chocolate Chip Muffins with Honey Frosting, 320–321
  Morning Honey Muffins, 151
  Pumpkin Pie Muffins, 318

multiple sclerosis, 36

mung beans, 40

muscle-up (exercise), 383–385

mushrooms
  Sautéed Kale with Bacon and Mushrooms, 252
  Winter Squash and Sausage Hash, 196

"yes" foods, 36

• N •

natrium glutamate, 159

natto, 118

natural fat, 73–74

navy beans, 40

negative affirmations, 25

nightshade food, 36

90-Day Primal Body Transformation
  day-by-day program, 465–480
  metabolic conditioning, 464
  overview, 459–460
  strength exercise routine, 461–463
  warm-up for, 464–465
  weekly schedule, 465

"no" foods
  30-Day Reset and, 60
  dairy products, 40–41
  grains and gluten, 39
  legumes, 40
  oils, 42
  potatoes, 41

"no" foods *(continued)*
  processed foods, 40
  sugar, 41
nori
  cellular damage
    protection, 26
  Seaweed with a Kick,
    267
  "yes" foods, 36
NutraSweet, 41, 131
nutrition
  density of, 157
  Paleo pyramid, 66–69
  sufficiency through,
    50–51
  USDA Food Guide
    Pyramid, 64–66
nuts
  calcium sources, 68
  choosing fats, 81
  fats for kids, 134
  food allergens, 53
  foundational foods for
    Paleo, 9
  Nutty Fruit Stackers, 274
  omega-6 to omega-3
    ratio, 72
  as travel snack, 123
  "yes" foods, 37

• O •

oats, 39, 76
oils
  choosing fats, 81
  "no" foods, 42
  olive oil, 26, 37, 207,
    287–288
  smoke point of, 86–87
  substitutions for, 128
  types of, 42, 73
okra, 36
olive, 81, 82

olive oil
  cellular damage
    protection, 26
  Cooked Olive Oil Mayo,
    288
  Olive Oil Mayo, 287
  Olive-Oil Braised
    Albacore, 207
  "yes" foods, 37
omega-6 to omega-3 fatty
    acid ratio, 72–73, 190
omelet, 144
OMG Chocolate Chip
    Cookies, 312
one-arm chin-up, 385–386
one-arm one-leg push-up,
    373–374
one-arm push-up, 368–370
one-arm row, 380
one-arm swing, 345–346
onion. *See also* shallots
  complex carbohydrates,
    74
  Immune-Building
    Vegetable Broth,
    162–163
  "yes" foods, 36
optimism, 7
orange, 37, 194, 291
oregano, 296
organ meats, 35, 79
osteoporosis, 110
outdoors, 24
overtraining, 105–106
oxidative energy system,
    437
oysters, 205

• P •

pain
  C-reactive protein and,
    110

impact of diet, 8
overtraining and, 105
pH of body, 52
Paleo
  ancestor diet, 10
  belief system changes,
    22
  blood sugar and, 16–17
  body design and, 10–11
  80-percent rule, 23
  exposure to outdoors, 24
  fitness in, 18–20, 28–31
  foundational foods for, 9
  genetics and, 20–21
  healthy cell creation, 51
  inflammation, 17–18
  intestinal changes from,
    15
  kitchen transformation,
    75–77
  as lifestyle, 8–9, 21
  mind-set for, 24–25
  nutritional sufficiency,
    50–51
  pH of body, 52
  science behind, 11–13
  skin issues, 15
  sleep quality, 16, 23
  socialization, 23–24
  stress, minimizing, 26–28
  transformation from,
    20–21, 53–54
  weight loss, 14–15
Paleo Big Three
  complex carbohydrates,
    74–75
  fat, 72–74
  overview, 69–70
  protein, 70–71
Paleo pyramid
  antinutrients and, 69
  calcium in, 68

fiber in, 67
overview, 66–67
vitamins and minerals in, 69
Paleo Ranch Dressing, 284
palm kernel oil, 42, 73
pancakes
    Almond Banana Pancakes, 150
    Mini Cinnamon Pancakes, 149
papaya, 37
paradigm, 22
Pareto principal, 98
Parkinson's disease, 110, 296
parsley, 296
parsnip, 36, 134, 251
pasta
    Lemon Cucumber Noodles with Cumin, 244
    substitutions for, 128
    Zucchini Pasta with Fire-Roasted Tomato Sauce, 236–237
pasture-raised animals, 78
peach
    Grilled Spiced Peaches, 270
    "yes" foods, 37
peanut oil, 42, 73
peanuts, 40, 53
pear
    Ginger-Fried Pears, 271
    "yes" foods, 37
peas, 40
pecans, 72
peppermint, 80, 253
pepperoni, 141
peppers
    complex carbohydrates, 74

Lunchbox Stuffed Peppers, 250
    Sausage-Stuffed Peppers, 221
pesto, 292
pH balance
    foundational foods for Paleo and, 9
    as health marker, 112
    importance of, 52
pheasant, 35
phosphagen energy system, 437
phytic acid, 64
pickles, 82
pineapple
    Coconut Shrimp with Sweet and Spicy Sauce, 203
    fruit consumption considerations, 44
    Pineapple and Mango Sweet Heat Chicken Wings, 219
    Pineapple Pork Ribs, 218
    "yes" foods, 37
pinto beans, 40, 118
pistachios, 72
pistol squat, 360–361
Pizza Frittata, 141
plantain, 36, 246
plum, 37
PMS (premenstrual syndrome), 52
poaching, 85, 121
polyunsaturated fat (PUFA), 74
pomegranate, 37
poppy seeds, 153
pork
    Breakfast Sausage Scramble, 143
    Cheater Pork Stew, 217

choosing, 79
    Citrus Carnitas, 197
    Grilled Eggs with Homemade Chorizo, 146–147
    Hearty Chili, 174
    Kalua Shredded Pork, 216
    Pineapple Pork Ribs, 218
    Slow Cooker BBQ Pulled Pork, 215
    Slow Cooker Pork and Sauerkraut, 212
    "yes" foods, 35
portions
    calories and, 47–48
    eating until satisfied, 48
    guidelines for, 49–50
    for kids, 134–135
    30-Day Reset and, 60
positive affirmations, 25, 59
postprandial blood sugar test, 109
potato
    "no" foods, 41
    substitutions for, 128
    vodka from, 46
poultry
    Chicken Cacciatora, 213
    Chicken Fennel Soup, 168
    Chicken Fingers, 193
    Chinese Chicken Salad, 186–187
    choosing, 78
    Club Sandwich Salad, 195
    Curried Chicken Salad, 179
    Deep Healing Chicken Broth, 161
    Easy Chicken Curry with Cabbage, 223

poultry *(continued)*
  Mango and Fennel
    Chicken Salad, 180
  Mango Coconut Chipotle
    Chicken, 214
  Pineapple and Mango
    Sweet Heat Chicken
    Wings, 219
  Slow Cooker Moroccan
    Apricot Chicken, 222
  Tandoori Chicken
    Thighs, 199
  Teriyaki-Turkey Meatball
    Soup, 172
  Thai Butternut Squash
    Soup, 173
  Thai Green Curry
    Chicken, 198
  Turkey Spinach Soup, 166
power exercises
  box jump, 418–419
  broad jump, 415–416
  double jerk, 420–421
  double snatch, 422–423
  jerk, 417–418
  overview, 411–413
  push press, 413–414
  strength exercise
    routine, 461–463
prana, 28
premenstrual syndrome
  (PMS), 52
processed food, 40
progress pictures, 460
proprioception, 449
prosciutto, 205
protease, 159
protein
  choosing, 78–79
  macronutrient
    sufficiency, 51
  in Paleo Big Three, 70–71

portion size, 49
portion size for kids, 135
vegetarian/vegan
  lifestyles and, 118
"yes" foods, 35
Provençal Veggie Soup,
  170
PUFA (polyunsaturated
  fat), 74
pulling exercises
  bodyweight row, 377–378
  chin-up, 378–379
  L-sit pull-up/chin-up,
    382–383
  muscle-up, 383–385
  one-arm chin-up,
    385–386
  one-arm row, 380
  overview, 99, 375–376
  pull-up, 381–382, 431
  strength exercise
    routine, 461–463
pumpkin
  healthy carbs for kids,
    134
  Pumpkin Cranberry
    Scones, 317
  Pumpkin Pie Muffins, 318
  Pumpkin Poppers, 319
  "yes" foods, 36
pushing exercises
  bench press, 369–371
  dip, 372
  handstand push-up,
    373–375
  military press, 367–368
  one-arm one-leg push-up,
    373–374
  one-arm push-up,
    368–370
  overview, 98–99, 363–365
  push press, 413–414

push-up, 365–367
strength exercise
  routine, 461–463

● *Q* ●

Qi, 28
quail, 35
quinoa, 39

● *R* ●

racked carry (exercise),
  392–393
racked lunge (exercise),
  358
racked squat (exercise),
  356–357
radish
  Vegetable Latkes, 243
  Vietnamese Cucumber
    Salad, 185
  "yes" foods, 36
rashes, 15
raspberries
  Berries and Whipped
    Coconut Cream,
    332–333
  fruit consumption
    considerations, 44
  Raspberry Cheesecake
    Bites, 254–255
  Raspberry Peppermint
    Sorbet, 253
  "yes" foods, 37
raw honey, 41, 82
raw sugar, 41, 308
RDA (recommended daily
  allowance), 65
rebounders, 56
recipe substitution, 128
repetitions (exercise), 454

restaurants, 120–121
rhubarb, 37
ribs, 218
rice
　Cauliflower Rice, 234
　"no" foods, 39
　substitutions for, 128
rice syrup, 41, 308
Roasted Oysters, 205
Roasted Red Pepper and
　Sweet Potato Soup,
　225
Roasted Rosemary
　Almonds, 262
roasting, 85, 121
rolling warm-up
　(exercise), 449–451
rosemary, 262
rum, 46, 127
ruminant animals, 190
rutabaga, 36
rye, 39

• S •

saccharin, 131
SAD (Standard American
　Diet), 117
safflower oil, 42, 73
sage, 265
salad
　Avocado and Egg Salad,
　177
　Chinese Chicken Salad,
　186–187
　Chopped Salad with
　Tahini Dressing, 184
　Cilantro Vinaigrette, 286
　Classic Cole Slaw, 188
　Curried Chicken Salad,
　179
　general discussion, 160

Kale with a Kick Salad,
　176
Mango and Fennel
　Chicken Salad, 180
Paleo Ranch Dressing,
　284
Simple Crab Salad, 181
Smooth and Creamy
　Avocado Dressing, 283
Sweet and Spicy
　Vinaigrette, 285
Tangy Carrot and Ginger
　Salad Dressing, 282
Turkish Chopped Salad,
　182
Tuscan Spinach Salad,
　178
Vietnamese Cucumber
　Salad, 185
Waldorf Tuna Salad, 183
salmon
　cellular damage
　protection, 26
　omega-6 to omega-3
　ratio, 72
　Salmon a L'Afrique du
　Nord, 208
salsa, 293
salt, 2
saturated fat, 73
sauces
　Basil and Walnut Pesto,
　292
　Cashew Butter Satay
　Sauce, 278
　Classic Stir-Fry Sauce, 281
　Cucumber Avocado
　Salsa, 293
　Moroccan Dipping
　Sauce, 279
　Orange Coconut
　Marinade, 291

Sri Lankan Curry Sauce,
　280
Tangy BBQ Sauce, 290
sauerkraut, 212
sausage
　Breakfast Sausage
　Scramble, 143
　Grilled Eggs with
　Homemade Chorizo,
　146–147
　Sausage-Stuffed Peppers,
　221
　Winter Squash and
　Sausage Hash, 196
　"yes" foods, 35
Sautéed Kale with Bacon
　and Mushrooms, 252
Sautéed Kohlrabi, 240
sautéing, 85, 121
scallops, 204
schmaltz, 81
seafood. See also
　individual seafood
　types
　calcium sources, 68
　cellular damage
　protection, 26
　Everything Seafood
　Seasoning, 299
　foundational foods for
　Paleo, 9
　purchasing, 79, 191
　Simple Crab Salad, 181
Seaweed with a Kick, 267
sedatives, 29
seeds
　choosing fats, 81
　fats for kids, 134
　foundational foods for
　Paleo, 9
　oils from, 42
　"yes" foods, 37

sensitivity to foods, 52–53
serotonin, 27, 59
sesame seeds, 72, 229
shallots
  Curried Cream of
    Broccoli Soup, 167
  Tomato Fennel Soup, 171
  "yes" foods, 36
shellfish
  food allergens, 53
  purchasing, 191
  Simple Crab Salad, 181
  "yes" foods, 35
short-cycle jerk
    (exercise), 420
shortening, 42, 73, 128
shrimp
  Coconut Shrimp with
    Sweet and Spicy
    Sauce, 203
  Creamy Red Shrimp and
    Tomato Curry, 224
  Grilled Buffalo Shrimp,
    202
  Orange Shrimp and Beef
    with Broccoli, 194
  purchasing, 191
side dishes
  Brussels Sprouts with
    Cranberries and
    Almonds, 241
  Cauliflower Rice, 234
  Cocoa Cauliflower, 235
  Creamy Kale, 230
  Creamy Spiced Broccoli,
    238
  holiday planning, 126
  Italian Broccoli, 239
  Kimchi, 242
  Lemon Cucumber
    Noodles with Cumin,
    244

Mashed Cauliflower, 233
Sautéed Kohlrabi, 240
Sesame Kale, 229
Spaghetti Squash
    Fritters, 232
Sweet Potato Shoestring
    Fries, 231
Vegetable Latkes, 243
Zucchini Pasta with
    Fire-Roasted Tomato
    Sauce, 236–237
sinus problems, 53
skin
  brushing, 56
  C-reactive protein and,
    110
  food sensitivities and, 53
  impact of diet, 7, 8, 15
  pH of body, 52
  proprioception and, 449
  30-Day Reset and, 55
  turmeric and, 296
sleep
  deprivation of, 17
  journaling, 61
  overtraining and, 105
  Paleo impact on, 16
  quality of, 23
slow cooking
  Beef Bone Broth, 211
  Cheater Pork Stew, 217
  Chicken Cacciatora, 213
  Creamy Red Shrimp and
    Tomato Curry, 224
  defined, 85
  Easy Chicken Curry with
    Cabbage, 223
  general discussion,
    209–210
  Kalua Shredded Pork,
    216

Mango Coconut Chipotle
    Chicken, 214
Meatloaf, 220
Pineapple and Mango
    Sweet Heat Chicken
    Wings, 219
Pineapple Pork Ribs, 218
Roasted Red Pepper and
    Sweet Potato Soup,
    225
Sausage-Stuffed Peppers,
    221
Slow Cooker BBQ Pulled
    Pork, 215
Slow Cooker Moroccan
    Apricot Chicken, 222
Slow Cooker Pork and
    Sauerkraut, 212
Slow-Roasted Rack of
    Lamb, 200
SMART (Specific,
    Measurable,
    Attainable, Relevant,
    Time-bound) goals, 97
smoke point, 86–87
Smooth and Creamy
    Avocado Dressing, 283
snacks
  Avocado Cups, 268
  Cocoa-Cinnamon
    Coconut Chips, 273
  Crispy Kale Chips, 261
  Fried Sage Leaves, 265
  Fudge Bombs, 272
  general discussion,
    259–260
  Ginger-Fried Pears, 271
  Grilled Spiced Peaches,
    270
  for kids, 130–132
  Meatball Poppers, 266
  Nutty Fruit Stackers, 274

Roasted Rosemary Almonds, 262
Seaweed with a Kick, 267
Southwest Deviled Eggs, 263
Sweet Potato Chips, 264
travel, 122–124
Tropical Mango Parfait, 269
snatch (exercise), 349–350
snow peas, 36
social events, 124–125
socialization, 23–24
soda, 38
sodium caseinate, 159
solanine, 41
sorbet, 253
sorghum, 39
soup
 Bacon Butternut Squash Soup, 169
 Chicken Fennel Soup, 168
 Coconut Curry Chowder, 164–165
 Curried Cream of Broccoli Soup, 167
 Deep Healing Chicken Broth, 161
 Hearty Chili, 174
 Immune-Building Vegetable Broth, 162–163
 Provençal Veggie Soup, 170
 purchasing, 158–160
 Roasted Red Pepper and Sweet Potato Soup, 225
 Teriyaki-Turkey Meatball Soup, 172
 Thai Butternut Squash Soup, 173

Tomato Fennel Soup, 171
 Turkey Spinach Soup, 166
 Watermelon Soup, 175
sour cream, 40
soy
 cleaning out kitchen, 76
 food allergens, 53
 misconceptions about, 22
soy milk, 119
soy protein, 159
soy sauce, 128
soybean oil, 42, 73
soybeans, 40
spaghetti squash
 complex carbohydrates, 74
 healthy carbs for kids, 134
 Spaghetti Squash Fritters, 232
 "yes" foods, 36
special occasions
 holidays, 125–128
 indulging, 128–129
 social events, 124–125
Specific, Measurable, Attainable, Relevant, Time-bound (SMART) goals, 97
speed, and power training, 412
spelt, 39
spices
 choosing, 80–81
 Dukkah, 301
 Everything Seafood Seasoning, 299
 Flame Out Blend, 304
 Garam Masala, 302
 Gremolata, 304

Grilling Spice Rub, 297
 healing powers of, 295–296
 homemade blends, 276
 Italian Seasoning, 300
 Morning Spice, 303
 Spiced Sweet Potato Fries, 247
 Spicy Stuffed Eggplant, 201
 Succulent Steak Seasoning, 298
 "yes" foods, 38
spinach
 calcium sources, 68
 complex carbohydrates, 74
 Mango and Fennel Chicken Salad, 180
 Roasted Oysters, 205
 Turkey Spinach Soup, 166
 Tuscan Spinach Salad, 178
 "yes" foods, 36
spine, 31
Splenda, 41, 131
sprinting, 102
sprouts, 36
squash, 36
squatting exercises
 benefits of, 351–352
 bodyweight squat, 354–355
 front squat, 359–360
 goblet lunge, 355–356
 goblet squat, 352–353
 overview, 100–101, 350–351
 pistol squat, 360–361
 racked lunge, 358
 racked squat, 356–357

squatting exercises
 (continued)
 strength exercise
 routine, 461–463
 strength training, 431
 thruster, 444
Sri Lankan Curry Sauce,
 280
Standard American Diet
 (SAD), 117
Star Fruit Magic Wands,
 256
starch, 76
steady-state cardio, 432
steaming, 85, 121
Stevia, 41
stir-frying, 85, 281
stock, 38
strawberries
 Berries and Whipped
 Coconut Cream,
 332–333
 Chocolate-Strawberry
 Crumble Bars, 316
 fruit consumption
 considerations, 44
 "yes" foods, 37
strength. *See also* power
 exercises
 benefits of, 90–91
 combining heavy weight
 and low reps, 430
 defined, 90
 determining personal
 definition of heavy,
 428
 developing, 92–93,
 364–365, 429–430
 exercise routine for,
 461–463
 exercises for, 431–432
 frequency of training,
 430–431

general discussion,
 425–426
 as health marker,
 107–108
 program simplicity, 20
 training for, 426–428
 types of, 427
 weight for training, 464
stress
 body reactions to, 26
 family meals and, 133
 food choices affected
 by, 27
 inflammation and, 17
 journaling, 62
 solutions for, 27–28
stroke, 296
Succulent Steak
 Seasoning, 298
sucralose, 41, 131, 308
sugar
 cycle of consumption, 43
 effects of transformation,
 58–59, 114
 foundational foods for
 Paleo and, 9
 fruit and, 36
 "no" foods, 41, 308
 stress and, 27
 substitutions for, 128
sugar snap peas, 36
summer squash
 complex carbohydrates,
 74
 Provençal Veggie Soup,
 170
 "yes" foods, 36
sun exposure, 24
sun-dried tomatoes, 83
sunflower oil, 42, 73
sunflower seeds, 72
sunlight, 59
sweat, 56

Sweet and Spicy
 Vinaigrette, 285
Sweet One, 131
sweet potato
 Anytime Waffles, 152
 Coconut Curry Chowder,
 164–165
 healthy carbs for kids,
 134
 Immune-Building
 Vegetable Broth,
 162–163
 Roasted Red Pepper and
 Sweet Potato Soup,
 225
 snacks, 122–123
 Spiced Sweet Potato
 Fries, 247
 Sweet Potato Chips, 264
 Sweet Potato Shoestring
 Fries, 231
 "yes" foods, 36
Sweet'N Low, 131
sweets
 Almond Cookies with
 Cinnamon Glaze,
 310–311
 Avocado Chocolate
 Bread, 328
 Banana Cacao Muffins,
 322
 Berries and Whipped
 Coconut Cream,
 332–333
 Blueberry Espresso
 Brownies, 326
 Chocolate Bacon
 Brownie Muffins, 323
 Chocolate Chip Cookie
 Dough Granola Bars,
 314
 Chocolate Ice Cream, 330

Chocolate Zucchini Bread, 327
Chocolate-Strawberry Crumble Bars, 316
Cinnamon Chocolate Chip Muffins with Honey Frosting, 320–321
Classic Apple Crisp, 315
Coco-Mango Ice Cream, 331
Coconut Chocolate Chip Cookies, 313
Cranberry Ginger Cookies, 309
general discussion, 307
Lemon Brownies with Coconut Lemon Glaze, 324–325
Maple Bacon Ice Cream, 329
OMG Chocolate Chip Cookies, 312
Pumpkin Cranberry Scones, 317
Pumpkin Pie Muffins, 318
Pumpkin Poppers, 319
swing (exercise)
one-arm, 345–346
standard, 343–345
swiss chard, 36

• T •

tacos, 192
tallow, 81
Tandoori Chicken Thighs, 199
tangerine, 37
Tangy BBQ Sauce, 290
Tangy Carrot and Ginger Salad Dressing, 282
taro root, 134
tea, 38, 83
teff, 39
tempeh, 40, 118
temperature conversion, 482–483
tequila, 46, 127
Teriyaki-Turkey Meatball Soup, 172
Thai Butternut Squash Soup, 173
Thai Green Curry Chicken, 198
Thai Rolled Omelet, 144
30-Day Reset
body cleansing from, 55–56
breaking habits, 55
guidelines for, 60–61
journaling, 61–62
overview, 54
planning for, 56–57
three-rep max, 107
thruster (exercise), 444
thyme, 296
thyroid dysfunction, 18
tofu, 40, 118
tomato
Avocado Cups, 268
canned, 38
complex carbohydrates, 74
Creamy Red Shrimp and Tomato Curry, 224
Eggs in Spicy Tomato Sauce, 145
Hearty Chili, 174
Machacado and Eggs, 148
Mark's Daily Apple Ketchup, 289
Provençal Veggie Soup, 170
sun-dried, 83
Tomato Fennel Soup, 171
"yes" foods, 36
Zucchini Pasta with Fire-Roasted Tomato Sauce, 236–237
tonic water, 46
trail mix, 246
trans fats, 42, 73
transformation from Paleo
capturing, 53–54
effects of carbohydrate reduction, 58
effects of sugar reduction, 58–59
overview, 20–21
travel, 121–124
treats for kids, 130–132
triglycerides
exercise and, 29
as health marker, 110–112
tropical fruit, 44
Tropical Mango Parfait, 269
tryptophan, 16
tuna, 183
turkey
choosing, 78
Teriyaki-Turkey Meatball Soup, 172
Turkey Spinach Soup, 166
"yes" foods, 35
Turkish Chopped Salad, 182
Turkish get-up (exercise), 406–410, 449
turmeric, 296
turnips, 36, 243

21-Day Primal Quick Start Program
day-by-day program, 455–459
overview, 448
warm-up for, 449–453
2-plus-1 rule, 132
two-arm waiter's carry (exercise), 393–394
two-point plank (exercise), 402–403

• U •

ugli fruit, 37
ulcerative colitis, 157
units of measure, 481–483
USDA Food Guide Pyramid, 64–66

• V •

veal, 35
vegan lifestyle, 118–119
vegetable oil, 42
vegetables. See also names of specific vegetables
calcium sources, 68
cellular damage protection, 26
choosing, 79–80
foundational foods for Paleo, 9
immune system and, 227
portion size, 49
portion size for kids, 134
Provençal Veggie Soup, 170
raw, 56
as travel snack, 122–123
2-plus-1 rule, 132
"yes" foods, 35–36
vegetarian lifestyle, 118–119
venison, 35
Vietnamese Cucumber Salad, 185
vinegar, 82
vitamin D, 24
vodka, 46, 127
volume conversion, 481
V-up (exercise), 397–399

• W •

waffles, 152
waiter's carry (exercise), 391–392
Waldorf Tuna Salad, 183
walking, 102
walnuts, 72, 292
warm-up, exercise
crawling, 451–453
90-Day Primal Body Transformation and, 464–465
rolling, 449–451
water
adding flavor to, 83
30-Day Reset and, 56, 60
tonic, 46
"yes" foods, 38
watercress, 36
watermelon
Raspberry Peppermint Sorbet, 253
Watermelon Soup, 175
"yes" foods, 37
weight conversion, 482
weight loss
by creating healthy cells, 21
impact of diet, 7, 14–15
as roadblock, 116
wheat
food allergens, 53
ingredients indicating presence of, 158–159
"no" foods, 39
whey protein, 160
whiskey, 46
white beans, 40
white potato, 41
Whole9, 2
wild animal meat, 71, 72, 79
wild boar, 35
windmill (exercise), 399–400
windshield wiper (exercise), 405–406
wine, 46, 127, 128
winter squash
healthy carbs for kids, 134
Winter Squash and Sausage Hash, 196
"yes" foods, 36
work capacity, 438

• Y •

yeast, 160
"yes" foods
fats, 37
flavorings, 38
fruit, 36–37
liquids, 38
overview, 34
proteins, 35

30-Day Reset and, 60
vegetables, 35–36
yoga
  stress relief through, 28
  30-Day Reset and, 56
yogurt
  "no" foods, 40
  substitutions for, 128
  vegetarian/vegan
    lifestyles and, 118
yucca, 36

• Z •

zucchini
  Chocolate Zucchini
    Bread, 327
  complex carbohydrates,
    74
  Provençal Veggie Soup,
    170
  Vegetable Latkes, 243

"yes" foods, 36
Zucchini Pasta with
  Fire-Roasted Tomato
  Sauce, 236–237
Zumba, 104

About the Authors

Patrick Flynn is a fitness minimalist, and he wants to help you to eat and exercise more deliberately. Pat believes the secret to a good exercise is simplicity and that any dietary or fitness regimen will improve in direct ratio to the number of things kept out of it that shouldn't be there.

Pat is the founder of ChroniclesOfStrength.com, a top 500 health and wellness blog focused on helping people find clarity in the world of weights through a "less is more" approach to fitness. Pat strips diet and exercise down to its fewest and most fundamental components, helping you separate the gold from the garbage and get going with what actually works for forging a leaner, harder, and healthier physique.

Pat writes mostly on minimalistic kettlebell and bodyweight training for strength, mobility, and fat loss. He also covers intermittent fasting, hormone optimization, sex, health, longevity, supplementation, and any other topic that he believes his readers will find somewhat useful.

For a free guide on kettlebell training for strength and fat loss, visit Pat's website at www.chroniclesofstrength.com. Pat also offers private online coaching. It's expensive, but word on the street is that it's worth it.

Adriana Harlan, originally from Rio de Janeiro, considers herself "one of the lucky people who get to live in Hawaii." Hawaii's warm weather enables her to surf, kitesurf, and dive, her three passions.

Several years ago, Adriana began having severe stomach and joint pains. After countless trips to doctors who provided no answers or relief, she finally decided to try a radical diet change and began eating Paleo. After four years of continuous research on the healing powers of nutrition, she no longer suffers from the nearly debilitating pains that prompted her lifestyle change.

Besides cooking and blogging, she works as an oceanographer and a web designer. Adriana also spends a lot of time on the beach training for kitesurfing competitions while her husband documents each day with video and photos.

Melissa Joulwan is the author of *Well Fed: Paleo Recipes for People Who Love to Eat* (Smudge Publishing, LLC) and the author of the recipes and Meal Map included in the New York Times Bestseller *It Starts With Food: Discover the Whole30 and Change Your Life in Unexpected Ways* (Victory Belt Publishing). Her recipes have appeared in *Paleo Magazine,* and she was a featured chef for U.S. Wellness Meats and Lava Lake Lamb. She also teaches Paleo cooking classes at the Whole Foods Culinary Center.

Melissa has been following a strict Paleo diet since 2009, when she underwent a thyroidectomy. In the aftermath of the surgery and recovery, she became particularly interested in how diet affects hormones, body composition, mood, and mental wellbeing. Her experiences are chronicled on the popular, award-winning blog The Clothes Make The Girl (www.theclothesmakethegirl.com), where she writes daily about the Paleo lifestyle, recipes, fitness training, yoga, meditation, and motivation.

Melissa is also a community ambassador for *Experience Life* magazine, a contributor to health and fitness periodicals, and a frequent presenter at Paleo conferences.

Dr. Kellyann Petrucci earned her bachelor's degree from Temple University, hosted her alma mater's Department of Public Health Intern Program, and mentored students entering the health field. She earned her master's degree from St. Joseph's University and Doctor of Chiropractic degree from Logan College of Chiropractic, where she served as the postgraduate chairperson. She enrolled in postgraduate coursework in Europe. She also studied naturopathic medicine at the College of Naturopathic Medicine, London. She is one of the few practitioners in the United States certified in biological medicine by the esteemed Dr. Thomas Rau, of the Paracelsus Klinik Lustmuhle, Switzerland.

During Dr. Kellyann's many years as a doctor/consultant at her thriving nutrition-based practice in the Philadelphia area, she's helped dozens of patients overcome major health issues while building the strongest, healthiest body possible. With years of research and observation, Dr. Kellyann learned that feeling and looking good came down to simple principles and food values that made an astonishing difference in people's lives. Dr. Kellyann found the principles of living Paleo to be the key for those who wished to open the door to losing weight, boosting immunity, and fighting aging. With the hundreds of Paleo successes she's seen thus far, Dr. Kellyann is committed more than ever to continuing to spread the Paleo lifestyle message.

Dr. Kellyann has written these health and lifestyle books: *Living Paleo For Dummies, Paleo Cookbook For Dummies,* and *Boost Your Immunity For Dummies* (all from Wiley). She appears on various news streams nationally and conducts workshops and seminars worldwide to help people feel and look their best. She is also the author of the popular website www.drkellyann.com, and gives daily news, tips, and inspiration on Twitter @drkellyann.

With her national Paleo door-to-door home delivery food service, www.livingpaleofoods.com, the busy mother of two sons is committed to making a Paleo lifestyle convenient for everyone, including the extremely busy!

Publisher's Acknowledgments

Compiler: Traci Cumbay

Senior Acquisitions Editor: Tracy Boggier

Project and Copy Editor: Victoria M. Adang

Technical Editor: Amy Kubal, MS, RD, LN

Art Coordinator: Alicia B. South

Project Coordinator: Erin Zeltner

Photographer: Rebekah Ulmer

Cover Images: ©iStock.com/maceofoto